The 1830s and 1840s are the formative years of modern public health in Britain, when the poor law bureaucrat Edwin Chadwick conceived his vision of public health through public works and began the campaign for the construction of the kinds of water and sewerage works that ultimately became standard components of urban infrastructure throughout the developed world. This book first explores that vision and campaign against the backdrop of the great "condition-of-England" questions of the period, of what rights and expectations working people could justifiably have in regard to political participation, food, shelter, and conditions of work. It examines the ways Chadwick's sanitarianism fit the political needs of the much hated Poor Law Commission and of Whig and Tory governments, each seeking some antidote to revolutionary Chartism. It then reviews the Chadwickians' efforts to solve the host of problems they met in trying to implement the sanitary idea: of what responsibilities central and local units of government, and private contractors, were to have; of how townspeople could be persuaded to embark on untried public technologies; of where the new public health experts were to come from; and of how elegant technical designs were to be fitted to the unique social, political, and geographic circumstances of individual towns.

Rejecting the view that Chadwick's program was a simple response to an obvious urban problem, Professor Hamlin argues that at the time a "public health" focusing narrowly on sanitary public works represented a retreat of public medicine from involvement with the great social issues of the industrial revolution. In exploring the views of medical men who were critical of Chadwick, Hamlin suggests the parameters of a public health that might have been, in which concern for health and well-being becomes the foundation of a public medicine that is a principal guarantor of social justice. This book offers modern public health professionals elements of a forgotten professional heritage that might be useful in responding to the bewildering range of health problems we now confront.

Public Health and Social Justice in the
Age of Chadwick

# Cambridge History of Medicine

Edited by

CHARLES ROSENBERG, Professor of History and Sociology of Science, University of Pennsylvania and COLIN JONES, University of Warwick

Other titles in the series:

*Continued on page following the index*

# Public Health and Social Justice in the Age of Chadwick

*Britain, 1800–1854*

CHRISTOPHER HAMLIN
*University of Notre Dame*

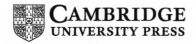
CAMBRIDGE
UNIVERSITY PRESS

PUBLISHED BY THE PRESS SYNDICATE OF THE UNIVERSITY OF CAMBRIDGE
The Pitt Building, Trumpington Street, Cambridge CB2 1RP, United Kingdom

CAMBRIDGE UNIVERSITY PRESS
The Edinburgh Building, Cambridge CB2 2RU, United Kingdom
40 West 20th Street, New York, NY 10011–4211, USA
10 Stamford Road, Oakleigh, Melbourne 3166, Australia

First published 1998

Printed in the United States of America

Typeset in Bembo

*Library of Congress Cataloging-in-Publication Data*
Hamlin, Christopher, 1951–
Public health and social justice in the age of Chadwick : Britain, 1800–1854 /
Christopher Hamlin.
p.    cm. – (Cambridge history of medicine)
Includes bibliographical references and index.
ISBN 0-521-58363-2 (hardcover)
1. Public health – Great Britain – History – 19th century.
2. Chadwick, Edwin, 1800–1890.   3. Sanitation – Great Britain –
History – 19th century.  I. Title.  II. Series.
[DNLM: – 1. Chadwick, Edwin, 1800–1890.  2. Public Health – history –
Great Britain.  3. Sanitation – history – Great Britain.    WA 11 FA1
H2p 1998]
RA485.H28    1998
362.1'0941'09034 – dc21
DNLM/DLC
for Library of Congress                                      98-20658
                                                              CIP

*A catalog record for this book is available from
the British Library*

ISBN 0 521 58363 2 hardback

# CONTENTS

# ILLUSTRATIONS

# ACKNOWLEDGMENTS

For their critical readings and much needed encouragement I thank Fern Hamlin, Elizabeth Hunt, Christopher Lawrence, John Pickstone, Mary Poovey, Charles Rosenberg, and Barbara Gutmann Rosenkrantz. I thank Peter Hennock for helping me to open the questions I address here and Liverpool University's Centre for the History of Social Policies and History Department for their hospitality in 1989–90. My thanks also to the able and endlessly patient staffs of the Public Records Office and the University College, London Archives Department, and to the National Science Foundation and the University of Notre Dame for their financial support.

# INTRODUCTION

Some years ago the school my daughters attended was found to be infested by cockroaches. This was reported to the appropriate authority and the problem took its place at the bottom of a long list, to be dealt with some months hence. One parent, however, had connections with the city public health department. A quiet word; an inspector arrived, looked, ordered immediate cleansing, and closed the school. That was Friday; Monday morning the roach-free school was open.

But what is this mysterious "public health"? Can the "public" even have a "health"? Surely "health" applies to individuals; aren't matters of the individual "private" not "public"? The term seems almost an oxymoron. Nonetheless, in many societies this "public health" has an authority to act on lives and property greater than that of any public agency save a fire department. But what are its boundaries, goals, justifications? Is it mainly an instrument with which a state guards those human goods that are its chief property? Or is it the institution through which we collectively secure our well-being?

What masquerades as an obscure offshoot of medicine or a marginal division of civil engineering is really a vast but unexamined part of our culture. Hidden beneath expertise and technology are our notions of what health is, of what problems have priority, of the conditions under which public authorities can or must act, even our notions of "decent" and "disgusting."[1] At its best public health is built of sound science and shared moral reflection. When we talk of it we are dealing in social philosophy, with ideas of liberty and responsibility, and even with the grand metaphysical questions of cosmology and causation.

Modern "public health" took shape in the nineteenth century. While it drew from many countries (and still differs from country to country in subtle and fascinating ways), it is usually seen to have come together in industrial revolution Britain in the 1830s and 1840s, at least so say the textbooks. There

---

1 For some of the conceptual problems see Roy Acheson and Elizabeth Fee, "Introduction," *A History of Education in Public Health: Health That Mocks the Doctors' Rules,* eds. Roy Acheson and Elizabeth Fee (Oxford: Oxford University Press, 1991), 1–14; Dorothy Porter, "Introduction," *The History of Public Health and the Modern State,* ed. Dorothy Porter (Amsterdam: Rudolpi, 1994), 1–44.

French traditions of statistics and medical topography and German traditions of medical police were blended by a group of statist philosopher-civil servants into an institution to respond to diseases, initially through the public structures of water supply and sewerage. Exported to the Continent, the colonies, and the rest of the world as they became urbanized and industrialized, British sanitary systems became the universal mark of adequate public provision for health.

When historians talk of public health they may mean one of three things – the actual state of the public's health, measured in mortality rates, filth in the streets, and so forth; or the institutions of Public Health; or finally some ideal PUBLIC HEALTH in whose name they condemn or congratulate the past. It is that ideal that is troublesome, for it implies that we can talk unproblematically about how far we are along the road to the ideal. Yet "public health" is not some eternal form; what "public" and "health" are to be, and how they are to be related, are political questions. Someone, somewhere, must say what aspects of whose health are the public's business, and equally what public businesses will be held accountable for their effects on health. What rights to what sorts of health will I, as one of a certain race, class, gender, nationality, and age, possess? For which of my illnesses is the polity, or other individuals or institutions, responsible; which will be judged acts of God or unavoidable products of natural systems (like markets)? The focus of nineteenth-century public health was epidemics of infectious disease, but other factors too affect health (depending of course on what one takes health to be). What of arcane toxins or violence or nutrition or forms of work, or even systems of political economy? On occasion, the missions of "public health" have been terrifyingly malleable: to its perpetrators, the Holocaust was a public health campaign, a matter of necessity and expediency.

Admit the unavoidability of determinations of which people have what rights to health and it becomes impossible to sustain the illusion of an ideal toward which all progressive public health is ever tending. The history of public health at that point ceases to be a subdivision of state growth or medical science and becomes part of the history of the acquisition of political rights or, if you will, the history of class struggle.

I

The focus of this study is the public health movement that arose in industrializing Britain in the 1830s and 1840s. Thanks to Charles Dickens, the scene is a common part of our historical imagination. It is a time of rapid change. People are on the move, from rural Ireland, the Scottish highlands, the newly enclosed English countryside, attracted to boom wages in new industry or expelled from the land by "improving" agriculturalists. Despite several years of abysmal harvests and epidemics, there are many more people – nine million in England and Wales in 1801, twice that fifty years later. Town populations double within two or three decades, infilling into cellars, spreading into new and cheap housing. Many now work in factories run by steam; and they work as extensions of automatic machines, power looms or self-acting mules. An age of benevolence, rooted in the elevation of sentiment and the presumption of a "moral economy" regulating social relations, gives way to an age of austere political economy, thriving on conflict and rooted in what are conceived the natural laws of human society, like those espoused by Ebenezer Scrooge. Exacerbating those changes are the twenty years of war with France between 1793 and 1815, which disrupt the economy and strengthen the forces of isolation and repression. Management of social relations by parish, parson, or justice of the peace gives way to policy-formulating royal commissions of statistician Benthamites. New breeds of religious seriousness set in: Unitarians and Anglican and dissenter evangelicals mix enthusiasm with intellect and challenge sensibilities and policies alike. It is also a time of some of the most profound social and political and scientific thinking: Paine, Coleridge, Bentham, Carlyle, Malthus, Burke, Darwin.

The political ranks too include truly able figures – concerned, diligent, well educated, honest: one thinks of Peel, Russell, and Palmerston. For the first third of the century governments (mostly Tory) fear to fiddle with the social and political "crises." Either the old makework English "constitution" is as good as it can be or there are just no clear solutions and interference will make matters worse. Getting their chance in the constitutional crisis of 1831, the Whigs broaden the franchise and redistribute the seats, but do not satisfy a literate and often militant working "class." For, above all, it is an age of incipient revolution. Nothing like France in 1789 or the Continent in 1848 ever quite happens – but it almost does on numerous occasions and in many places, in Ireland, London, Lancashire, South Wales, the West Riding.[2]

In the midst of this change is the lawyer Edwin Chadwick, "the bureaucratic radical," disciple of the archutilitarian Jeremy Bentham, author of the

2 Such a portrait might be drawn from many sources. Among those I have found most useful are Benjamin Disraeli, *Sybil, or the Two Nations,* with an introduction by Walter Sichel (London: Oxford University Press, 1926); Maxine Berg, *The Machinery Question and the Making of Political Economy, 1815–1848* (Cambridge: Cambridge University Press, 1980); Boyd Hilton, *The Age of Atonement: The Influence of Evangelicalism on Social and Economic Thought, 1785–1865* (Oxford: Clarendon Press, 1988); Gertrude Himmelfarb, *The Idea of Poverty: England in the Early Industrial Age* (New York: Random House, 1985); Paul Mantoux, *The Industrial Revolution in the Eighteenth Century: An Outline of the Beginnings of the Modern Factory System in England* (Chicago: University of Chicago Press, 1983); E. P. Thompson, *The Making of the English Working Class* (Harmondsworth, U.K.: Penguin, 1968); Llewellyn Woodward, *The Age of Reform, 1815–1870,* 2d ed. (Oxford: Clarendon Press, 1962); Anand Chitnis, *The Scottish Enlightenment and Early Victorian English Society* (London: Croom Helm, 1986); William Ashworth, *The Genesis of Modern British Town Planning: A Study in Economic and Social History of the Nineteenth and Twentieth Centuries* (London: Routledge and Kegan Paul, 1954); Graeme Davison, "The City as a Natural System: Theories of Urban Society in Early-Nineteenth-Century Britain," *The Pursuit of Urban History,* eds. D. Fraser and A. Sutcliffe, 349–70 (London: Edward Arnold, 1983).

famous *Report on the Sanitary Condition of the Labouring Population* (1842), written while he was secretary to the commission administering the new poor law. On the basis of his report the first modern public health agency, the General Board of Health, was founded in 1848, with the mission of promoting the magnificent *systems* of urban infrastructure that Chadwick dreamed of. Chadwick was a hydraulic thinker, imagining a constant flow of water sweeping rapidly and continuously through towns, cleaning everything, carrying all wastes to be used for beneficent purposes in the countryside. Chadwick led the board until 1854, when he was deposed: Culture, institutions, even nature resisted the systems his tutelary state would impose.

Nonetheless there followed a great age of sanitary improvement, lasting until the First World War. Sanitation became a social movement, focused on liquidating readily identifiable targets (like "all manner of filth," that awful entity at which Victorians loved to shudder) or intangible yet easily imagined targets, like the wisps of malignity that backed up through sewers or later those monad armies, the germs, which being "beings," were surely no less willfully hostile than the host of a rival nation or of a colony in the making.[3] It was a time of impressive investment in environmental quality: in water supply, waste disposal, smooth clean streets, ventilated and roomier dwellings, public green space. Remarkably these were democratic or leveling technologies, bringing to all what had been available only to the wealthy. Indeed, sanitary reform has been seen as the most profoundly humanitarian of reforms, the proof of society's recognition that human health matters. Its central tenet, the filth theory of disease, is seen as a courageous advance over the "comfortable belief" that deadly disease was but the appropriate end for "the unfit and superfluous, the paupers and the weaklings."[4]

## II

There are many problems – of who, why, and how – in understanding why modern public health should emerge in Britain in the 1830s and 1840s. One might argue that public health appears where one would least expect it.

First, ideology: Those who effected state growth were against it. They embarked on a great campaign of public investment in disease-preventing public works in a cultural climate that minimized the range of problems considered public.[5] The mix of liberal political economy with more or less Malthusianism championed the truly free person who, acting in the marketplace

---

3  See the character Mr. Firedamp in Thomas Love Peacock, *Crotchet Castle* (1831), Peacock, *Nightmare Abbey/Crotchet Castle,* ed. Raymond Wright (Harmondsworth, U.K.: Penguin, 1969), 139.
4  R. A. Lewis, *Edwin Chadwick and the Public Health Movement, 1832–1854* (London: Longmans, Green, 1952), 42.
5  David Roberts, *Victorian Origins of the British Welfare State* (1960; reprint, Hamden, Conn.: Archon Books, 1969), 100–101.

(less so in the polity), made the world. Free people took care of their own health. True, many political economists recognized a sphere of appropriate state regulation. They did not agree what belonged in it, nor did a duty to *regulate* some markets (in water, roads, sewers, railways, gas, perhaps houses and food) imply a responsibility to *provide* those services. For most this sphere was small. Such a perspective had little in common with the Continental tradition of medical police, the most prominent version of a public health. A medical police conceived human bodies as state resources to be managed for state ends.[6] Medical police concerns were the product of worries about depopulation; from the perspective of early-nineteenth-century British Malthusianism there were already too many people. If humans are not assets, the status of fatal disease as a public problem is ambiguous at best.

Considerations of what a state is to do assume the existence of a viable state. Compared to Prussia, Austria, or France, early-nineteenth-century Britain was hardly a state. Quite different institutions and perspectives prevailed in Scotland and Ireland from those of England and Wales; with regard to many matters relevant to public health, England was more an agglomeration of counties, parishes, and common law courts than a state. Much is said of the nineteenth-century "revolution in government"; of paper-shuffling clerks at Whitehall and roving bands of expert inspectors promulgating new standards of health, welfare, and accountability; enforcing rules; offering the necessary legal, financial, medical, or technical expertise.[7] The century did produce a modern state, but it did so through dealing with public health and similar matters, not as a precondition for dealing with them. Bureaucracy-driven France or science-driven Germany would seem a likelier place for a great public health movement.

Third, public health was the product of odd coalitions. Joining the Benthamite policy analysts were the strangest of bedfellows, the evangelical Christians. Beyond wondering how someone like the seventh earl of Shaftesbury, transfixed with the imminence of the last days and the world's sinfulness, could have worked with the ruthlessly secular and obsessively bureaucratic utilitarian Edwin Chadwick lies the question of how the evangelicals came to put faith in sewers and water.[8] Evangelicals, like political economists, varied greatly in

6 George Rosen, "Cameralism and the Concept of Medical Police," "The Fate of the Concept of Medical Police, 1780–1890," "Economic and Social Policy in the Development of Public Health," in his *From Medical Police to Social Medicine: Essays on the History of Health Care,* 120–41, 142–58, 176–200 (New York: Science History, 1974).

7 Oliver MacDonagh, "The Nineteenth Century Revolution in Government: A Reappraisal," *Historical Journal* 1 (1958): 52–67. For a review of recent literature see Roy M. MacLeod, *Government and Expertise: Specialists, Administrators, and Professionals, 1860–1919,* ed. Roy M. MacLeod (Cambridge: Cambridge University Press, 1988), 1–24. See also S. E. Finer, "The Transmission of Benthamite Ideas, 1820–1850," *Studies in the Growth of Nineteenth-Century Government,* ed. Gillian Sutherland (Totowa, N.J.: Rowman & Littlefield, 1972), 11–32.

8 J. L. Hammond and Barbara Hammond, *Lord Shaftesbury,* 3d ed. (London: Constable and Co., 1925); Lewis, *Chadwick,* 183.

outlook. In general their worry was for the souls of the industrial proletariat. Public solutions, like a right to public aid or "improvement" via water-and-drainage projects, treated symptoms and were distractions, postponing the time when each individual had to reckon with divine will. The very harshness of making a living was providential; it reinforced the call to virtue. Some stressed the charitable bonds between people at different social stations. They insisted that these be personal; to substitute bricks, pipes, and bureaucrats for Christian love seemed not only inappropriate but retrogressive, inasmuch as it endorsed false notions of autonomy and unrealistic and inappropriate political and social expectations.[9] It is true that on many questions of social policy – education, prison and poor law reform, opposition to slavery – coalitions of philosophical radicals and evangelicals had been politically effective. The two groups had common social origins in middle-class dissent, their spiritual journeys were often parallel, they held in common a belief in the possibility of thorough-going human reformation (though they appealed to very different sources to warrant those beliefs). But to find them involved in big government and sanitation is at first glance surprising.[10]

Fourth, medicine, the profession one might expect to lead in public health, did not, and was in no condition to do so. A united, if still not unified medical profession was only achieved in 1858. By then there were plenty of job-hungry practitioners to form the rank and file of public health, many of them medical officers to poor law unions.[11] They did take command, but by then public health was already mainly an institution of local government and in-frastructure, which they could only minimally reshape.[12]

Had there been agreement about the causes of disease, medical leadership might have been less crucial. Yet with regard to what disease meant, what caused it, how to prevent it, there was only the vaguest consensus. Yes, environment affected health, but which elements of environment were responsible for which diseases in which degrees? Attributions of disease (or damage to the "constitution") to environmental factors were often so general as to be unfalsifiable; specific allegations (e.g., Chadwick's claim that "all smell is disease") were falsified repeatedly yet not abandoned. Hence those who would appeal to medical theory got nothing solid from it. The very possibility of

9 David Roberts, *Paternalism in Early Victorian England* (New Brunswick, N.J.: Rutgers University Press, 1979), 7–8.

10 M. C. Buer, *Health, Wealth, and Population in the Early Days of the Industrial Revolution* (London: Routledge, 1926), 45; Raymond Cowherd, *Political Economists and the English Poor Laws: A Historical Study of the Influence of Classical Economics on the Formation of Social Welfare Policy* (Athens: Ohio University Press, 1977), 89.

11 Jeanne Peterson, *The Medical Profession in Mid-Victorian London* (Berkeley: University of California Press, 1978); Anne Digby, *Making a Medical Living: Doctors and Patients in the English Market for Medicine, 1720–1911* (Cambridge: Cambridge University Press, 1994), 50.

12 Dorothy Watkin, "The English Revolution in Social Medicine, 1889–1911" (Ph.D. diss., University of London, 1984); Steven J. Novak, "Professionalism and Bureaucracy: English Doctors and the Victorian Public Health Administration," *Journal of Social History* 6 (1973): 440–62.

epidemiological research was hampered by insufficient data. Causes of death registration was established in England only in 1837 and was hardly straight-forward even then; what morbidity data were available reflected all the accidents of a system of medical care based in dispensaries and charity hospitals.[13]

Finally, consider the kind of public health that arose in Britain, one preoccupied with water and wastes. It is difficult to acknowledge a need to explain this for it remains a central and uncontroversial part of public health. The water and sewage technologies the sanitarians developed quickly became one of the most widely diffused technological complexes in human history. They so exemplify development and decency (not to mention health) that many of us judge places mainly on "sanitary" grounds: be the inhabitants dull, rude, even brutal, so long as they have proper restrooms they are civilized (nor, conversely, will genuine humanity or conversational brilliance compensate for bad toilets).

That we no longer see this achievement as revolutionary shows only how well the revolutionaries "black boxed" it. A world in which modern sanitation would have been rejected is unthinkable – the overflowing privy transcends ideology, calling only for a minimally competent engineer.[14] Not so in 1840, however. This course of urban evolution would be questioned on grounds of principle (that it was no business of government to discipline defecation) and on grounds of practicality. Water and sewerage systems are prodigiously expensive, and in the 1840s had no "track record" of successful performance – and who would pay for the retrofit of urban Britain?[15] In the best of circumstances, public actions are hard to explain, the more so when they require long effort and large expenditure, involve layers of complex choices (on everything from soil mechanics to property law), are taken to secure a future barely imaginable, and are done more or less voluntarily through quasi-democratic local institutions, rather than as mandates of an authoritarian state.

Moreover, the sanitarian's gaze belies our stereotypical Victorian's refinement: It is on excrement. One can perhaps understand how that fastidiousness might have led them to see muck as a public problem, but not one to talk about in public. Yet talk they did, and endlessly – in euphemisms, but with great earnestness. On it they leveled their exacting empiricism. Consider Jo-

13 Christopher Hamlin, "Could You Starve to Death in England in 1839? The Chadwick-Farr Controversy and the Loss of the 'Social' in Public Health," *American Journal of Public Health 85*, no. 6 (1995): 856–66.

14 Bruno Latour, *Science in Action: How to Follow Scientists and Engineers Through Society* (Cambridge, Mass.: Harvard University Press, 1987).

15 In the summer of 1838 at the very beginning of the sanitary movement, one of Chadwick's friends, James Mitchell, advised him that the idea of a public health based on new sewerage was ludicrously impracticable: "To remedy this [lack of drainage] is far beyond the powers of anybody to effect. The expense would be enormous. Who is to bear this expense?" ("On the Districts in Which Fever at Present Prevails," *Poor Law Commission [PLC]–Bethnal Green Correspondence*, June 1838. Public Record Office [PRO] MH 12/684).

seph Pritchard of the Wigan Working Classes Public Health Association (founded May 1848), who classified "certain districts . . . according to the degree of privy accommodation afforded. . . . Out of a large number of privies observed there were

> Rather filthy 2
> Filthy 10
> Very filthy 45
> Exceedingly filthy 7
> Disgustingly filthy 26[16]

What can be the need for so careful a discrimination; how, we wonder, does he decide? Far from being indecent, dung and dirt were polite conversation – not so food and wages, as we shall see.

## III

How we are to explain these anomalies? The dominant paradigm of British public health history appeals to the logic of rational state growth. It took shape in the 1950s. The welfare state had triumphed. The new National Health, no less than the Allied victory, seemed both the climax of a great struggle and the proof of progress. Chadwick is properly central in it: In 1952 appeared the two great biographies of him – Samuel Finer's *Life* and R. A. Lewis's treatment of his years in public health. These were followed by Royston Lambert's study of Chadwick's successor John Simon and by many detailed studies of state growth. As usually told, this story is one of the triumph of empirical science, accountable government, and even compassion over ignorance, apathy, and corruption. The perspective is plain in David Roberts's title, *Victorian Origins of the Welfare State*, or Ruth Hodgkinson's *The Origins of the National Health Service*, whose true subject is its subtitle: *The Medical Services of the New Poor Law*. Such titles were not publishers' anachronisms; they reflected the larger story of which public health was a part.[17]

---

16 Quoted in G. T. Clark, *Preliminary Inquiry into the Sewerage, Drainage, and Supply of Water, and Sanitary Condition of the Inhabitants of the Town of Wigan*, 1849, 3, 8– 9.

17 S. E. Finer, *The Life and Times of Sir Edwin Chadwick* (London: Methuen, 1952); Lewis, *Chadwick*; Royston Lambert, *Sir John Simon and English Social Administration* (London: McGibbon and Kee, 1965); Ruth G. Hodgkinson, *The Origins of the National Health Service: The Medical Services of the New Poor Law, 1834–1871* (London: Wellcome Historical Medical Library, 1967); Roberts, *Victorian Origins*; Oliver MacDonagh, *Early Victorian Government, 1830–1870* (London: Weidenfeld and Nicolson, 1977), 130–152. For the persistence of this tradition see Anthony S. Wohl, *Endangered Lives: Public Health in Victorian Britain* (Cambridge, Mass.: Harvard University Press, 1983); Virginia Berridge, "Health and Medicine," *The Cambridge Social History of Britain, 1750–1950*, Vol. 3, *Social Agencies and Institutions,* ed. F. M. L. Thompson (Cambridge: Cambridge University Press, 1990), 171–242. This perspective similarly characterizes much American writing on the history of public health (e.g., John Duffy, *The Sanitarians: A History of American Public Health* [Urbana: University of Illinois Press, 1990]). George Rosen, crusading for the new social medicine, identified a larger

At the risk of sacrilege let me caricature that paradigm with a tale I will title "The Sanitarian's Progress." First was St. Jeremy the Bentham, who told of the government that must come. After Jeremy had prophesied he gained as a disciple the young lawyer Edwin, a journalist's son, from Rochdale, in Lancashire. After saintly Jeremy's death, Edwin roamed far to expose the evils of the land, to heal them with the balm of right bureaucracy, and to speak of the sanitary kingdom to come. But though he brought good to the people, he was hated by the rich.[18] When he entered the capital he was set upon by the water seller, Mr. "Filthy-Stein" (for thus he drank his beer), Mr. "Fair-a-See" (who saw no filth; all was fair), and all the lawyers of the (Inner) Temple, who scattered confusion across the land and then preyed upon the confused. And when he went to baptize the poor with pure soft water, to flush their sins away through pipe sewers, and to fertilize the new garden with sewer manure, they turned on him. In 1854 he was betrayed by the politicians and left office forever. Yet his followers, especially Simon, who was his Paul, spread the word of Edwin about the health that could be, and the sewers and waterworks were built, and disease and squalor were banished from the land.

If public health is understood in this way, its history is pretty well done. Here Chadwick the discoverer is but the vehicle of truth. Carried on the current of empirical social science, he can do no other in leading the way to sanitary salvation. Our only job will be to chart that salvation in town after town. Everywhere the plot will be similar, with the same "parish pump" irrelevance, a contest between right–wrong, good–bad, clean–dirty, honest–corrupt, moral–immoral, progressive–reactionary, harmony–discord, change–stagnation.

But what we need from history has changed. Given the fragility of contemporary civil and urban life, we are in no position to celebrate an achievement; our problem is to solve the puzzle of how to live together in healthy, diverse communities. The old paradigm admits no real puzzles or possibilities. It is a winner's story; the very success of the winner's choices makes them unproblematic. Health did improve during that great age of public health. Yet to make that progress its own explanation, to say that the public health reformers did what they did because it was "progressive" to do so, is at best perilously close to making an event the cause of its own happening. That paradigm also omits real alternatives. The Chadwick biographers, like the

domain for public health than did most of the writers on Britain but was no more willing to see that scope as contingent and negotiated (Rosen, "What Is Social Medicine? A Genetic Analysis of the Concept," *Bulletin of the History of Medicine 21* [1947]: 674–733). For a critique of this perspective see Paul Richards, "State Formation and Class Struggle," *Capitalism, State Formation, and Marxist Theory,* ed. Philip Corrigan (London: Quartet, 1980), 49–78; Adrian Wilson, "The Politics of Medical Improvement in Early Hanoverian London," *The Medical Enlightenment of the Eighteenth Century,* eds. Andrew Cunningham and Roger French, 4–39 (Cambridge: Cambridge University Press, 1990).

18 Hammond and Hammond, *Lord Shaftesbury,* 155.

gospel writers, speak only for the protagonist. Few others receive even the gift of voice, much less an opportunity to defend or explain themselves. We don't even learn much about the protagonist, for ultimately such accounts offer no explanation beyond invocations of grace (true observation) and destiny (necessary solutions). Politics and power appear as obstacles to truth, rather than as forums for reconciling differences or expressing public will. This leaves us without a clue as to *how* the winners finally won (for the game is clearly political), yet ironically it strengthens the simple appeal to truth, which remains as the only possible explanation.

The vision of the inexorable progress of science and health is usually founded in an appeal to "conditions," the idea that public health activity is driven by public health need. Filling our narratives are overflowing privies and windowless cellars, descriptions drawn from any of the many social investigations of the period. Accompanying them are death tolls of epidemic diseases ascribed to these conditions. Often historians move from descriptions of such conditions to the conclusion that those conditions demanded remedies and that they were therefore provided, more or less expeditiously. Given enough disease, as with cholera in 1832, the responsible authorities will correlate it with various factors, say urban squalor. Through trial and error, they home in on its true causes and take ever more effective action. Thus one historian writes that "drainage and water were needed by everybody (why not food and work, one might ask), and their regulation if not their provision entailed local responsibility for public services." Another writes: "The growth of an industrial and urban society brought serious social abuses which . . . forced the English to establish effective central departments. Child labor and unhealthy slums, in conjunction with negligent JP's and town councils, led inevitably to factory inspectors and a central Board of Health."[19]

Yet the historian's imperative has no teeth. Of course conditions were deplorable, but their deplorability tells us nothing about who responded to them and how. The need was not always met; the responsibility had to be recognized to be acted upon. Not everybody, not in Britain, not in Europe, not in the rest of the world, not then, not now, had or has drains and water, whether one calls these luxuries or necessities. Communities and states tolerate different degrees of environmental unpleasantness, different levels of preventable mortality.

The recognition that conditions do not determine responses is necessary if we are to avoid falling under the rhetorical spell cast by sanitarians a century and a half ago.[20] When we write that water or drains were "needed" or

---

19 Ursula R. Q. Henriques, *Before the Welfare State: Social Administration in Early Industrial Britain* (London: Longman, 1979), 117; Roberts, *Victorian Origins*, 316–17; cf. ibid., 215; MacDonagh, *Early Victorian Government*, 133–34.

20 As I write this a storm has just swept down leaves and branches to clog the drains, leaving a great pool of stagnant water that the surveyors of highways (or the modern equivalent) will not soon

explain the public health movement in terms of mortality rates or muck in the streets, we allow the sanitary reformers to control their own history, to lead us by the nose down the small-bore pipe sewer. Conditions do not bring us to the realm of motives, strategies, interests, ideologies, and power. Then as now, an appeal to empiricism (and health crisis) can circumvent messy political and ethical questions: "Our investigators have found a crisis; we must launch cadres of experts to analyze and solve it!" To read these documents as their creators wanted them read is to learn little about them or about the politics of making a public health. For some, the real interest is in conditions and the sanitarians will be our only witnesses. Nonetheless, to accept their accounts as explanations is to float right by the great puzzle of how people come to take particular steps to improve health and well-being.

Until we press these criticisms further we will be unable to integrate the history of public health into the rest of history. Remarkably, we do not read other areas of Victorian social policy so naively: the reformers' briefs for a punitive poor law, or a debilitating industrial regime, or an intrusive police force, or a didactic system of education.[21] There we see ideology all too

get around to clearing. Up and down the street are squashed squirrels (occasionally a small raccoon or rabbit) in various stages of putrefaction, mixed in with decaying vegetable matter. The rain has been heavy and I can watch the overflow sewers disgorge raw sewage into the river. When I walk in the nearest nature preserve (our equivalent to the Victorians' public walks), I am across the river from the sewage plant, and the stench is usually overpowering. By my own back fence is a heap of festering matter (I call it a compost heap) from which swarms of tiny insects rise. A tub of dog dung, collected from the lawn, awaits the weekly visit of the scavenger. Within the house dog hair and dust lie matted in the carpets; the bath tub leaks sometimes (as does the basement wall), leaving puddles of stagnant water on the concrete floor; and a Victorian sanitarian would shudder at the iridescent fluid in our sump or at the diaper pail in the baby's room. I do not suggest that any (or all) of these constitutes as serious a threat to health as the conditions nineteenth-century sanitary investigators regularly encountered (on the other hand, I live in a pleasant middle-class neighborhood; there are places in this and most modern cities much more similar to what the Victorians described). What I want to suggest is the degree to which it was not conditions that were at issue, but perceptions of them. The battle was over public sensibilities. The frequent expressions of outrage of townsfolk on reading the inspectors' descriptions of their streets, yards, and houses are better understood not as denials of fact or as perverse love of filth, but as the different perceptions of insider and outsider. See Buer, *Health, Wealth, and Population,* 239; Warwick Anderson, "Excremental Colonialism: Public Health and the Poetics of Pollution," *Critical Inquiry 21* (1995): 640–69.

21 We have come to accept divergent explanations of this sort for two kinds of reasons, I think. The first is simply that we have adopted most of Chadwick's environmental sensibilities: a place without piped-in water, water closets, and pipe sewers is virtually unthinkable. We do not accept his sensibilities about the revolutionary poor, and hence see ideology behind his workhouses and police states. The second reason is that history of public health has for most scholars been an obscure province of history of medicine, which in turn is (more so than modern medical historians care to admit) an obscure province of history of science. Finer, Lewis, and Lambert were not historians of medicine, yet historians of medicine and science have taken possession of their topic in a way that social, cultural, and political historians have not. The comfort of historians of science with idioms of discovery and problem solving (and with platonized entities like the "Nature" that science discloses) has a good deal to do with the prominence of this scientism. Much the same essentialism is characteristic of the history of medicine in general, a human activity that is somehow structured by or even determined by a natural thing, "disease." See Charles Rosenberg, "Intro-

clearly: we are skeptical of their "facts," alert to their specious arguments. Yet often the same people were solving the real problems of public health and promulgating the programs of social control. Chadwick is the exemplar. Historians of public health see him very differently than historians of the poor law. Those wanting to write about both have been puzzled. Were there two Chadwicks? – the wicked uncle Edwin who would enforce the workhouse test and force seduced girls to take full responsibility for illegitimate children, and the benign stranger who would "pipe" the rats and filth away, leaving cleanliness and good?[22]

## IV

How then to make Chadwick more than a deus ex machina to sweep the dung from the stage of history? By appreciating that the early Victorians invented one public health among many. Their sanitary movement was not a systematic campaign to eliminate excess mortality. Its concern was with *some aspects* of the health of *some* people: working-class men of working age. Women, infants, children, and the aged were largely ignored (or, in essence, made part of the environment that affected the male worker). It tended, moreover, to represent those men in terms of their houses, streets, drains, or towns: The condition of Chadwick's man could be reduced to the rate at which his sewage flowed down a tube and the volume of air that passed his nose, and secondarily to the tidiness of his cottage (and prettiness of his wife), but only slightly to the temperature of his dwelling, the adequacy of his clothing, and the quality and quantity of the aliment that vanished down his esophagus.[23]

duction: Framing Disease: Illness, Society, and History," *Framing Disease: Studies in Cultural History,* eds. Charles Rosenberg and Janet Golden (New Brunswick, N.J.: Rutgers University Press, 1992), xv–xxvi.

22 Among the few who have tried to give a consistent reading to both areas of social reform are A. P. Donajgrodzki and David Roberts. Roberts defends the reformers, seeing the problems of rural crime, pauperism, and a textile industry that required nimble children as as real and valid as the problems of infectious disease and finding Chadwick's empirical approach to the latter as rational and just as his empirical approaches to the former. To Donajgrodzki what unites these reforms is the need to mold into docility a dangerous working class. "The early Victorians . . . were almost obsessively interested in discovering the bases of social order" and with a "social police." This was as true for secularist, rationalist Benthamites as for traditional Tories and evangelicals. Donajgrodzki finds need to "reconcile the apparently inconsistent impulses in early Victorian social reform," sometimes "benevolent" and sometimes "coercive," but argues that "far from being inconsistent" these were "mutually supportive phases in the control of the poor." His Chadwick is "neither liberal and individualistic, and even less, collectivist." Chadwick's "new institutional means were . . . to assert tutelary control over the working class" (Roberts, *Victorian Origins*; A. P. Donajgrodzki, " 'Social Police' and the Bureaucratic Elite: A Vision of Order in the Age of Reform," *Social Control in Nineteenth Century Britain,* ed. A. P. Donajgrodzki [London: Croom Helm, 1977]: 51–76; see also MacDonagh, *Early Victorian Government,* 151, 175; but see Roberts, *Paternalism,* 188, 207).

23 The work of cultural historians interested in representations of bodies has been suggestive. See Mary Poovey, *Making a Social Body: British Cultural Formation 1830–1864* (Chicago: University of

In this public health some parts of the environment (like sewer design) became part of medicine, while others, like diet and workplace, disappeared.[24]

Often only one other option to Chadwick's initiative is recognized: one can sewer or one can do nothing, the position of a "complacent school" of gloomy Malthusians who saw "in the operations of misery and disease the workings of beneficent natural laws."[25] Yet there was another position, one (at the risk of anachronism) to the "Left" of Chadwick, a position that viewed as pathological the totality of social and economic conditions in which the industrial revolution had left many poor people. This is not simply a position in principle. It was occupied, but by poorly organized groups who often disagreed with one another on fundamental issues: Chartists, Tory radicals, anti–corn law leaguers, factory reformers, new poor law opponents, and some medical men, including union medical officers, Edinburgh general practitioners, and even some prestigious metropolitan surgeons and physicians. To members of these groups the idea that some facet of industrialization and urbanization – whether overwork, trade cycles, or tariffs – killed people was by no means a comfortable belief; it was, on the contrary, absolutely unacceptable. There was here the raw material for making health as prominent a criterion for the assessment of public policy as, say, economics has become. That did not happen. Chadwick and company rejected work, wages, and food to focus on water and filth, arguably the greatest "technical fix" in history.

To present Chadwick's public health critically, as another bit of asphalt to hold the ideology together, is not necessarily to disparage the Victorian sanitary achievement or even the ideal world it envisioned. On the contrary, in towns across Britain the vision of a healthful urban environment unleashed vast public energy. The structural changes produced, particularly those hidden underground, far surpassed in expense and perseverance what we have done in the way of truly public works, and we can, I think, only look in awe at what they did and hope to find some way of living up to their example. But in a time of such flux and social experimentation, of so many and such powerful thinkers, we have a right to expect more. So a long line of social critics have argued, from Carlyle and Marx and Morris on to E. P. Thompson. Yet while recognizing the many ways early industrialism harmed health, they did

Chicago Press, 1995); Catherine Gallagher, "The Body Versus the Social Body in the Works of Thomas Malthus and Henry Mayhew," *The Making of the Modern Body: Sexuality and Society in the Nineteenth Century,* eds. Catherine Gallagher and Thomas Laqueur (Berkeley: University of California Press, 1987), 83–106; David Armstrong, *The Political Economy of the Body* (Cambridge: Cambridge University Press, 1983); Mitchell Dean, *The Constitution of Poverty: Toward a Genealogy of Liberal Governance* (London: Routledge, 1991), ch. 4.

24 Among the most interesting exclusions, because they were given much attention in the public health literature, were matters of alcohol abuse and housing (Brian Harrison, *Drink and the Victorians: The Temperance Question in England 1815–1872* [Pittsburgh: University of Pittsburgh Press, 1971], 355, 360; Anthony Wohl, *The Eternal Slum: Housing and Social Policy in Victorian London* [London: Edward Arnold, 1977], 5–7).

25 Lewis, *Chadwick,* 62.

not criticize it in terms of "public health": Others had already coopted the term. Hence my passionate ambivalence. I see that first part of the nineteenth century as a crucial time, not just for Britain but for the industrial world.

It is important to take stock of both the great deal that was accomplished and the great deal that might have been. The crises we face today, particularly with regard to health, welfare, quality of life and surroundings, are at least as acute as those in early industrial Britain. We know, I think, that to solve them we must invest in the public good; yet often local polities cannot find the will to improve schools, increase access to health care, remove toxic wastes, augment safety. The pervasive decay of public life and the ease with which we become inured to it make clear that we cannot count on reaching a level of intolerability that will once-and-for-all impel us to fix things. On the contrary, as Chadwick and others knew, there is a cycle of degradation: The worse things get, the worse we get.

Grappling with those problems requires a usable past that reopens possibility. We must bring to consciousness all the ways social arrangements affect health, must keep in mind the close link of health to human rights, must avoid a history that reifies a peculiar and restricted public health as part of the inexorable growth of the problem-solving state.

### V

My focus here is the "what" of public health: the founding of an enterprise that is in the main a product of Chadwick's influence. Mostly I shall be concerned with the drama of the 1840s about what public actions were to be taken in the name of health. In a later work I plan to focus on the "how": how that definition became laws, professional authority, structures, and even modes of social relation during the second half of the nineteenth century. Two caveats: The book is not a history of the physical and psychological well-being of the British populace during the period, the sort of project carried out in the able works of F. B. Smith or Anne Hardy. I also avoid some topics that certainly belong to the history of public health as an institution: the statistical movement, the cholera epidemics, the struggles to reform both water supply and interment practices in the metropolis.[26] They are well handled elsewhere and would take us too far from the main line of narrative.

My thesis is simple: public health in Britain in the first half of the nineteenth century involved two transforming questions. The first is William Coleman's question of how broad "public health" was to be, of how the moral economy

---

26  See, for example, F. B. Smith, *The People's Health, 1830–1910* (New York: Holmes & Meier, 1979); Anne Hardy, *Epidemic Streets: Infectious Disease and the Rise of Preventive Medicine* (Oxford: Clarendon Press, 1993); Michael Durey, *The Return of the Plague: British Society and Cholera, 1831–2* (Dublin: Gill and MacMillan, 1979); John M. Eyler, *Victorian Social Medicine: The Ideas and Methods of William Farr* (Baltimore: Johns Hopkins University Press, 1979).

of medicine was to mesh with the political economy of industrial capitalism.[27] Here Chadwick narrowed public health, casting out all factors that affected health save water and sewers, which were politically innocuous. The second is Foucault's question of what power relations would be embodied in sanitary works.[28] In the name of efficiency and science, Chadwick sought control over sanitary systems; to others central control seemed to make water and sewers into vast disciplinary networks linking all to the central state. They, in the name of liberty and practicality, would make sanitation a mode of community self-expression.

Chapters 1 and 2 explore the "public health" that might have been, the representation of the problems of the industrial revolution as problems of health, and the ambivalence of medical men to that situation. Chapters 3–7 focus on Edwin Chadwick's public health activities from 1832 to 1845: his creation of a concept of "sanitary condition" and his equating of public health with "sanitation." Chapters 8–10 examine efforts to find a constituency for sanitation and to market it to towns, and consider the reasons for Chadwick's downfall in 1854.

27 William Coleman, *Death Is a Social Disease: Public Health and Political Economy in Early Industrial France* (Madison: University of Wisconsin Press, 1982).
28 Michel Foucault, *Discipline and Punish: The Birth of the Prison,* trans. Alan Sheridan (New York: Vintage, 1979). It may also be called Daniel Boorstin's question (*The Americans: The Democratic Experience* [New York: Vintage, 1974]).

# 1

## Health as Money

In November 1823 a letter appeared under the heading "Mothers Suckling Their Infants at Guildford Treadmill" in Alexander Burnett's *Medical Advisor and Guide to Health and Long Life,* a quasi-popular, quasi-professional, and quasi-radical journal. It alluded to an earlier letter to the *Morning Post* alleging that a mother, confined in Guildford jail for inability to support her illegitimate baby, was being forced to walk the treadmill while nursing the child. The correspondent wrote that there were "*now toiling at Guildford tread-wheel, two mothers giving suck, their infants each no more than two months old, who from the diminution of the mother's milk, produced by the exhausting nature of their labour, are in a state of starvation, which, combined with the exposure to the cold, cause them to be incessantly crying.*" The letter set off a spate of denials and reassertions. "M." wrote that treadmill stints had been short and had now stopped, and that the mothers were healthy and under special care from the governor's wife. "Academicus" replied, reasserting that the babies suffered from "hunger and cold; that the milk of both the mothers was diminished by the labour," and asking "if any *nutriment* could be *sufficient* to counteract the tendency of their toil to diminish the supply of milk." That writer asserted that "no language is adequate to the task of depicting in its true colours the antisocial and barbarous enormity of which the magistrates who committed *mothers giving suck* to the tread wheel have been guilty." When the Surrey magistrates protested, *The Medical Advisor* called them "women haters."[1]

The episode is eloquent in its very ambiguity. It is certainly vivid: a vast unceasing machine; a tiny and frail human, a mother, the epitome of humanness. But what exactly is the crucial issue – the treadmill, the hunger, or the motherhood – and what is the case doing in a medical journal? No one says

---

1 "Mothers Suckling Their Infants at Guildford Treadmill," 27; "M," "Mothers Suckling Their Infants at Guildford Treadmill," 54; "Academicus," "Mothers Giving Suck at the Guildford Treadmill," 70–72 (italics in original); "Onslow and Drummond, Surrey Magistrates and Woman Haters," 118–19; "The Tread Wheel," 254, all in *Medical Advisor and Guide to Health and Long Life 1* (1823). The spontaneous outrage is probably phony; the exposé coincided with parliamentary consideration of an antitreadmill bill.

the women are ill or bothers to investigate the starvation claim. Clearly there is an affront to feeling; we sympathize. But "barbarous enormity" asks for outrage, not just sympathy: A wrong has been done to a body; rights have been violated. "You can't treat her that way," we are invited to shout.

Bodies are the business of medicine, but they are also the matrix in which are written the rights a society allots to people of various genders, races, and classes: bodies embody. That medicine should embrace such political matters was apparently clear to Burnett's readers. It was also clear how medical men were to react to those events: without explanation or argument, they will know that what is going on is not simply inhumane, but also wrong and medically unacceptable. They will know this as professionals, not as do-gooders. In so many words he says this to the Surrey magistrates, who "must go again to school, and become doctors, before they can oppose our medical opinion."[2] He also finds no need to explain why these are *public* medical matters. He assumes medicine has an authority (and duty) to intervene and outlines an odd public health through which it does so: publicity. When the newspaper reports reach "the breakfast tables of *high authority,*" and they "consider our *medical* arguments upon the subject, and . . . consult with their *own* medical friends upon the truth and justice of them . . . their assistance (which would soon decide the affair) will not be wanting."[3] Doctors may not openly or officially take responsibility for the nation's health, but quiet words with powerful clients will do the trick.

### I

At Guildford jail, food, work, warmth, infant care, freedom, behavior, class, and gender combined to constitute the problem Burnett was addressing. These matters may seem to belong more to social welfare, social policy, or even socialism than to medicine. Yet at the time they were part of a medical agenda, though by no means exclusive to it. Because they were matters of political and social relations, they were inescapably public, and their consideration in a medical context can rightly be said to represent a kind of public health.

It is a public health that does not figure much in conventional histories, however. With regard to Britain, these typically emphasize a process that begins with the cholera of 1832, or in 1838, when three doctors, Neil Arnott, J. P. Kay, and Thomas Southwood Smith, set out to discover the cause of fever in the East End of London and find it to be filth. Edwin Chadwick, secretary of the Poor Law Commission, who has sent them on their mission, makes their findings the germ of his great *Report on the Sanitary Condition of*

---

2 "Tread-Mill – Holme Sumner, and the *Medical Advisor*," ibid., 117–18. On withered breast imagery see Jutta Schwarzkopf, *Women in the Chartist Movement* (New York: St. Martin's Press, 1991), 91.
3 "Mothers Suckling Their Infants," 27.

*the Labouring Population* of 1842. Modern public health follows, but half a century earlier – "hardly a glimmer of intelligent public interest."[4]

Yet this is a winner's designation. If one takes concern for the common health as a defining feature of community, then all communities have some sort of public health. But that only begs the question, for "health" and "public" can be construed in many ways. What happened in the 1830s was not a beginning but the kind of revolutionary change that obliterates an earlier landscape. In reading the fossil record we recognize that which has descended to the public health of the present – quarantine boards and vaccination campaigns – much more readily than that which has not. When some of what has not survived has been intentionally effaced from professional memory it is all the harder.

When historians look back from Chadwick, they have usually focused on a loose band of urban medical men, active from the 1760s through the first decade of the new century, who were conspicuous for their interest in the public aspects of infectious disease. Many of them were Edinburgh-educated dissenters or Quakers: John Ferriar and Thomas Percival of Manchester, John Haygarth of Chester, James Currie and Matthew Dodson of Liverpool, John Lettsom and William Fothergill in London. Cut off from the normal routes to medical prestige – particularly the Royal College of Physicians and its Oxbridge clientele – they cultivated alternate paths to prominence. They pressed both for a more energetic response to infectious diseases (through fever hospitals, for example) and for the sorts of structural reforms of streets, houses, and sewers that would be urged by later sanitarians.[5] But while they are seen as doing what Chadwick would do, they did it less well, because their science was primitive; because they were too few and too isolated; because unlike the righteous, rational, and responsible Victorians, the corrupt Georgian public was too apathetic and disorganized; because there was no powerful state to back them up.

Yet it is misleading to see these as the happy few, an advance guard of the public health to come – first, because while they may have concentrated on sanitary matters more than their colleagues, their ideas, proposals, and activities were not outlandish at the time; second, because whatever the similarities

---

4 John Simon, *English Sanitary Institutions, Reviewed in Their Course of Development, and in Some of Their Political and Social Relations* (London: Cassell and Co., 1890), 178.
5 R. A. Lewis, *Edwin Chadwick and the Public Health Movement, 1832–1854* (London: Longmans, Green, 1952), 36; Francis Lobo, "John Haygarth, Smallpox, and Religious Dissent in Eighteenth-Century England," *The Medical Enlightenment of the Eighteenth Century,* eds. Andrew Cunningham and Roger French, 217–53 (Cambridge: Cambridge University Press, 1990); Robert Kilpatrick, " 'Living in the Light': Dispensaries, Philanthropy and Medical Reform in Late Eighteenth Century London," ibid., 254–80. The importance of eighteenth-century hygiene is argued in M. C. Buer, *Health, Wealth, and Population in the Early Days of the Industrial Revolution* (London: Routledge, 1926); M. Dorothy George, *London Life in the Eighteenth Century* (1925; reprint.: New York: Harper Torchbooks, 1965).

between their public medicine and Chadwick's, the differences are greater.[6] He and they were on opposite sides of a great gulf in medical and social thought; health and disease fit into society very differently in the 1780s than in the 1830s.

Even though it had begun to change, the profession of which these pioneers were members was one rooted in parish and market town more than in hospital, slum, or dispensary, much less laboratory or dissecting room. Its most important characteristic was a focus on health, on chronic states of being, more than on disease. Health, in turn, insofar as it was a public matter, belonged to the sphere of justice, dispensed with a fatherly and magisterial hand, mindful of "natural feelings." Medicine was part of the expression of humane sentiment, the cultivation of morality, the maintenance of social equilibrium.

In this medicine the chief causes of disease were the absence of the causes of health. Because these were interchangeable to a degree, and because most of them were purchasable, they may be styled *currencies of health*. With reference to the poor, central medical concerns included hunger (and its relation to wages, food prices, and population), exhaustion (and its relation to new forms of work), and mental depression and anxiety (related to economic security, social mobility, and conditions of living). Combinations of these led to chronic diseases, like dyspepsia, scrofula, consumption, various bronchial problems, and perhaps to fever, which might through the mechanism of contagion become epidemic. They were seen also to lead to drunkenness, indolence, domestic violence, irreligion, and unacceptable sexual and political activity.

Most importantly, this was a medicine driven by the client's own sense of well-being. One did not stop in periodically to be physically examined, tested, and told one was diseased; one interrogated one's own well-being, found something amiss, and consulted some learned person(s), whose advice might be taken or ignored. As is evident from many of the recommendations those persons gave – travel, change your diet, change your work, take three months at a spa – this was mainly a medicine for persons of means.[7] Yet some of the habits of practice carried over in the treatment of the poor, who had a sub-

6 Among modern scholars aspects of this transformation are discussed in several works by John Pickstone: *Medicine and Industrial Society: A History of Hospital Development in Manchester and Its Region, 1752–1946* (Manchester: Manchester University Press, 1985), ch. 2–3; "Ferriar's Fever to Kay's Cholera: Disease and Social Structure in Cottonopolis," *History of Science 22* (1984): 401–19; "Dearth, Dirt, and Fever Epidemics: Rewriting the History of British 'Public Health,' 1780–1850," *Epidemics and Ideas: Essays on the Historical Perception of Pestilence*, eds. Terence Ranger and Paul Slack, 125–48 (Cambridge: Cambridge University Press, 1992); "Ways of Knowing: Towards a Historical Sociology of Science, Technology, and Medicine" *British Journal for the History of Science 26* (1993): 433–58.

7 Dorothy Porter and Roy Porter, *Patient's Progress: Doctors and Doctoring in Eighteenth-Century England* (Stanford, Calif.: Stanford University Press, 1989); Anne Digby, *Making a Medical Living: Doctors and Patients in the English Market for Medicine, 1720–1911* (Cambridge: Cambridge University Press, 1994), 199–223.

jectivity to be recognized, if it could not always be fully respected. That is evident in the dispensary movement, probably in medical services under the old poor law, and even in the response to epidemic fever. The new fever hospitals were concerned not only with isolation of contagious bodies but with prevention and convalescence, indeed with the totality of factors that affected the incidence of fever.

In short, medicine had a place in the "moral economy" described by E. P. Thompson. It complemented church and magistracy in maintaining a harmonious and stable society. It was hardly a liberal vision. Yet to radical critics of industrialism it could be a liberating one, simply because it assumed that centuries of constitutional tradition, from the Saxons through the dissolution of the monasteries and the Glorious Revolution, gave every Englishman a birthright of political (and biological) rights, which the institutions of society must recognize and protect. The parish had an obligation to the parishioner, whether the need was food or physick. That the ideal was seldom realized is less important than that it was recognized and could serve as a political re-source. Indeed, it underlay the odd Tory–radical coalition of the 1830s. How-ever much they might disagree on democracy or property, a segment of ultra Tories, including the likes of Benjamin Disraeli and Robert Southey as well as the factory reformers Michael Sadler and Richard Oastler, could agree with materialists like Richard Carlile or labor organizers like William Lovett that liberal industrialism was outrageous in acting as if the world ran on contracts and self-interest rather than Christian duty and constitutional obligation.[8]

It was a passionate and powerful cause, especially among those who gen-uinely straddled the poles of Tory and radical like the populist critic William Cobbett and the medical politician Thomas Wakley. But theirs was the losing side. It lost for many reasons – in part because of disagreement on fundamental issues, in part because of the great and growing power of the liberal indus-trialists, but in part also because of the fear of the governing classes. For it was a time of crisis: Nearly a quarter century of war between 1790 and 1815; periodic demographic, climatic, and economic shocks – the Highland clear-ances, runs of bad harvests in the early 1790s and the late 1810s, the cycles of industrial capitalism. All this was made even more worrisome by the pro-foundly unsettling philosophies of the new Jacobinism on the one side and the new political economy on the other. Behind this lay worries about "pop-ulation": according to Thomas Malthus, Britain, like every nation, populated itself to capacity. The poor did not *have* problems: They *were* a "problem"; in their very existence they were their own (and everyone else's) problem.[9]

8 E. P. Thompson, *The Making of the English Working Class* (Harmondsworth, U.K.: Penguin, 1968), 377–84, 836–37. On the problem of the term "radical" see Gertrude Himmelfarb, *The Idea of Poverty: England in the Early Industrial Age* (New York: Random House, 1985), 33–41, 230. On the importance of contracts in the new society see Thomas Haskell, "Capitalism and the Origins of the Humanitarian Sensibility," *American Historical Review 90* (1985): 339–61, 547–66.
9 Himmelfarb, *Idea of Poverty*, 129.

Guaranteeing their health and that of their offspring would make conditions worse. Wages would fall; lives would gravitate to the squalid level of the Irish peasantry. They must learn prudence. That fear was not restricted to the few occasions of violent confrontation: too many people seemed unwilling to behave properly, to defer to institutions that defined their place in the world, institutions themselves rapidly changing. Thus, the mid-1790s to the late 1830s, years of the heart of the industrial revolution and the beginnings of a "revolution in government," was a period of political counterrevolution.

But in medicine long-held conventions of explanation and intervention did not shift as quickly as society and ideology were shifting beneath them.[10] Accordingly, a medicine that had been consonant with social and economic sensibilities in the eighteenth century became dissonant. By the 1830s, while the old medicine might still be quite adequate for cultivating the constitutions of dowager duchesses at Bath, it was no longer fit to be seen in *public*. As Chadwick would discover, in the hands of dispensary doctors, or parish surgeons, or the new poor law union medical officers he established in 1834, it could be threatening. The great political questions were now social. More and more people lived now as an industrial proletariat, their welfare dictated by the rise and fall of the demand for labor in the experimental factories of industrial capitalism. The cash nexus promised nothing beyond minimal survival to some abstract quantity of labor, yet here was a venerable authority saying that these were not adequate conditions for something called "health," which was by no means infinitely negotiable. Instead of asking how long *could* people work, and on what wages, and with what housing, medical men would ask how long *should* they work. Like the ultra Tories, they answered with talk of the "constitution," a term they used in a curiously similar way, as the unchallengeable standard with which they would judge the appropriateness of any new arrangements proposed.[11]

The public health of the thirties and forties would evolve not from medicine, but from religion, poor law, and police. These were admittedly tutelary institutions, intended to suppress old habits and inclinations and cultivate new ones, and to instill a new kind of work discipline. In Chadwick's world the

10 On the power of the medical and surgical establishment see Adrian Desmond, *The Politics of Evolution: Morphology, Medicine and Reform in Radical London* (Chicago: University of Chicago Press, 1989). In the 1820s the Royal College of Surgeons of Edinburgh still saw classicism rather than new science as the route to professional status and aped the physicians in requiring theses of its students (Lisa Rosner, *Medical Education in the Age of Improvement: Edinburgh Students and Apprentices 1760–1825* [Edinburgh: Edinburgh University Press, 1991], 101–2). While the church and even many evangelicals went along with the new political economy, many doctors did not, see R. A. Soloway, *Prelates and the People: Ecclesiastical and Social Thought in England, 1783–1852* (London: Routledge and Kegan Paul, 1969); Boyd Hilton, *The Age of Atonement, the Influence of Evangelicalism on Social and Economic Thought, 1785–1865* (Oxford: Clarendon Press, 1988).
11 Roy Porter, "Gout: Framing and Fantasizing Disease, "*Bulletin of the History of Medicine 68* (1994): 1–28.

old moral economy had been swallowed up by a natural economy: not feelings, but natural laws that enforced responsibility would guide social interaction and public policy. Needed was a medicine of control, not balance. If garden variety humans were unsuited to the new factories, they might be trained or "reprogrammed." The metaphor is no anachronism. Locke's psychological models modified by Scottish philosophers saw the human as an adaptable machine. Hence, change the environment: Renew the air, change the water, replace the litter in the cage, broadcast round the clock lectures on political economy, and a reliable animal machine would walk out.

The template for Chadwick's public health and for other tutelary social reform programs was the prison reform movement of the late-eighteenth and early-nineteenth centuries. Prison reform has its own "Chadwick" in the Bedfordshire sheriff John Howard, who spent twenty years from the 1770s until his death in 1790 touring prisons, jails, bridewells, and schools, British and foreign. Traditionally, Howard has been a Dickensian hero, embodying the sentimental humanitarianism of the eighteenth century yet anticipating the social inquiry of the nineteenth. In the warehouse jails of the eighteenth century he found dirt, disease, cruelty, corruption, and a lack of accountability, findings that have been taken as both necessary and sufficient causes for reform. But more recent historians have challenged that image. Though Howard-inspired reforms improved welfare, they were prompted less by sympathy than fear and were undertaken less to aid the distressed and mistreated than to control minds and to establish a society in which free people would behave reliably. It was not prison but prisoner that needed reforming. This is all the clearer of Howard's successors, secular utilitarians like Jeremy Bentham as well as enthusiastic evangelicals like Hannah More. Treadmills, or silent systems, or readings from Scripture, were reforms because they enhanced control.[12]

One may ask, however, what is essentially medical about such matters, and how can prison reform be a foundation for a public health. To be sure, it is easy to find medical metaphors for any reform movement – a prison is a place of therapy for unsociable souls, which fits the unfit to return to society. Yet from the outset, both the language prison reformers used and the problems they addressed were often recognizably medical. In 1750 London's Newgate Prison had been rebuilt after an "assizes" fever in which officials of the court – judges, lawyers, jurymen – were infected with a deadly fever by prisoners in the dock, who had generated and gestated that fever in prison awaiting trial. Despite their relative infrequency, assizes fevers had a large place in fever

12 Michael Ignatieff, *A Just Measure of Pain: The Penitentiary in the Industrial Revolution, 1750–1850* (New York: Pantheon, 1978); Robin Evans, *The Fabrication of Virtue: English Prison Architecture, 1750–1840* (Cambridge: Cambridge University Press, 1982); Margaret DeLacy, *Prison Reform in Lancashire, 1700–1850: A Study in Local Administration* (Stanford, Calif.: Stanford University Press, 1986).

lore. They violated order; here was the retribution of the unjust on the just.[13] Since the fever contagion was widely held to be either rebreathed air or some dense exhalation associated with it, assizes fevers could be prevented by taking control of the air. Ventilation would dilute contagion to harmlessness.[14]

But there was also a "contagion" of vice; bad habits were as catching as jail fever. To a remarkable degree, inmates ran the unreformed jails, allocating space, goods and services, privileges and responsibilities. In doing so they mingled "promiscuously," depraved housebreakers corrupting honest debtors or reformable youths. "Moral contagion" was no mere metaphor in a Lockean psychology in which mental activity was physical. An act of will could no more stop the sights and sounds of prison from impacting on the sensorium than it could stop a falling meteorite.[15] Just as the medium of fever was air, the media of moral contagia were visual and aural, actions seen, corrupting words heard.

As we move via the concept of contagion between fever on the one hand and criminality and insubordination on the other, we begin to sense how readily belief in an infinitely alterable human could underwrite a public health. And if criminality was a diseased response to environmental stimuli, so too radical political activity, pub frequenting (even if temperate), even living in a cellar or a crowded house. To see those who end up in prisons or workhouses or Liverpool cellars as diseased minds/bodies was to dehumanize them. The very fact that they existed in those pathogenic force fields proved that they were not simply the makers of rational if unacceptable decisions, and the longer they remained the worse they got. Ironically, the attribution of social problems to environmentally caused disease did not stop many social reformers from continuing to see them as sin: even if unacceptable ways of being were the vector sum of what one saw, heard, and breathed, one was still responsible for doing right. Chadwick, famous for regarding disease as the cause of pauperism, is reputed to have said that there was no such thing as an innocent pauper.[16]

The way to cure these diseases was a public architecture that permitted control of all stimuli. In the "reformed" prisons of the 1820s prisoners served their sentences in silence; they wore blinders and took their religion in stalls

---

13 Evans, *The Fabrication of Virtue*, 95–97.
14 These ideas were most fully developed in the work of the clergyman–physiologist Stephen Hales and popularized by the satirist–physician John Arbuthnot. In the years around 1750 Hales oversaw installation of his wind-powered ventilating machines at several English jails. See Evans, *Fabrication of Virtue*, 97–102; Hales, *A Treatise on Ventilators*, 2 vols. (London: Manby, 1753), II, 21–45.
15 Ignatieff, *A Just Measure of Pain*, 60; Evans, *The Fabrication of Virtue*, 115.
16 Raymond Cowherd, *Political Economists and the English Poor Laws: A Historical Study of the Influence of Classical Economics on the Formation of Social Welfare Policy* (Athens: Ohio University Press, 1977), 23. This issue of determinism versus free will was one of the central issues over which the followers of Robert Owen battled with the establishment (John F. C. Harrison, *Quest for the New Moral World: Robert Owen and the Owenites in Britain and America* (New York: Scribner, 1969).

to prevent the interchange of glances. Reading matter and visits were reduced; the chaplain's sermon was to be the only item to enter the brain.[17] Similarly, the workhouse was to be no mere homeless shelter but a semioticist's playground of reminders, exhortations, carrots and sticks. The water and sewer networks of Chadwick's sanitarians were likewise a "total institution" that would both make "civilized" behavior attractive and possible and civilize directly through *force* of habit (a term that resonated powerfully in this post-Newtonian world).

All these institutions were machines to enforce healthy, moral lives. They might be seen as establishing the minimum conditions of true freedom (health and morality would follow as rational uses of that freedom) or, leaving freedom aside, acting as determinants of such lives. The standards were exacting. As Foucault has suggested, in this era of "disciplines" every valued attribute that one might but had not yet acquired marked a failure. It was not enough not to be a thief, one had also to be sober, industrious, thrifty, regular, politically docile, monogamous.[18] Not to be so was, in effect, to be diseased as well as immoral and criminal. And in a competitive world those standards were continually receding: One was never moral enough, industrious enough.

None of this happened without a struggle. As the Guildford treadmill case illustrates, there was conflict over who would own "reform." In Burnett's view it was the "humanitarian" reforms that had culminated in the treadmill that required reform. The persistence into the 1840s of traditional medical thinking accounts for Chadwick's efforts to marginalize medicine. An acceptable public health could be created only by jettisoning the great issues of wages, hours, and rights, to which both medical men and radicals would apply concepts of constitution. His public health would focus on the acute diseases of populations, like cholera and fever.[19] These it would attribute to remediable components of the environment, not to the crumbling constitutions of poor persons. The medicine that reentered public health in the 1860s was more compatible with the commodification of industrial work. It was disease-centered, focusing more on cases than on persons.

Both Chadwick and his successor John Simon legitimated their conceptions of public health with history. Theirs was a history of scientific discovery rather than one of public healths changing to meet new political climates. Looking at the period preceding "scientific" public health, Simon found only "fluffy"

---

17  Ignatieff, *A Just Measure of Pain*, 213.
18  Michel Foucault, *Discipline and Punish: The Birth of the Prison*, trans. Alan Sheridan (New York: Vintage, 1979), 176–83. See also Charles Bahmueller, *The National Charity Company: Jeremy Bentham's Silent Revolution* (Berkeley: University of California Press, 1981), 1–2; Evans, *The Fabrication of Virtue*, 115–16: "Vice [i.e., "proclivity for sensual pleasures"] after all was never reasonable – it had to be some kind of mental malfunction."
19  Himmelfarb (*Idea of Poverty,* 220) notes Cobbett's loathing of the totalizing implications of the very word "population."

generalizations.[20] The political medicine of Burnett has been invisible. Its terms and assumptions were discarded and ridiculed and now seem not quite medical. It was never institutionalized. Still, given the record of involvement of medical men in public questions, which, in turn, were often articulated as questions of health and medicine, it is appropriate to think of a pre-Chadwickian paradigm, characterizing public health in Britain from roughly 1790 to 1840. This chapter shows the great social issues as significantly medical; the next shows how medical thought was significantly social.

## II

For most of the first half of the century, the struggle between the moral economy and its naturalistic successor was between the legacies of two Thomases, Malthus and Paine, the authors, respectively, of the *Essay on Population* (1798) and the *Rights of Man* (1791). "Legacies," not "followers," is the right word, for however much their ideas were criticized, these two transformed the way people talked and thought.[21] Even those who would rebut them found themselves working with the assumptions, concepts, terms, and modes of argument of these master thinkers; in appealing to an English constitution, many of those Tories who abhorred the seditious, atheistical, and banned Paine were nevertheless thinking about the "rights of man." Typically, the clash between these traditions belongs to the history of political ideas and class relations. But it belongs also to the history of ideas about health.

What Malthus published in 1798 was the "population principle," the idea that always and everywhere the human population strained against the limits of subsistence. An age of plenty for the many was illusory. To say that the struggle for survival was continual and inescapable was tantamount to broadcasting the idea that nature itself condemned all but a few to lives of permanent suboptimality. While it may seem obvious, it is important to note that this condition was defined mainly in terms of health. To be sure, overpopulation led to immorality and crime, but its principal manifestations were starvation, disease, and death.

Underlying Malthus's deductions was a commonsense pathology stressing factors that sapped "vitality" and led to exhaustion or "starvation" (broadly conceived as privation of any of the "necessaries of life"). For Malthus disease was simple and lawlike. It was nature's "terrible corrective" to overpopulation. Disease might occur episodically, but over the long term the level of disease was a function of the level of deprivation (precisely the opposite of the ar-

20 Simon, *English Sanitary Institutions,* 175. Simon does lay claim to eighteenth-century humanitarianism (i.e., the antislavery movement) but does not find much that is medically significant.
21 Himmelfarb, *The Idea of Poverty,* 99–101, 126; Mitchell Dean, *The Constitution of Poverty: Toward a Genealogy of Liberal Governance* (London: Routledge, 1991).

gument Chadwick would make). In the second and later editions of the *Essay on Population*, Malthus complemented the axiomatic character of the population principle with empirical investigations of the checks to overpopulation in various times and places. Disease, with war and famine, were the main "positive checks" (as distinct from the "preventive" check of late marriage). Thus in "more populous countries, particularly those abounding in great towns and manufactures, an insufficient supply of food can seldom continue long without producing epidemics, either in the shape of great and ravaging plagues, or of less violent, though more constant, sickness."[22] In Scotland, the "endemic and epidemic diseases . . . fall chiefly, as is usual, on the poor. The scurvy is in some places extremely troublesome and inveterate; and in others it arises to a contagious leprosy, the effects of which are always dreadful, and not unfrequently mortal. One writer calls it the scourge and bane of human nature. It is generally attributed to cold and wet situations, meager and unwholesome food, impure air from damp and crowded houses, indolent habits, and the want of attention to cleanliness." In Ireland, "the checks to the population . . . arise from the diseases occasioned by squalid poverty, by damp and wretched cabins, by bad and insufficient clothing, by the filth of their persons, and occasional want."[23]

Within this framework, there was no threshold between health and disease. The natural growth of population forced "the lower classes of people to subsist nearly on the smallest quantity of food that will support life." The only threshold was alive or dead. At the Malthusian maximum toward which societies gravitated, a grim equilibrium existed with new bodies coming along at the same rate as the existing bodies slid into death.

Malthus saw no need to appeal to learned medicine to support these claims, for nothing he said about disease was controversial. It seemed obvious, even truistic, that disease was deadlier to the weak than to the strong. He did not worry whether diseases were caused by miasms or contagia, or whether the effects of hunger could be distinguished from those of dwelling in crowded houses surrounded by filth, or whether poverty directly generated disease or simply augmented the number of victims.[24] He simply assumed that people

---

22  T. R. Malthus, *An Essay on the Principle of Population; or A View of Its Past and Present Effects on Human Happiness; With an Inquiry into Our Prospects Respecting the Future Removal or Mitigation of the Evils Which It Occasions. The Version Published in 1803, with the Variora of 1806, 1807, 1817, and 1826*, 2 vols., ed. Patricia James (Cambridge: Cambridge University Press/Royal Economic Society, 1989), bk. 1, ch. 6, 72. "Terrible corrective" is from Thomas Short's 1750 *Essay on Air*.

23  Malthus, *Essay*, bk. 2, ch. 12, 288, 292.

24  "The causes of most of our diseases appear to us to be so mysterious, and probably are really so various, that it would be rashness to lay too much stress on any single one: but it will not perhaps be too much to say that *among* these causes, we ought certainly to rank crowded houses, and insufficient or unwholesome food, which are the natural consequences of an increase of populations faster than the accommodations of a country with respect to habitations and food will allow." "How little soever force we may be disposed to attribute to the effects of the principle of population in the actual production of disorders, we cannot avoid allowing their force as predisposing

lived as well as nature permitted. Surely they would not pack into small dwellings or remain dirty if they had alternatives, any more than they would remain hungry if they had food. (Chadwick, by contrast, would treat such practices as indulgence of "habits.") Malthus saw little point in blaming the poor for being poor: Nature itself was so powerful an enforcer that society's chastisement was scarcely necessary.[25]

Many of Malthus's legatees did blame the poor. They saw Malthus's work not just as a diagnosis of the forces that govern populations, but as a guide to policy (and even as an ideological bludgeon).[26] The jump from description to application and exhortation was short: it was hard to make "redundant population" sound neutral. Read in the context of a political economy of individualism, the population principle explained why the poor law didn't work and how to fix it. It accounted for revolutionary discontent, exhausting factory conditions yet low wages, and the "demoralization" of the working classes. All were due to the presence of too many people, existing within (and because of) an environment that irresponsibly shielded them from the consequences of their irresponsible reproduction. The only solution was to train people to live within the disciplines nature imposed.

To Paine's legatees, like William Cobbett and Michael Sadler, the condition of England was not a matter of demographics but of rights. Hardly surprising to find squalor when the people were being systematically deprived of their

---

causes to the reception of contagion, and as giving very great additional force to the extensiveness and fatality of its ravages." Ibid., bk. 2, ch. 13, 297–99.

25 Because he saw the population problem as natural tragedy rather than culpable act, Malthus could be sympathetic with the plight of the poor, and particularly of poor women. At the beginning of the *Essay*, he notes that "among those unfortunate females with which all great towns abound, more real distress and aggravated misery are perhaps to be found than in any other department of human life" (ibid., bk. 1, ch. 2, 18). He appreciated also that the "preventive check" – control of reproduction through late marriage – was unlikely to operate unless a minimum level of well-being existed. Hopeless desperation did not facilitate prudence; epidemics, far from slowing population growth, could foster rapid growth of a miserable population. Thus, as well as providing a rationale for abolishing the poor law, Malthusian theory also provided a rationale for a "safety net" guaranteeing that minimal level of services that would permit a poor person to determine how best to improve his or her life. Yet at the same time Malthus does see the principle of population as having an edificatory function: "As dirt, squalid poverty, and indolence are in the highest degree unfavourable to happiness and virtue, it seems a benevolent dispensation that such a state should . . . produce disease and death, as a beacon to others to avoid splitting on the same rock" (ibid., bk. 4, ch. 1), in James Bonar, *Malthus and His Work* (New York: Augustus M. Kelley, 1966), 320.

26 At least in the *Essay*, Malthus was concerned mainly with a general description of populations. Note that in his appeal to natural theology, he does not blame individuals or societies. While the poor are victims, it is "we" as a population which has increased faster than subsistence: "In the history of every epidemic it has almost invariably been observed that the lower classes of people, whose food was poor and insufficient, and who lived crowded together in small and dirty houses, were the principal victims. In what other manner can nature point out to us, that if we increase too fast for the means of subsistence, so as to render it necessary for a considerable part of the society to live in this miserable manner, we have offended against one of her laws." Malthus, *Essay*, vol. 2, bk. 4, ch. 1, 89.

rights. In the old days yeoman farmers had held commoner's rights to the land, but two centuries of enclosure acts had chased them off to the towns or transformed them into hired laborers. In the case of artisans, the old "statutes of laborers" or the laws on commerce in certain goods had allowed the trades to control their numbers, their work processes, their wages. But Parliament no longer enforced apprenticeship laws, and free artisans were fast becoming wage laborers. And finally, having taken the land and the rights of artisans to control their trades, Parliament proposed to curtail or even eliminate their right to parish relief, all in the name of population crisis. The solution: Settle the people on the land, uphold the artisans' control of their trades, and squalor would vanish.[27]

The issue of the most sustained clash of these perspectives, from the 1790s to the establishment of the Poor Law Board in 1847, was poor law reform. What exactly the English poor law crisis was depended on whom you asked, and when: it included many problems, problematic to different groups of people. The old poor law, the infamous (or famous) "act of Elizabeth" of 1607, established a right to relief from the parish in which they held legal residence (normally the parish of their birth) for those in distress. The nature and extent of this relief were worked out locally, by parish overseers and by county magistrates, to whom their rulings could be appealed. Usually, relief involved small cash payments, medical care, and supplements to wages. To Pitt's government in the late 1790s, the crisis was simply that too many people were not getting the relief they needed.

By the teens and twenties, the issue had become more complex, involving the determination of legal settlement and therefore of responsibility; the equitable distribution of rates in an era when commerce and industry were supplanting agriculture; the effect of rating on investment in workers' housing; and the conflicting orders of rigid overseers and sentimental magistrates. The focus, however, was the (apparently) rapidly rising cost of relief and its "demoralizing" effect.[28] To almost all in the reform camp – pragmatists like Robert Peel and Lord John Russell, evangelicals like Thomas Chalmers, Malthusians like Robert Slaney and Richard Sumner, philosophical radicals like Lord Brougham, Edwin Chadwick, and Francis Place – reform meant lowering costs by disciplining the poor, who were too many (they had bred irresponsibly), too lazy (parish relief was too easy to obtain), and too improvident (in good times they failed to plan for bad).[29] Remarkably, the cyclicity

27 Herman Ausubel, "William Cobbett and Malthusianism," *Journal of the History of Ideas 13* (1952): 250–56; Thompson, *Making of the English Working Class*, passim; Himmelfarb, *The Idea of Poverty*, 183, 208.

28 Quite what the total costs of relief were was not clear. Some modern historians have maintained that after rising quickly in the 1790s, the poor rates rose and fell with trade cycles, but were basically stable during the period (Cowherd, *Political Economists*, 173–75). The legal status of poor relief was quite different in Scotland and Ireland. There were crises there too during the period.

29 Here too one finds a coalition of evangelicals with political economists: Cowherd, *Political Econ-*

of demand for labor, though recognized, was suppressed: It might seem to excuse the worker for not finding work.[30] While poverty had been seen as the normal state of those who worked to live, "pauperism," a willingness to declare oneself dependent, was now seen as a social sickness, a moral failing, even a crime – the languages were integrated and interchangeable.[31] The readiest cure was a simple act of eradication, suggested Malthus: children born after a certain date were to have no right of support if they became destitute.

From the late teens to the midtwenties it seemed that Malthus's logic must prevail, but it did not. Instead, the young Benthamite barrister Edwin Chadwick suggested an automatic deterrence mechanism to the Royal Commission on the Poor Laws of 1832. Make the pain of pauperism greater than the pain of poverty. Require all those who would elect the status of pauper to leave all their worldly goods and enter an unpleasant workhouse. Make "relief" cease to relieve and you would end the dependence on relief.

For Chadwick this "lesser eligibility" principle belonged to economics, not medicine. Yet Bentham's analysis, like Malthus's, lent itself to medicalization. Bentham sought to maximize pleasure; his heavily sensory concept of pleasure was not far from a broad and common concept of health (as physical, mental, and even social well-being); "pain" and "disease" were their respective opposites. The practical problem, then, was to make an environment more painful than life outside. With regard to some of those currencies of health – freedom, drink, access to sexual relations, contact with friends and family, decisions about what was to be done with the remains of deceased relatives – that pain could be exacted simply by putting up walls and enforcing rules. For others – housing, food, heat, clothing, medical care, and work – administrators faced continual decisions about rationing. Not only had the package of conditions they provided to be worse than what independent laborers were tolerating (individual components had to be at least as bad); there had to be grades of increasing severity to distinguish the workhouse, with its more or less innocent orphans and aged, from the bridewell or reformatory, and in turn from the penitentiary.[32] Since contemporary economic policy did not

*omists*, 32; J. R. Poynter, *Society and Pauperism: English Ideas on Poor Relief, 1795–1834* (London: Routledge and Kegan Paul, 1969), 228–29; Graham Wallis, *The Life of Francis Place, 1771–1854,* 4th ed. (London: George Allen and Unwin, 1925), 166–67, 332.

30 Cowherd, *Political Economists,* 163, 170, 198–99, 238; Nicholas C. Edsall, *The Anti-Poor Law Movement, 1833–44* (Manchester: Manchester University Press, 1971), 48; Ursula R. Q. Henriques, *Before the Welfare State: Social Administration in Early Industrial Britain* (London: Longman, 1979), 33; Lewis, *Chadwick,* 25; Poynter, *Society and Pauperism,* 304. See Bahmueller, *National Charity Company,* 132, for Bentham's views.

31 Cowherd, *Political Economists,* 2, 268; Ignatieff, *Just Measure of Pain,* 210–14.

32 Thus the embarrassment of finding that prison regulations on working hours and mealtimes were more generous than common practices in factories (*Reasons in Favour of Sir Robert Peel's Bill, for Ameliorating the Condition of Children Employed in Cotton Factories; Comprehending a Summary View of the Evidence in Support of the Bill, Taken before the Lords' Committees in the Present Session of Parliament* [London: Clowes, 1819], 9). See also Himmelfarb, *The Idea of Poverty,* 164.

guarantee that wages would be sufficient for any particular standard of living, it was never quite clear what environment had to be created to achieve "less eligibility."

One could not say one was trying to create unhealthiness – the public wanted its workhouses to be humane as well as deterrent, to provide for genuine health needs while discouraging people from using that provision. One could emphasize those pains that were not so directly related to health, like loss of one's home or one's freedom to socialize; one could also promote an objective medicine of acute diseases over a subjective medicine of chronic conditions; or one could try to exclude medicine altogether and keep the whole issue of pauperism within the realm of economics: The poor were to choose between two sets of incentives, not between two unhealthful environments.

We can see the profound impact of Malthusianism on the health aspects of poor relief policies by comparing Chadwick's deterrent workhouse with Jeremy Bentham's pre-Malthus "Pauper Panopticon" (1797), often seen as its model. Like Chadwick's, Bentham's institution was to deter pauperism, but not at the expense of health or natality. Married couples would sleep together behind curtains. The health of mothers and children would be ensured by incentives. "For every woman who dies in child bed" workhouse administrators would be charged "head-money." The nurse most successful in lowering the rate of infant mortality would get a premium. Sex (within marriage) would be encouraged through experiments to discover the earliest age at which a satisfactory sexual relationship was possible.[33] The workhouse diet was to be the lowest that would sustain health, not just life (the diet of agricultural laborers in the Scottish Highlands was seen as the minimum). In short, the poor had the right to health through good diet, ventilation, warmth, and cleanliness (and as we shall see, freedom from unhealthy work). So much was the workhouse to be a place of health that Bentham hoped it would attract paying guests.[34]

33  "Nature shows the commencement of the ability – nature shows the commencement of the desire. – How long must the ability continue useless? How long must the desire be a source of vexation, instead of enjoyment?" This was to be understood in terms of maximizing happiness: "The maximum enjoyment gives the maximum of clear happiness. But the longer the *duration* of any source of enjoyment . . . the greater the *sum* of enjoyment." Bentham saw this as a greater problem for rich than for poor, yet "even in this class . . . the number of years thus lost, must, upon any calculation, or rather without any calculation, leave a blank much to be regretted in the book of life." Bentham, "Outline of a Work Entitled Pauper Management Improved," *The Works of Jeremy Bentham Published under the Superintendence of His Executor, John Bowring*, 11 vols. (Edinburgh: William Tait, 1843), vol. 8, 437; cf. 381, 391, 425; Bahmueller, *National Charity Company*, 171–72. Precedent for premiums for nurses came from the eighteenth-century philanthropist Jonas Hanway (Cowherd, *Political Economists*, 3). Bentham himself was quickly persuaded by Malthus (Bahmueller, *National Charity Company*, 96, 101).

34  Bentham, "Pauper Management," 387, 430, 421–22. Bentham, like Chadwick, would define dis-

How much had things changed by the 1830s! The separation of the sexes was a key principle of the workhouse.[35] It was both a punitive and a therapeutic measure, a way to make workhouse life less appealing than life outside and an effective preventive of "redundant" population. Notions of subsistence diet in the 1830s generally contained less meat and variety than they had in the 1790s, and work had to be found that was more tedious, painful, and futile than what was available in the labor market outside.

Of those currencies of health, food was the most controversial. One could not go without it; in excess, however, it could compensate to some degree for inadequate heat and clothing.[36] Food costs dominated the household budgets of the poor, who also faced the continual problem of what to buy and how to distribute food among family members. During the period dietary expectations were falling. Diets that shocked Malthus and led, he believed, to disease were rich compared to those which were taken as normal by social investigators in the thirties and forties. Obvious starvations were rare, in part because those with little food often had more prominent diseases. But if doctors had little to say about starvation, coroner's juries or the mayors of towns in distress, like Stockport in 1842, were less reticent: Starvation, caused not by nature but by policy, was a public health problem.[37]

Hence getting a minimal diet was no easy task for administrators of workhouses and prisons (they would sometimes admit that it was impossible and insist the other costs would compensate for an actual improvement in diet). There was little in the way of a science of nutrition, yet much speculation as to what persons might be kept alive on, and a good deal of hope in this age of agricultural revolution that new cheap foods for the poor might be found. Bentham had celebrated the experiments of the American expatriate Count Rumford, who exemplified his maxim that incentives for efficiency must be vested in those who could produce it. Rumford had contracted to support the Bavarian poor and enriched himself serving them "Rumford soup."[38] Chadwick, too, took up the problem of workhouse diets immediately on

ease as a condition independent of diet: "If there be no disease in any instance . . . the *smallest* allowance is preferable as being the least *expensive*" (quoted in Bahmueller, *National Charity Company*, 145–46).

35 John Knott, *Popular Opposition to the 1834 New Poor Law* (New York: St. Martin's Press, 1986), 110.

36 As we shall see in chapters 4 and 9, the sanitarians would argue that good air could compensate for lack of food.

37 Malthus, *Essay*, 290; Bahmueller, *National Charity Company*, 36–37; W. Cooke Taylor, *Notes of a Tour in the Manufacturing Districts of Lancashire* [1842], 3d ed., with a new introduction by W. H. Chaloner (New York: Augustus M. Kelley, 1968), 31, 201–4, 216; Knott, *Popular Opposition*, 230.

38 Poynter, *Society and Pauperism*, 86, 90–91, 133; Knott, *Popular Opposition*, 140; Bahmueller, *National Charity Company*, 36–37, 70–72. As the contractor running the Lambeth poorhouse, Charles Mott, later assistant poor law commissioner, exemplified this approach in practice (Cowherd, *Political Economists*, 233).

becoming secretary to the administrative Poor Law Commission (PLC) in 1834. From research on prisons, he concluded that less food was healthier than more.

But no matter what they chose to feed their inmates, administrators of deterrent institutions were always vulnerable to the charge that the diet was too rich, a claim which seemed warranted if anyone outside seemed to be getting by on less. Defending Guildford jail in the House of Commons, Holme Sumner M.P. noted that Mrs. Loder, the treadmill-climbing mother, had actually gained weight in jail. While this might meet the charge of harsh treatment, it invited the countercharge that such treatment would hardly deter her "irresponsible" behavior.[39] In the same year such charges led to a reduction of the diet of Millbank prisoners to gruel, bread, and weak soup. During the winter of 1823, there were thirty-one deaths from scurvy and four hundred prisoners diseased; the prison had to be closed.[40]

The working-class press, and its Tory supporters like the *Times,* insisted on translating economics back into health. To them, the logic was unmistakable. If, in the ordinary economy, people sometimes starved and the poor died disproportionately of epidemic and endemic diseases, and if workhouse life must be less attractive, it followed that more must starve and die in the workhouse. That this seemed to happen was confirmed by the fact some people who went into such institutions never came out again. Hence the common view of workhouses as places of "starvation and infanticide," institutions that both reflected the operation of Malthus's principle and wielded it to instill social discipline.[41]

Poor law administrators were in no position to refute such charges unequivocally. Deterrence required brinkmanship. Always, the poor must be made to see the workhouse as the last straw, a pain one embraced in the face of imminent death. The successful workhouse was the empty workhouse, noted the assistant poor law commissioner Charles Mott.[42] Deterrence worked. Investigators of the trade distress in Stockport in 1841–42 found that

---

39 "She declared that she was better fed, and had more care taken of her, and was altogether more comfortable during her imprisonment, than she had ever been before; that she had gained health and strength during the time she was subject to work on the wheel; and on her leaving the prison, expressed much apprehension that she should not fare as well on her return home" (*Hansard's Parliamentary Debates, new series [ns] 10,* 5 March 1824, 763–64).

40 DeLacy, *Prison Reform,* 178–80, 187; Ignatieff, *A Just Measure of Pain,* 175–78. "Penitentiary at Millbank," *Lancet, i* (April 1823): 95–100; Richard Baron Howard, *An Inquiry into the Morbid Effects of Deficiency of Food Chiefly with Reference to Their Occurrence amongst the Destitute Poor* (London: Simpkin, Marshall, and Co, 1839), 47, 56.

41 Henriques, *Before the Welfare State,* 52; Edsall, *The Anti–Poor Law Movement,* 21; Alfred [George Kydd], *The History of the Factory Movement from the Year 1802, to the Enactment of the Ten Hours' Bill in 1847,* 2 vols. (London: Simpkin, Marshall, and Co., 1857), vol. I, 72. According to the *Manchester and Salford Advertiser,* the poor law amendment act should have been called an act "for better encouragement of seduction, and the propagation of bastardy and infanticide" (Knott, *Popular Opposition,* 93, 137–41, 232–34).

42 Alfred, *History,* I, 77. On Mott, see Cowherd, *Political Economists,* 233.

people starved rather than declare themselves paupers, and from fear as much as pride.[43]

The poor then heard conflicting messages – on the one hand, that the workhouse was worse than life outside; on the other, that it was healthful. The "redundant population" they heard much about was no theoretical abstraction, but they. Chadwick himself was no Malthusian, but many PLC staffers were. The workhouse seemed but a means to force them into the maw of industrial capitalism, which in turn seemed an ongoing experiment to find the minimum conditions of human survival. To Cobbett, the new poor law was simply a way to compel workers to "live on lower wages and poorer quality food." The result was pervasive distrust.[44] When Chadwick said he was doing something for your own good, the opposite was probably true. On the grounds that no rational person became ill simply to be dependent on the state, Malthus endorsed charitable dispensaries, hospitals (though not population-encouraging foundling hospitals), and poor law medical care. But since many of those the medical charities were to relieve believed these "burking houses" existed to make them, dead or alive, teaching materials or experimental subjects, that endorsement backfired.[45] Likewise, however healthy the new foodstuffs, they were despised and feared. Just as hospitals were burking houses, new foods were likely poisons, if those who were so emphatic about having you eat them were the same Malthusians who saw *your* existence as *their* main problem.[46]

This conflict over how the provision of the necessaries of life and health was to be made compatible with the natural market is exemplified in the "Marcus" affair. In late 1838 *On Populousness*, a series of essays by one "Marcus," appeared. These seemed to advocate a state system of infanticide of newborns in excess of two per pauper couple, for the purpose of reducing

---

43 Knott, *Popular Opposition*, 232; Taylor, *Lancashire*, 42.

44 Quoted in Knott, *Popular Opposition*, 252. The factory system was described in much the same way. Cf. James McNish of Glasgow, to Sadler Committee, objecting to "the whole aim and end of their [lives] being tried by the one calculation of upon how little can life and the motion of a pair of hands be supported. The depression of living human beings to the material level of the lowest kind of factory furniture, is an act of the grossest blasphemy" (in Alfred, *History*, I, 310–12). And some poor law reformers, like Joseph Townsend, openly fueled such fears; Townsend advised that hunger was the strongest social control: Able to " 'tame the fiercest animals, it will teach decency and civility, obedience and subjection, to the most brutish, the most obstinate, and the most perverse' " (quoted in Bahmueller, *National Charity Company*, 79–80, 90).

45 Kenneth Smith, *The Malthusian Controversy* (London: Routledge and Kegan Paul, 1951), 64–45; Henriques, *Before the Welfare State*, 50–51, 56; Poynter, *Society and Pauperism*, 284–86; W. P. Alison put the issue clearly, arguing that the "true and consistent economist" must object to all poor relief (*Observations on the Management of the Poor in Scotland, and Its Effects on the Health of Great Towns*, 2d ed. [Edinburgh: Blackwood, 1840], 41–42). On Chadwick's views see M. W. Flinn, "Medical Services under the New Poor Law," *The New Poor Law in the Nineteenth Century*, ed. Derek Fraser, 45–66 (London: Macmillan,1976); and Cowherd, *Political Economists*, 251.

46 On "burking houses" see Knott, *Popular Opposition*, 262–64; and Ruth Richardson, *Death, Dissection, and the Destitute* (London: Penguin, 1988).

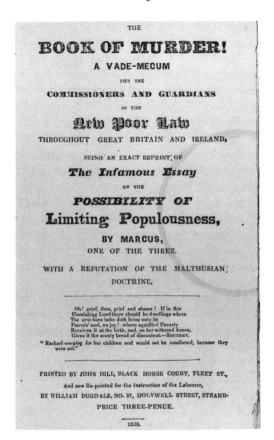

THE

# BOOK OF MURDER!

### A VADE-MECUM

FOR THE

#### COMMISSIONERS AND GUARDIANS

OF THE

## 𝕹𝖊𝖜 𝕻𝖔𝖔𝖗 𝕷𝖆𝖜

THROUGHOUT GREAT BRITAIN AND IRELAND,

BEING AN EXACT REPRINT, OF

### *The Infamous Essay*

ON THE

#### **POSSIBILITY OF**

## Limiting Populousness,

### BY MARCUS,

ONE OF THE THREE.

WITH A REFUTATION OF THE MALTHUSIAN
DOCTRINE.

Oh! grief, then, grief and shame! If in this
Flourishing Land there should be dwellings where
The new-born babe doth bring unto its
Parents' soul, no joy! where squallied Poverty
Receives it at the birth, and, on her withered knees,
Gives it the scanty bread of discontent.—SOUTHEY.
"Rachael weeping for her children and would not be comforted, because they
were not."

PRINTED BY JOHN HILL, BLACK HORSE COURT, FLEET ST.,

And now Re-printed for the Instruction of the Labourer,

BY WILLIAM DUGDALE, NO. 37, HOLYWELL STREET, STRAND-

PRICE THREE-PENCE.

1839.

Working-class editions of "Marcus's" essays of the fall of 1838 exploring the viability of a program of state-administered infanticide illustrate the political sensitivity of the health, the welfare, and, indeed, the very existence of the poor in the late 1830s.

the redundant population. The Reverend Joseph Rayner Stephens, a leader of the northern anti–poor law movement, implied that the essays were from the Poor Law Commission. Despite Stephens's arrest for fomenting insurrection, the radical press reprinted the texts under the titles *The Book of Murder!* and *Child Murder* and reiterated Stephens's insinuations.[47]

47 *Marcus on Populousness* (London: John Hill, 1838); *Child Murder!!! A Reprint, Word for Word, of the Infamous Production by Marcus Advocating the Murder of the Children of the Poor* (London: Thomas White, 1839); *The Book of Murder! A Vade-Mecum for the Commissioners and Guardians of the New Poor Law throughout Great Britain and Ireland, Being an Exact Reprint of the Infamous Essay on the Possibility of Limiting Populousness, by Marcus, One of the Three. With a Refutation of the Malthusian Doctrine* (London: William Dugdale, 1839). See also Cowherd, *Political Economists*, 175; Knott,

What is key here is how these pamphlets were read in an environment in which the health, and indeed the very existence, of working-class people were flash points of conflict. To the editors of the *Book of Murder* it seemed plain that the pamphlets were a testing of the waters. The new poor law was in "perfect harmony" with "the Murder Book!" The bureaucracy to implement "painless extinction" was already in place in the system of births registration begun a year earlier (significantly, the Poor Law Commission had been among the most enthusiastic supporters of registration). The proposal for systematic infanticide seemed to extend the existing practice of not prosecuting infanticide aggressively. It also seemed of a piece with the transfer under the new poor law of responsibility for illegitimate children from fathers to mothers. One rationale for that change had been to discourage women who were considering nonmarital pregnancy. Yet since nothing in the law gave women the legal power or social resources needed to make that freedom of choice real, the transfer was as much "a premium on the pursuit of male lust" as a disincentive to women.[48] Surely such policies were intended either to force desperate mothers to do the reducing of the population with their own hands or, alternatively, to encourage illegitimacy as means of supplying cheap child labor to the factories of the North.[49] Chadwick, after all, was principal author of the 1833 factory act which, by restricting children's working hours, led to the working of children in relays, and thereby increased the demand for child labor. Genocidal intentions also explained the organization of the workhouse, in which inmates were "imprisoned, half or wholly starved, separated the husband from the wife (no more infants to be allowed to them – mark the coincidence!) the wife from the husband, the parents from the children!" In fact, the population principle was incorrect, the editors insisted; only under capitalism, where profit, not need, governed production, was there a food shortage.[50]

### III

Along with lack of food, exhausting work was the other great threat to health. In Jeremy Bentham's Pauper Panopticon, work was to be a healthful diver-

---

*Popular Opposition*, 237–42; Edsall, *The Anti–Poor Law Movement*, 189. There is no evidence that "Marcus" was connected with the Poor Law Commission. The Chartists were in fact guilty of a gross, though understandable, misreading. For contemporary views on infanticide see Smith, *The Malthusian Controversy*, 192, 316; L. Rose, *The Massacre of the Innocents* (London: Routledge and Kegan Paul, 1980).

48 The other main rationale was the endless paternity litigation under the old poor law, as parishes sought to belabor one another with the burden of support. Even more than the workhouse, the new poor law's bastardy clauses were repugnant to the poor. Schwarzkopf, *Women in the Chartist Movement*, 45, 56, 104; Knott, *Popular Opposition*, 272–73.

49 Alfred, *History*, I, 54, 68–70; Edsall, *The Anti–Poor Law Movement*, 21.

50 *The Book of Murder!*, 3–6.

sion: "No unhealthy occupations, no excessive labour, so much as permitted – Employments of different kinds, out-door and in-door, hard work and light work, sitting work, and moving work, alternating – and operating, with reference to each other, in the way of recreation." Piecework was to be disallowed since it encouraged overwork.[51] Naive in the 1790s, such a proposal was risible in the 1830s. How would such a workhouse deter? Who would work long hours in the mines, mills, and fields with such a prospect?

Food and work were clearly related but in paradoxical ways: lack of food limited work, yet the way to more food was more work – fourteen-hour workdays for children was a matter not of cruelty but of survival, maintained defenders of the factory. That work affected health was no new discovery. As with food, there were two levels of issues. On the one hand were questions of which forms of work harmed health, and how seriously, and whether that harm could be prevented. But there was also a broader question of whether that harm was truly a problem, or alternatively, like poverty and famine, simply a natural concomitant of the life one was destined to lead. Could a laborer, a weaver, or a Sheffield metal grinder really expect the same level of health as the gentlefolk?

This was the great age of factory legislation. In 1802 the elder Sir Robert Peel, himself a cotton manufacturer, secured passage of a bill to protect pauper apprentices in the new cotton industry. As the industry grew and moved from remote streamsides to towns, the child workers were no longer orphan "apprentices." Concern arose again in 1816, and a relatively ineffective act to protect all child textile workers passed in 1819. In 1830 Richard Oastler, an estate manager, alerted the public to the scandal of "Yorkshire slavery," the unchristian destruction and deformation of children working twelve or more hours daily in textile factories. Oastler's exposé led to renewed demand for a ten hour day for children (and, by extension, for adults). An 1831 select committee investigation chaired by the Tory M.P. Michael Sadler amplified that outrage, and to deflect it the Whig government quickly established a royal commission with Chadwick and Southwood Smith as chief members. Its reports led in 1833 to an act reducing children's work to nine hours, instituting inspection and education, but facilitating the working of shifts. An 1842 act, founded in the reports of another Royal Commission on the Labor of Children in Mines and Manufactories, extended regulation of children's (and women's) hours and working conditions to mines. Finally in 1847 Parliament passed the sort of ten hours' act the movement had long fought for.

Proposals for workday reductions did not arise from careful analyses of which trades had the longest hours, hardest work, or greatest mortality rate; the factory campaigns reflected a mix of astute politics and powerful journalism. Though some claimed it as the traditional workday, ten hours was an

---

51 Bentham, "Pauper Management," 431, also 382–83.

arbitrary figure; it was by no means clear that knocking a couple of hours off the workday in a process that was inherently debilitating would significantly improve workers' health. Instead, "ten hours" was to be the cause that would demonstrate the power of the workers over a Parliament that had sold them out in the Reform Act of 1832 and then in the new poor law of 1834. In the North both the anti–new poor law movement, and Chartism, whose goal was the expansion of democracy, overlapped significantly with the ten hours' campaign.[52] Similarly, for many manufacturers the issue of interference was more important than any particular length of workday.

While shudders of sympathy and outrage fanned the flames of factory reform, medicine provided the fuel of authority. The majority of medical men who involved themselves in the factory question did so on the side of regulation. They translated that outrage into physiology. Three groups of medical men were involved. Most remarkable is the virtually unanimous testimony in the select committees of 1816 and 1832 of the metropolitan medical elite, professors of surgery or anatomy at the London hospitals and holders of key positions in the Royal Colleges of Physicians and Surgeons, men like Astley Cooper, Sir Anthony Carlisle, Sir Gilbert Blane, Sir B. C. Brodie, Sir Charles Bell, and J. H. Green. For the most part they knew nothing of life in factories and spoke from theory and general experience.[53] Second were less prestigious practitioners from factory towns, like John Boutflower and Thomas Bill, surgeons of Bolton and Manchester, respectively, in 1816–19, and in 1832 Samuel Smith and Charles Turner Thackrah of Leeds. Besides those who testified, others signed petitions or wrote short reports for inclusion in partisan pamphlets. The few medical witnesses who testified against legislation in 1816–19 were also local practitioners.[54] Finally, there were a few whom it is best to

---

52  Edsall, *Popular Opposition, 56–57*; Ann Robson, *On Higher Than Commercial Grounds: The Factory Controversy, 1830–1853* (New York: Garland, 1985), 18.

53  In 1816–19 these included Matthew Baillie, Sir Gilbert Blane, Astley Cooper, Sir Anthony Carlisle, Christopher Pemberton, and Sir George Leman Tuthill. Cooper, Carlisle, and Tuthill appeared before Sadler's committee, as did Sir Charles Bell, professor of anatomy at the Royal College of Surgeons; Sir William Blizard, surgeon to the London Hospital; James Blundell, lecturer in surgery and midwifery at Guy's; Sir B. C. Brodie, surgeon at St. George's and Royal Surgeon; John Elliotson, professor of medicine at University College; J. H. Green, professor of anatomy at King's College; G. J. Guthrie, surgeon of the Westminster Hospital; Charles Ashton Key and John Morgan, Guy's surgeons; Benjamin Travers, St. Thomas's surgeon; and Peter M. Roget, who had briefly practiced in Manchester. Cf. Ure's contempt (*The Philosophy of Manufactures: or an Exposition of the Scientific, Moral, and Commercial Economy of the Factory System of Great Britain* [London: Charles Knight, 1835; reprint: New York: Augustus M. Kelley, 1967], 374).

54  Robert Gray, "Medical Men, Industrial Labour and the State in Britain, 1830–1850," *Social History 16* (1991): 19–43; Charles Wing, *Evils of the Factory System Demonstrated by Parliamentary Evidence* (London: Saunders and Otley, 1837), clxvi–clxxi; *Information Concerning the State of Children Employed in Cotton Factories Printed for the Use of the Members of Both Houses of Parliament* (Manchester: J. Gleave, 1818; reprint, New York: Cass, 1972). See *Answers to Certain Objections Made to Sir Robert Peel's Bill, for Ameliorating the Condition of Children Employed in Cotton Factories* (Manchester: R. and W. Dean, 1819; reprint, New York: Arno, 1972), 67, for a list of Manchester area medical petitioners for reduced hours.

call "medical activists." In their view better health required far-reaching social and/or political reform. J. H. Farre, for example, who had practiced on the slave plantations of Barbados, saw an inherent opposition between medicine and political economy. The Bury surgeons Matthew Fletcher and Peter McDouall were both Chartist leaders; McDouall edited (and probably wrote most of) a Chartist newspaper that is noteworthy in representing social injustice in terms of health.[55]

Why did medical men flock to this position? Particularly for Bolton or Leeds practitioners to denounce the factory took courage. Pressure was brought to bear. The three surgeons of the Leeds infirmary would not endorse even the mild claim that "scrofulous diseases are greatly aggravated by overworking, and that the tendency to scrofula itself may probably be produced by it."[56] At least two medical men who had petitioned in favor of Peel's 1818 bill recanted and testified against it after receiving visits from manufacturers (even then they would not say that long labor was healthy for children; they simply didn't know whether it was harmful or not).[57] Yet medical men do not rush to professional suicide; their involvement surely delineates both the profession's self-image and the networks within which its members pursued their careers. They had more to gain from calling attention to the constitutional delicacies of children than they had to lose from offending factory owners.

What was it in factories that so harmed children's health? Most dramatic, of course, were accidents – clothes caught in whirring machines; fingers, arms, heads pulled in and off. This was only a marginal issue, however, both in 1816–19 and in 1832–33. More important was factory work itself as a debilitating influence undermining "health" or "constitution." Phrases like "injury to health" or "damage to the constitution" appear in the testimony of almost all the medical witnesses. Sir Charles Bell's answer was typical: Like the other metropolitan medics, he was asked whether, on the basis of "general principles," his "extensive practice," and his "studies," he thought there were "injurious consequences" of factory work. Bell replied that it "would be very injurious to the constitution, and engender a variety of diseases; the great disease, emphatically using that word, is scrofula: where there is a want of exercise, deficient ventilation, depression of mind, and want of interest in the occupations, I should say, especially in young persons, scrofula, in its hundred

---

55 On McDouall see Gray, "Medical Men." On Fletcher see Alfred, *History*, I, 260, 270; Knott, *Popular Opposition*, 91, 98, 272–73. On medical radicalism see Ian Inkster, "Marginal Men: Aspects of the Social Role of the Medical Community in Sheffield, 1790–1850," *Health Care and Popular Medicine in Nineteenth Century England: Essays in the Social History of Medicine,* eds. John Woodward and David Richards, 128–63 (London: Croom Helm, 1977), esp. 145.

56 Alfred, *History,* I, 340–41.

57 See especially W. J. Wilson and Gavin Hamilton, quoted in Wing, *Evils of the Factory System,* cxxvii-clxv.

forms, would be the consequence."[58] As Bell indicates, the damage done by factory work did not show up as a specific disease. Workers were pale, sickly, and scrawny, or as the Leeds surgeon Samuel Smith put it, "out of condition . . . there is no actual disease present, yet there is a continual tendency to disease. There is a diminished power in the body of resisting the attack of disease. . . . There is never a year passes, but I see several instances where children are in the act of being worn to death by thus working in factories." His colleague Charles Thackrah called them "strangers to health. They live, 'tis true, but this life is not full life. With many it is but a state of lingering disease."[59]

Most witnesses saw no clear boundary between impaired health and actual disease: to diagnose a disease was both to indicate the severity of the impairment and to identify particular physiological processes involved. The chief diagnoses applied to factory children were scrofula (terminating in consumption) and rickets. These were seen as interrelated and, as Bell's "scrofula, in its hundred forms," suggests, were more theoretical pathological processes than empirical clinical entities.[60] Interestingly, though 1817–19 were fever years, the factories were not seen as hotbeds of fever.[61]

One component of health was normal growth. However debilitating factory work might be for adults, it was particularly harmful to children because they were growing. It was here the rickets diagnosis entered as a general term for the skeletal deformations of childhood. Far more than learned lectures on the constitution, skeletal deformations were the keystone of Sadler's case. The appearance, even more than the testimony, of a parade of "monsters" – those with hunchbacks or deformed shoulders – indicted the factory in a way that sallow complexions or consumption statistics could not. (Among the chief

58 Ibid., 112.
59 Smith, quoted in ibid., 214; Thackrah in *The Justice, Humanity, and Policy of Restricting the Hours of Children and Young Persons in the Mills and Factories of the United Kingdom* (Leeds: R. Inchbold, 1833), 55.
60 Green gave the fullest description while admitting that it was "scarcely possible to present in any brief summary the many dire effects of scrofulous disease, but we may mention, first, that the mesenteric glands are often the seat of disease, favoured by the irritation of unwholesome and ill-digested food, shewing itself in weakness, emaciation, protuberant abdomen, and slow fever. Next, the absorbent glands about the neck, the inflammatory swelling, excited, perhaps, by variations of temperature; for the particular seat of the disease, or its development in any particular organ, may be determined by accidental circumstances. Then we find that the disease attacks the skin in the form of scaly eruptions, cracks, stops, ulcerations, and slowly suppurating tubercles. Again, that the eyes become affected in the various forms of scrofulous ophthalmy, and often end in blindness, or the bones, and especially the joints, become diseased, terminating in caries of the spine and white swellings. Then, that the internal viscera are affected with tubercles, as the liver, brain, spleen etc. And, lastly, that the lungs become the seat of this destructive disease in the form of that incurable complaint of our climate, pulmonary consumption" (quoted in Wing, *Evils of the Factory System*, 154).
61 But see W. Sharp, quoted in ibid., 207–8.

concerns of Chadwick's commission was to show that these deformities were atypical.)

The metropolitan surgeons and anatomists attributed these deformities to the repeated motion of machine tending or to long periods of standing during the years when the bones were malleable. Gravity alone could stunt growth, noted Key of Guy's: "We know . . . that a body, if kept in a horizontal position for a great length of time, will grow very fast; and . . . that if a contrary course is pursued, and the body is kept for a great length of time in an erect posture, a contrary effect will be produced."[62] In addition "peculiarities of the womanly make" made women less able to bear long standing than men and were said to cause particular harm to girls in puberty: a narrowing of the pelvis, which made childbirth difficult.[63] Again, the image of factory work preventing motherhood (or killing mothers) was ripe for the publicist. Beyond this, factory work was held on the one hand to accelerate puberty and stimulate sexual desire in girls and on the other to hamper conception. These assertions arose as the medical men grappled with a contradiction: if factory girls were so promiscuous (it was taken for granted they were), why was there not a high illegitimacy rate among them? Thus, through a process mainly physical, the factory girl acquired the physiology (and habits and inclinations) of the prostitute.[64]

That it was plausible to think that standing before a mule could "harlotize" a girl through some train of cause and effect makes clear how fragile was this constitution. The agents that affected it need not be particularly exotic. What made cotton spinning so unhealthy was not exposure to contagia or strange dusts, but simply heat and stale air: in a hot, humid atmosphere full of concentrated human exhalations, the body, its pores clogged with sweat, could not replenish itself with "that which is of a vital character"; such conditions were "most pernicious to human existence."[65] This bad air struck the nervous system, inducing "irritability . . . excitability of the feeling, and a certain busy play of the ideas when the mind is roused, together with that state of the mind generally which constitutes fretfulness and discontent." It sapped the "solid strength of the mind"; "fretful minds" were as much a product of the

62  Ibid., 173; also 116.
63  Blundell, quoted in ibid., 124. On difficult childbirth see Alfred, *History*, I, 181. For this reason the age of female puberty was a key issue. See John Roberton, "An Inquiry Respecting the Period of Puberty in Women," *North of England Medical Journal* 1 (1830): 69–85, 179–91.
64  Thus Blundell asserted that "ill health and sexual profligacy tend to produce sterility," though he believed that in factories "means preventive of impregnation are more likely to be generally known and practised by young persons" (in Wing, *Evils of the Factory System*, 125). Carlisle explicitly made the connection with the physiological characteristics of prostitutes (in ibid.,140; see also Blizard, 118, for a physiological explanation; Alfred, *History*, I, 185). See also Gray, "Medical Men"; [W. R. Greg], *An Enquiry into the State of the Manufacturing Population and the Causes and Cures of the Evils Therein Existing* (London: Ridgway, 1831), 25.
65  Blizard, quoted in Wing, *Evils of the Factory System,* 115.

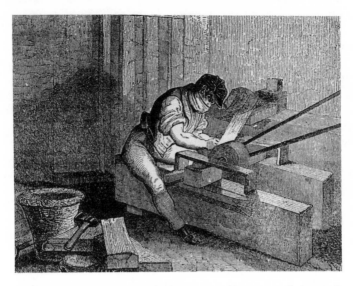

Early-nineteenth-century medical practitioners were puzzled as to how to respond to hazardous trades, like the metal grinding depicted here, which, with the division of labor and the development of capitalist production, became nearly universally fatal (from Knight's Pictorial Gallery of the Arts, 1851).

factory as "feeble bodies."[66] Revolutionary activism in northern towns was attributable to factory heat and air; so too, according to Farre, was spiritual deterioration, for that heat and air excited "in the *animal* part of the mind, gloomy and discontented trains of thought, which disturb and destroy human happiness. . . . The reflecting spiritual mind gradually becomes debased; and unless education interpose to meet the difficulties of the case, the being is necessarily ruined, both for present and for future life."[67] Constitutional fragility might be hereditary. Arguing from the failure of confined animals to breed successfully, Carlisle thought factory children would be "unfit to carry on a succeeding generation of healthy and vigourous human beings; . . . for there is nothing more hereditary than family tendencies, particularly tendencies engendered by such habits as are hurtful to the first formations of animal structures."[68]

It is evident that these pathological conditions were not diseases in the usual sense of temporary and accidental fluctuations from some normal health. What was being described was nothing other than the systematic destruction of bodies, physically, socially, spiritually. Ultimately that destruction could be

66 Blundell, quoted in ibid., 126.
67 Farre, quoted in ibid., 150.
68 Carlisle and Brodie, quoted in ibid., 134–35, 128.

measured in class-specific mortality rates, highest for workers, lowest for the wealthy. That recognition appears most starkly in what is probably the most thorough occupational disease case study of the period, on "grinder's asthma," by Arnold Knight, physician to the Sheffield General Infirmary. Dry grinders (working on forks) were apprenticed at fourteen, were experiencing symptoms by twenty, were dead by thirty-two. The grinders themselves called it asthma, noted Knight, because they did not like to admit that it was almost invariably fatal. Hoods and filters had been tried and rejected as cumbersome or ineffective. There might be hope for patients if they could follow some other trade, but they were trapped by their craft; the only way to acquire the capital to move to other work was longer hours of grinding: you could kill yourself saving yourself. The patient could "never with strict propriety be said to be cured; indeed, when he has once been affected, the remainder of his life can be considered only as 'one long disease.' " Possibly a legislative solution could be found, but Knight was not hopeful.[69]

While one might admit that factories destroyed health, where was one to look for modes of production that promoted it? Did health entail abolishing factories or only modifying them? At least in broad terms the medical men (again we are talking more of elite metropolitans than proletarian provincials) made quite plain the conceptions of "man," "nature," and "society" that were the basis of their conceptions of physiology and pathology. Health was balance, a dynamic equilibrium manifest in a set of relations among organs, faculties, appetites, and environment. These relations evolved gradually in accord with the greater laws of nature. "Man can do no more than he is allowed or permitted to do by nature, and in attempting to transgress the bounds Providence has pointed out for him, he abridges his life in the exact proportion in which he transgresses the laws of nature and the Divine command," asserted Farre.[70] Night work, for example, was "contrary to what nature seems to warrant."[71] Not surprisingly health was characteristic of country, not of town, life.

69  Arnold Knight, "On the Grinders' Asthma," *North of England Medical Journal* 1 (1830): 85–91, 167–79. Knight included a controlled clinical follow-up study comparing 250 grinders with 250 artisans in other trades. On Knight see Ian Inkster, "Marginal Men," 143–47.
70  Farre, quoted in Wing, *Evils of the Factory System*, 146. There was much reference in the 1816–19 controversy to "the laws of animal life" which were "to be set aside by algebraical inferences and calculations." *Answers to Certain Objections made to Sir Robert Peel's Bill*, 7; Sincere Friends of Industry, to the Mutual Advantage of Master and Labourer, *Remarks on the Objections Which Have Been Urged against the Principle of Sir Robert Peel's Bill* ([London]: 1818; reprint, New York: Arno, 1972); Alfred, *History*, I, 117.
71  Blizard in Wing, *Evils of the Factory System*, 115; see also Blundell, ibid., 121. Carlisle held that hours of work should vary with season. This was a "law of animal nature; . . . we never offend against those laws without being punished. . . . In the winter season the whole animal creation requires greater rest . . . and if, in an artificial state, men or animals are compelled to labour an equal number of hours in the winter season, as in the summer season, it would . . . be decidedly injurious to their health. . . . The whole creation, man, animals, birds, fishes, and even insects, rise, if they be day creatures, with the rising of the sun, and go to rest with the setting sun" (ibid.,133).

From this perspective, the factory seemed wildly destabilizing, maximizing the one good of capital growth at the expense of all others. With greater or lesser degrees of discomfort, some medical men found themselves identifying political economy as the problem, and, in effect, seeing the need to cultivate a political medicine that would counteract its authority in public affairs. Farre was most forthright: "The result is so inevitable, that I view it as a species of infanticide, and a very cruel, because lingering, species of infanticide . . . [and] the only safeguard . . . consists in opposing this principle of political economy by the medical voice, whenever it trenches on vital economy." In the factory system "the profit . . . gained is death to the child," and medical men could "never assent to life being balanced against wealth." The Manchester obstetrician John Roberton held that "the nature of their present employment renders existence itself in thousands of instances, in every great town, one long disease." The hygienist J. B. Davis maintained that "the *division of labour*, on which our modern superiority so much depends . . . has been carried further than the great pliability of the human constitution will allow; and . . . our manufactories and workshops have become the prolific sources of deformity, sickness, and death."[72]

But while it was all very well to talk of balance, what justified locating the fulcrum in the bucolic Georgian parish? Why could not free laborers be allowed to seek their own equilibrium? While some defenders of the factory, like Andrew Ure, the main target of Karl Marx's sarcasm, depicted factory children romping through their day, not all denied the harmfulness of factory work.[73] They denied only that a *public health* problem existed for which they were to blame. Some held that the problem was not *public* since wages paid to free laborers compensated for injury to their health. Others held that no *problem* existed: life itself was fatal; there might be no balance, just an inescapable trade-off.

For them, the question was what one (particularly one of a certain class) could justifiably expect from life. As an anonymous pamphleteer explained:

> The miner is doomed, day after day, to inhale the most insalubrious of atmospheres; the hand-weaver, from morning till night, toils in a low-roofed and damp workshop; the man who is employed in a chemical work is exposed to [injurious] vapours . . . even agricultural labourers, by being forced to encounter all the inclemencies of our changeable climate, often become the victims of rheumatism and its kindred maladies. . . . In these and in innumerable other cases, the labouring classes are surrounded with circumstances inseparable from their employment, which appear to be unfavourable to prolonged and uninterrupted health.

72 Farre quoted in ibid., 148–50; Roberton quoted in Alfred, *History*, I, 186; J. B. Davis, *A Popular Manual of the Art of Preserving Health* (London: Whittaker, 1836), 73. See also Gray, "Medical Men," 35.
73 Ure, *Philosophy of Manufactures,* 301.

To recognize that a mode of work was "prejudicial to the well-being of the bodily constitution and that there are some employments more favourable to uniform and lasting health" than others did not warrant public action. It might be quite true "that long confinement is not so beneficial to health as a shorter period would be; that a high temperature is less salubrious than a moderate and regular one; and that children reared in the country would in general be more healthy than persons of the same age who are long confined in factories," but no one could guarantee that all lives must meet some ideal standard of health.[74]

It had to be recognized, argued the ultraliberal Leeds publisher and manufacturer Edward Baines, that work, as the means to survival, was also the means of health: "Food cannot be obtained without toil, but toil is a less evil than hunger: clothing cannot be made without exertion and application, but these are to be endured rather than nakedness. *A physician might, if so disposed, get up a case against any employment of civilized or savage life, sufficient to excite public sympathy and abhorrence;* but so long as men cannot live without working, they must work in spite of inconvenience." Were we to "abandon every occupation which may accelerate . . . disease or decay, the most indispensable occupations of civilized men must be given up. . . . *A man who hesitated in his choice of a trade till he found one which was free from all objection, would starve before he had decided how he should live.*" The complaint, Baines maintained, was about the human condition − the "evil[s] of our destiny as men" − and not about particular occupations.[75] That work was pain was hardly a novel observation to anyone who had read far enough in Genesis.

The chief "medical writer" on whom Baines and most others relied for information on occupational health was the Leeds surgeon Charles Turner Thackrah, author of *The Effects of the Arts, Trades, and Professions and of the Civic States and Habits of Living, on Health and Longevity* (1832), the authoritative work in English on occupational health. One might expect a work on this topic from a Leeds surgeon in 1832 to be profoundly political, but though he testified to Sadler's committee that factory labor injured children and spoke in favor of the ten hours' bill at a local meeting, Thackrah was more interested in cultivating the vineyard of academic medicine than that of radical politics. In a debate dominated by speculation, he carried out substantial research, both epidemiological (e.g., inquiring whether workers in particular occupations customarily reached old age) and pathological (with his "pulmometer" Thackrah distinguished variations in the respiratory power of workers in different occupations). He sided with neither masters nor men; he was as likely to denounce the gratuitous bad habits of workers as the neglect of employers

74 *An Inquiry into the Principle of the Bill Now Pending in Parliament for Imposing Certain Restrictions on Cotton Factories* (London: Baldwin, Craddock and Joy, 1818), 7, 10.
75 Baines, *History of the Cotton Manufacture of Great Britain*, 2d ed., with a new introduction by W. H. Chaloner (New York: Augustus M. Kelley, 1966), 454–55.

(he did, however, find Yorkshire woolen mills far healthier than Lancashire cotton mills). Both sides in the factory question appealed to his book, though Chadwick ignored it in the *Sanitary Report*.[76]

Though he found a few occupations (like butchering) positively healthy, Thackrah saw much work as an assault on health: "Though health is directly attacked, and finally destroyed, by many occupations, it is much more frequently undermined. By close attention, and continued labour, the nervous system is depressed; the digestive organs are disordered; the circulation and respiration are rendered irregular; in a word, all the systems become progressively impaired, and vitality seems at length exhausted. Life is worn out by excess of labour." " 'Worn out' is as often applied to a workman as a coachhorse," he added, "and frequently with equal propriety." This destruction might not be reflected in occupational mortality rates, since weak workers left or were dismissed before their work-induced consumptions killed them. Thackrah had trouble tracing those who had left textile mills but did note that there were few old spinners. On the vexed question of how hard one need work, Thackrah too took refuge in the ambiguity of "balance." He thought that in some cases workers' greed led them to work too long. Their incomes were too high; they had cultivated "artificial wants." The solution was a return to that other standby, "nature." "We must reduce our unnecessary expense, and devote one-fourth of the day to recreation, if we wish to live comfortably, and attain the age of man."[77]

Somewhere between the truism that life was hard with only death to look forward to and the view that most humans were experiencing only a fraction of the years and well-being properly theirs was a need for some consensus about what sort of life a working person could expect: this, and not the number of hours children (or even adults) ought to or might be allowed to work, was the essential issue. Other than the economists, who would judge the activity against the standard of capital growth, medical men came closest to offering an alternative standard and means of analysis to answer that question: Religion, law, politics, philosophy had neither the unanimity, nor the authority, nor the methodology. It was within a largely medical context that answers were sought to the questions of which aspects of factory work – hours and wages, age of workers, their postures or motions, mill ventilation, the social interaction among workers, even their trips from home to mill and back

76 C. T. Thackrah, *The Effects of the Arts, Trades, and Professions and of the Civic States and Habits of Living, on Health and Longevity: With Suggestions for the Removal of Many of the Agents Which Produce Disease, and Shorten the Duration of Life*, 2d ed. (London: Longmans, Rees, Orme, Brown; 1832), 203–10. On the relative salubrity of woolen mills, cf. Henriques, *Before the Welfare State*, 73. For contrasting uses of Thackrah's work see [R. H. Greg], *The Factory Question, Considered in Relation to Its Effects on the Health and Morals of Those Employed in Factories* (London: J. Ridgway, 1837; reprint, New York: Arno, 1972), 27; M. T. Sadler quoted in Alfred, *History*, I, 167.

77 Thackrah, like many proponents of factory legislation, hoped that limiting hours would restrict output, producing higher prices and allowing constant wages (Thackrah, *Effects*, 203–10).

– led to which deteriorations of health and morals: fever, consumption, orthopedic deformities, mental dullness or irrational excitability, precocious sexual activity, depression and demoralization, even suicide.[78]

Yet most medical men – Farre, Fletcher, and McDouall are exceptions – navigated very delicately when they approached the borders of their discipline. Many of the medical men speaking on the factory question in 1831–32 prefaced their remarks by stating that they were speaking "merely" as medical men (and perhaps also on behalf of "humanity"). Thus the Bradford surgeon William Sharp: "As to the policy of the measure I presume not to give an opinion . . . that is not within my province; but as I see a great deal of the effects of working children in this way, I think I am capable of giving a decided opinion upon this question; *and my opinion decidedly is,* THAT TEN HOURS IS THE EXTREME THAT CHILDREN OUGHT TO BE WORKED." They would then follow such a preface with graphic details of physiological destruction. One can take the "merely" as sincere, an admission that considerations of health and humanity ultimately are not authoritative, and that others must decide what the state is to do. Or one can read it as false deference, an assertion that while the medical man cannot invoke authority beyond his discipline, there is no need to do so: The verdict of medicine is final and absolute.[79] There seems no way of plumbing this ambivalence. It is likely a prudent ambivalence, and probably a realistic one: One of the truths of medical practice, as Knight recognized, is that there is much that is wrong that one cannot change.

## IV

It is worth asking why, given the significant involvement of medical men grappling with straightforwardly medical issues, factory reform (and equally the population–food–poor law issues) are not usually seen to belong to medical history or even to the history of public health, but to political, labor, and social history. It is not that the medical men of the day lacked authority and were not listened to – we will see Chadwick, principal author of the 1833 factory commission reports, torturing the evidence of his medical subcommissioners, which confirmed much of the Sadler testimony. He could not refute it, felt unable to ignore it; distort it he could and did.[80]

---

78  On suicide see F. Bisset Hawkins, *Elements of Medical Statistics with a New Introduction by James H. Cassedy* (Canton, Mass.: Science History, 1989), 108–14.

79  *The Justice, Humanity, and Policy of Restricting the Hours of Children,* 68–69. See the similar qualifications of Thackrah, *Effects,* 54. In chapter 3 we shall see Chadwick exploiting this qualification to neutralize medical opinion.

80  Henriques, *Before the Welfare State,* 84–88; Wing, *Evils of the Factory System,* xxviii–xxix. On the links between social history and the history of occupational health see Paul Weindling, "Linking Self Help and Medical Science: The Social History of Occupational Health," *The Social History of Occupational Health,* ed. Paul Weindling (London: Croom Helm, 1985), 2–31.

Part of the reason is that the identity and intellectual content of medicine changed; the public health of the 1870s was an emasculated form of the still-born political medicine of a half century earlier. The "last hurrah" of this political medicine is the first volume of *Capital*. For Marx, a concept of human health was the bedrock for economic analysis. To produce, the worker had to live and to reproduce. Health then (or the labor unit of value, if you like), was the ultimate commodity – food, energy, money, capital all translated into health.[81] From that concept came the central idea of surplus labor, the recognition of how "dead labour" or "capital" can only live "vampire-like . . . by sucking living labour, and lives the more, the more labour it sucks." Capital sucked living labor through long hours. "By the unlimited extension of the working day, you may in one day use up a quantity of labour-power greater than I can restore in three." If, working a day of "normal length" (one that allowed the laborer to recover fully from the destruction of work), a laborer's working life was thirty years, those long hours would extract that thirty years' labor in only ten. Yet the laborer received only a third of the labor value, just what was necessary to keep him alive for that ten years; the other two-thirds, sucked up by capital, was "surplus value."[82]

This was no mere theory, Marx insisted: It was confirmed by medical testimony. There was the case, for example, of Mary Anne Walkley, seamstress, milliner, who died in June 1863, aged twenty, having worked sixteen-and-a-half-hour days in a sweatshop. A coroner's jury attributed her death to apoplexy "accelerated by overwork." He cited the prominent sanitarian B. W. Richardson, on blacksmithing, which, "unobjectionable as a branch of human industry, is made by mere excess of work, the destroyer of the man. He can strike so many blows per day, walk so many steps, breathe so many breaths, produce so much work, and live an average, say of fifty years; he is made to strike so many more blows, to walk so many more steps, to breathe so many more breaths per day. . . . He meets the effort; the result is, that producing for a limited time a fourth more work, he dies at 37 for 50."[83] Marx took evidence from a number of investigations in the early 1860s of industries in which child labor was still unregulated. He appealed to medical men both for explanations of the physiology of exhaustion and for expressions of outrage at this "sacrifice" of children. He recognized food, work, and money as currencies of health and spoke of the "coining of children's blood

---

81 E.g., in Labor "a definite quantity of human muscle, nerve, brain, etc., is wasted, and these require to be restored." "The minimum limit of the value of labour-power is determined by the value of the commodities, without the daily supply of which the labourer cannot renew his vital energy, consequently by the value of those means of subsistence that are physically indispensable" (Karl Marx, *Capital: A Critical Analysis of Capitalist Production, trans. from the 3rd German edition by Samuel Moore and Edward Aveling*, ed. Frederick Engels, 3 vols. [New York: International Publishing Co., 1939], I, 149–51, 217).
82 Ibid., 216–17, 243. The vampire metaphor recurs (cf. 230).
83 Ibid., 239–41.

into capital." He also knew of the testimony of "the most distinguished physicians and surgeons in London" to the Sadler committee.[84] (Indeed, had he looked at more of the medical literature he would have found the concept of surplus value in all but name.[85]) Repeatedly he borrowed motifs and arguments from the medical testimony of the teens and early thirties, only substituting "capital" for "the factory": In "its were-wolf hunger for surplus-labour, capital oversteps not only the moral, but even the merely physical maximum bounds of the working day. It usurps the time for growth, development and healthy maintenance of the body. It steals the time required for the consumption of fresh air and sunlight. . . . It reduces the sound sleep needed for the restoration, reparation, refreshment of the bodily powers to just so many hours of torpor as the revival of an organism, absolutely exhausted, renders essential." Ultimately, the effects of capital were "the premature exhaustion and death of this labour-power itself."[86]

Yet, remarkably, he did not see himself as writing on health or medicine. Nor do we. Marx belongs to economics and politics, medicine belongs to science. By the late 1860s a chasm had already opened. What was plain to Farre – that health was the antithesis of capitalism, and medicine the obvious institutional and intellectual basis to counter it – eludes Marx. In part the reason is that medicine had changed. What remained of the earlier tradition was now tangential. That health was a commodity had nothing to do with the business of medicine.


V

We may finally ask why, if all these social issues – prison administration, poor law reform, acceptable work – were discussed as matters of health, this political medicine or public health was stillborn. That question can be examined from the perspectives both of the medical profession and of their erstwhile allies: those working-class radicals critical of the factories and new poor laws of liberal industrialism.

---

84  Ibid., 230, 242, 256, 265–66. See also his discussions of food, 670–81. In particular he notes the involvement of "Dr. Farre, Sir A. Carlisle, Sir B. Brodie, Sir C. Bell, Mr. Guthrie, etc.," and singles out Farre, who "expressed himself still more coarsely."

85  E.g., an anonymous London dispensary practitioner in 1844: "The severe training and heavy work they perform cause them to use up their three score years and ten in little more than half the time – like the clock, the faster it goes, the sooner it runs down. The best machine can but perform the quantum of its duty. . . . Without adequate food, the human frame, though a machine of wonderful construction, and surprising power, quickly wears out" ("The Health of the Metropolis," *People's Medical Advisor Containing Original Essays on Subjects of the Most Vital Importance to All Classes 1* [1844]: 81–83). See also R. H. Tawney, in the introduction to William Lovett, *Life and Struggles of William Lovett in His Pursuit of Bread, Knowledge, and Freedom with Some Account of the Different Associations He Belonged To and Of the Opinions He Entertained*, 2 vols. (New York: Knopf, 1920), I, xix–xx.

86  *Capital*, I, 249–50.

While the radical press gives attention to starvation and exhaustion, it gives much more to democracy and civic rights. For many and very understandable reasons radicals were unwilling to be medicalized. It was one thing to denounce the destruction of the bodies of children (and women), quite another to say that those men who sought liberty as well as bread were cases for the pathologist. They also had reason to distrust bureaucracies of dependence, however benevolent: Paternalism always wanted something in return, usually passivity. Although its main demands were political – a broader franchise, secret ballots, annual parliaments – the Chartist movement that took shape in the summer of 1838 was crowded, especially in the North, with "bread and cheese" Chartists, those most victimized by the trade depression, violent haters of the new poor law and passionate proponents of "ten hours." In retrospect one cannot fairly say whether political or economic considerations were the more important for any of these people; one can get a sense, however, of how the two sets of concerns went together: power.[87] The way to improve the people's health was not a blanket of charity, but control over taxes, labor laws, tariffs, relief policies.

But medical men were ambivalent too. An ambitious profession might well have seized this opportunity to become general purpose social experts, the healers of this disease of class, but the doctors did not. Perhaps it was that there was no satisfactory framework within which medicine could be applied to such problems. Yet political economists, with no official framework or even any professional organization, profoundly influenced policy. In the framework coming into existence at the time – the inspectorial state – medicine would be underrepresented. The dissection inspectors were medical men, but none of the factory inspectors was, and only one assistant poor law commissioner.[88] They sacrificed a great deal in failing to take this opportunity. In poor law administration, rather than asserting that they were the ultimate professional authorities responsible for the physical and mental well-being of humans, medical men, as parish or union medical officers, accepted a subservient status, kowtowing to the instructions of even the most boorish vestries. While the profession campaigned to make sure that posts went to qualified practitioners, it shrank from the great public matters of food, work, and child care.[89]

The reasons for their failure are many. Medicine was, as has been mentioned, a poorly united, overcrowded, and squabbling set of professions. Yet

87 Knott does point out that Fergus O'Connor saw Chartism as including a full health care policy (*Popular Opposition*, 141; see also 145–46, 247, 273). This was certainly Cobbett's view (Ignatieff, *A Just Measure of Pain*, 164–65).
88 This was James Phillips Kay. Frank Mort (*Dangerous Sexualities: Medico–Moral Politics in England Since 1830* [London: Routledge and Kegan Paul, 1987], 27) sees Kay as exemplifying a large movement; Kay seems isolated to me.
89 As we shall see in chapter 3 there were many exceptions. Chadwick certainly thought the poor law medical officers had far too much to say on these issues.

two underlying factors also warrant consideration: the official identity of medicine in Britain and the character of medical practice and knowledge. Medicine was, with the church and law, one of the three medieval professions. For the other two, a public role was unavoidable, since both professions were state establishments. The priest in the Church of England was in many domains a ruler, not only of spiritual affairs, but of much education and charity as well. Often the only educated person in the area, the clergyman was the magistrate, responsible for everything from repairing bridges to determining paternity (some even served as road surveyors, one as public scavenger).[90] The law, too, was both a public institution and a profession that "manned" that institution. In common law, to plead, write briefs, or judge was to establish the rights and obligations of the state. But to practice medicine was not to make health policy: medicine was a private profession. It sought state protection, but for an activity carried out in private consultations, and which had little direct impact on the state. Medical men advised, they did not dictate or rule. Such professional self-concept characterizes the testimony of the medical elite in the Sadler hearings: they could identify what was wrong but lacked any sort of precedent or authority to have it stopped. Any county magistrate, however ill-educated, would have had little hesitation deciding matters on which the most learned physician, however convinced and committed, would only advise.[91]

Moreover, the focus of medicine, at least traditional medicine, was person, not policy, and balance, not perpetual and disorienting change. Client-initiated consultations to resolve client-defined health problems had nothing to do with policy. Even this balance was idiosyncratic: however acutely one might recognize damaged constitutions and infer their causes, traditional medicine was no trustworthy basis for pronouncing on minimum conditions of work, food, housing for people in general, precisely because it did not recognize people *in general*. The sheer multiplicity of those causes also tended to undermine the importance attached to any one of them; Ure justifiably complained of the "plasticity of the medical mind."[92] That concreteness of medical practice had also much to do with a lack of enthusiasm for "population" and the other abstractions of the political economists. In some of those (Malthusian) abstractions people were problems; disease was cure. Yet political econ-

90  Brian Keith-Lucas, *The Unreformed Local Government System* (London: Croom Helm, 1980), 89.
91  Mort's notion of a "statist putsch [that] was intimately bound up with medics' own desire for enhanced status and authority" seems overstated. While there is significant medical involvement in social issues there was no move toward a "medocracy." It is intriguing that, as Mort notes, medical men did claim "intellectual monopoly over key explanations of human affairs and social progress, notably over the rapid cultural transformations taking place within urban society." Medicine may well have "rubbed shoulders with moral philosophy and political economy" but showed great unwillingness to take command in these arenas (Mort, *Dangerous Sexualities*, 27).
92  Ure, *Philosophy of Manufactures*, 374.

omists did not attend at the bedsides of those whose diseases were induced by poverty.

These traditions of medical thinking are the subject of the next chapter, for we only make sense of what Chadwick did in fabricating public health by understanding the fabric from which he cut it.

# 2

## A Political Medicine

The great social issues of the first half of the nineteenth century – hunger, public order, population, and conditions of work – were stated as issues of health. It is almost inevitable that medical men would have been asked to comment on them, yet as we have seen, the profession made no effort to become public guardians of the people's health. There were good reasons to keep old client-based networks; moreover, medicine was ill-equipped to colonize. It was a crowded and divided profession: physicians, surgeons, and apothecaries (and increasingly those general practitioners qualified as apothecaries and in surgery) squabbled for status and practice. English qualifications vied with Scottish. Significantly, expansion into social policy occurred only after the medical reforms of 1858, and then quickly.

Understandable, yet nonetheless remarkable, this unwillingness, for just as the social issues of the day were significantly medical, so medical theory was significantly social, more alert to social causes of disease than any we have had since. One speaks with caution of the "medical theory" of the period, for it was a time of great competition among medical systems, of controversies on everything from proper fever therapy to the very essence of life. All the same, one can identify a broad framework of common concepts. For example, hygiene was central. Mind and body were seen as integrated. Each affected the other; both were affected by environment, broadly understood as the totality of physical, biological, hereditary, social, and psychological conditions of life. Because, in some way, most of these conditions could be altered, such a medicine was a source of great hope. With the rise of disease-centered pathology in the second half of the nineteenth century, this framework gradually faded, and it has been insufficiently understood or appreciated by most historians. I discuss first general concepts of physiology, pathology, and etiology. The second half of the chapter focuses on the application of this medicine to the social crises of industrializing Britain.

I

Eighteenth-century medical theory is deep water indeed, but it is necessary to wade in to clarify terms like "fever," "miasm," "contagion," and so on. To immerse ourselves in its strangeness let us dive into what one might expect to be a treatise on public health, Charles Collignon's *Medicina Politica, or Reflections on the Art of Physic As Inseparably Connected with the Prosperity of the State* (1765). Collignon, Cambridge anatomy professor, argued that the healthy mind required the healthy body and that "the well-being, prosperity, and stability of *empires* [are] greatly dependent on the Health of *Individuals*." The individuals he had in mind were not the poor but the wealthy, and in this humanitarian age one of the illnesses they might suffer was insensitivity to sentiment. By repairing the constitution, medicine could nurture appropriate feelings of pity and compassion; it could "destroy the acquired propensities, that inflame to an opposite behaviour: a behaviour found in pride or passion, arising . . . from reiterated fullness, provoking to peevishness, and not allowing a proper attention to human sufferings." Jealously, ambition, pride were likewise expressions of humoral imbalance: "What is ambition," asked Collignon, "but a more protracted paroxysm, of an existing mischievous insanity?" Religion could take root only in the healthy; irreligion was a sign of illness: "In proportion to the readiness with which some constitutions are inclined to sudden commotion of the blood beyond others, arises the propriety to more frequent offenses; against decency and duty. . . . The keeping in due temper the fluids, and solids of the Body . . . this I say has a natural aptitude to lay us open to the conviction of religious truths, and to make us pliant to be directed in our behaviour, by its laws."[1] A powerful medicine indeed to gentle the Georgian rake!

Collignon's goal is clearly social: he will use regimen to regulate class relations, just as Chadwickian sanitarians would use water and sewers. Both believed that through expert management of the environment, health, outlook, and behavior could be utterly altered. Yet in the nineteenth century the focus would be the pathological poor, while Collignon will practice his art on the bloated and callous gentry.

Clearly, Collignon's conception of disease is different from ours. Legatees of the germ theory, we tend to see it as an invasion of the body's integrity. An uninvaded body may be declared healthy regardless of its owner's subjective view of its condition. We see disease as a narrow and specific entity, health a broad and vague range of unproblematic states of being. Collignon's notion of cause was equally far from the causes medical men would appeal to a century later in the early days of the germ theory: diseases arose from "baleful

1 Charles Collignon, *Medicina Politica, or Reflections on the Art of Physic as Inseparably Connected with the Prosperity of the State* (London: J. Bentham, 1765), 18, 28, 34.

vicissitudes of heat and cold, moisture and drought; from internal Passions and external violence; from errors of Judgment, and excess of Indulgence."[2] Like most of his contemporaries, Collignon saw health as more than the absence of disease. He viewed disease physiologically, as an imbalance of some crucial internal commodity (e.g., vitality) or in some crucial internal process (e.g., circulation or elimination). The physician's job was the fine tuning of each individual's constitution to climate, diet, activity. Here health was narrow and disease broad. Not only was the "health point" different for each person, but it was always changing with season, age, accidents of circumstance. Since constitutions can be out of tune in greater or lesser degrees, one can be more or less diseased; there is thus a continuum between health and nonhealth.[3] Since constitutions are integrated, one expects illness to manifest itself throughout the person, as much in mind as in bowels, muscles, and bones. Any state of unhealthiness might require medical attention; many delicate persons spent much of their lives at Bath and like spas under close medical management. In practice, of course, one did not speak of a "disease" until the deviation from health passed some vague threshold and took on some definite form or course.[4]

2 Ibid., 8. DeLacy, following Riley, distinguishes between a neo-Hippocratic and a Galenical school in the eighteenth century. On this dichotomy Collignon is clearly a Galenist, as one would expect from his Oxbridge connection. Even if such a dichotomy can be demonstrated as reflecting distinct schools of thought and not merely different contexts of application and explanation, both positions still conceive the body as subject to environmental forces, behaving in a comprehensible and lawlike fashion, be they closer or more distant (Margaret DeLacy, "Influenza Research and the Medical Profession in Eighteenth-Century Britain," *Albion* 25 [1993]: 37–63; James C. Riley, *The Eighteenth Century Campaign to Avoid Disease* [London: Macmillan, 1987]; Charles Rosenberg, "Medical Text and Social Context: Explaining William Buchan's Domestic Medicine," *Bulletin of the History of Medicine* 57 [1983]: 22–42).

3 Parr defines "disease" as "that condition of the human body, in which the actions of life and health proper to it are not performed, or performed imperfectly. According to this definition the disease consists in disordered or impeded functions; and these form, in our view, its essence. By these it is defined; by these distinguished" (Bartholmew Parr, *London Medical Dictionary; Including under Distinct Heads, Every Branch of Medicine, viz. Anatomy, Physiology, and Pathology, the Practice of Physick and Surgery, Therapeutics and Materia Medica; with Whatever Relates to Medicine in Natural Philosophy, Chemistry, and Natural History* [Philadelphia: Mitchell, Ames, and White; 1819], s.v. "Causa," 381). Cf. Copland's definition of "health" as "uninjured . . . vitality endowment," with corresponding harmony of function and wholeness of structure. When disease occurs, "energies of the vital principle become depressed, excited, exhausted, or otherwise altered" (in James Copland, *A Dictionary of Practical Medicine, Comprising General Pathology*, 3 vols. [London: Longman, 1858], vol. I, 557; s.v. "Disease: the Causation and Doctrine of"). Significantly, Chadwick's mentor Bentham used a modern definition of health in justifying the deterrent workhouse: "Health being the mere *negation* of *disease*, if there be no disease in any instance . . . as far as health is concerned the *smallest* allowance is preferable as being *least expensive*" ("Outline of a Work Entitled Pauper Management Improved," *The Works of Jeremy Bentham Published under the Superintendence of His Executor, John Bowring* , 11 vols. [Edinburgh: William Tait, 1843], vol. 8, 387).

4 Parr, *London Medical Dictionary*, s.v. "Hygidion." Parr wrote that "many changes may take place, without inducing a lesion of the functions, and, of course, a disease." On the social basis of this medicine see N. D. Jewson, "The Disappearance of the Sick-Man from Medical Cosmology, 1770–1870," *Sociology* 10 (1976): 225–44.

Within such a physiological approach, a disease exists only in the diseased individual. One may diagnose it as belonging to a species, but that in no way denies the inviolate individuality of *this* disease in *this* person. Its causes too were unique. Frequently they were events in the sufferer's personal history: what had she been eating; had he had bad news recently; was the family living in clean, airy conditions; were they working too hard? The many systems of disease classification were mainly ways of organizing knowledge for teaching and communication. "Systems are the work of our own minds," wrote the medical lexicographer Parr: "nature advances by almost imperceptible shades." To name a disease, even to talk of its seed or "germ," did not necessarily imply that each disease was genetically unique, the consequence of a specific unique cause.[5] Epidemics, it is true, were often seen as distinct entities, but the distinctiveness might lie in time or place (e.g., the plague of 1666) more than in assumptions of a mobile and persistent entity that periodically reappeared to engender the same effect.

While Collignon is evidently a Galenist (he talks of humors rather than fibers or ferments or vitality), had he drawn on Boerhaave's atoms, or written slightly later and emphasized nervous energy or vitality, he would have been addressing the same sorts of problems in similar ways. Even a pathology of lesions, physical injuries to tissues, such as would be imported from France in the early nineteenth century, could accommodate such a conception of disease.

Ancient Galenic conventions of causal explanation also suggested what strategies, public and private, might prevent such diseases. Contemporary textbook writers explained that a disease was the product of many different kinds of conditions or events, divided into two classes.[6] The "proximate cause" of disease was the lesion or faulty process most closely associated with the disease itself.[7] "Remote causes," on the other hand, were further subdivided as "ex-

---

5 Parr, *London Medical Dictionary*, II, 29, s.v. "Nosology"; I, 381, s.v. "Causa."
6 The views both that scientific progress would lead to the recognition of a specific cause for each disease and that all cases of a given disease need have the same cause(s) seemed not only philosophically unwarranted, but implausible, and even downright erroneous. See Whitley Stokes, quoted by Alfred Hudson: " 'This supposition of a *single cause* of the effects we witness, is quite unsupported by nature. Every animal, every plant, every rock, requires for its production the co-operation of many causes that we know and most probably of many more that we have not yet discovered' " (Hudson, "An Inquiry into the Sources and Mode of Action of the Poison of Fever," in William Davidson and Alfred Hudson, *Essays on the Sources and Mode of Action of Fever* [Philadelphia: A. Waldie, 1841], 108). Charles Williams argued that causation was fundamentally more complicated in medicine than in the "simpler" physical sciences: "In most cases there is not that uniform and constant relation between these as causes, and the diseases as effects, which we might expect from the analogy of causation in the simpler sciences" (Charles Williams, *Principles of Medicine Comprising General Pathology and Therapeutics*, edited with an introduction by Meredith Clymer [Philadelphia: Lea and Blanchard, 1848], 20–21.
7 With the advance of pathological anatomy and redefinition of disease as lesion, talk of proximate cause became redundant and confusing. Yet well into the nineteenth century disease was still an entity interpreted by the physician from the account and appearance of the patient and this hidden

citing" or "predisposing." "Predisposing causes" were all the forces that could alter the constitution; one's predisposition was the summation of one's exposure to such causes. Writing in 1827, the Manchester obstetrician John Roberton explained the concept: "Previous to the commencement of any disease, there is a state of predisposition, which fits or prepares the system for being acted upon, by the morbific cause. This applies as well for diseases which operate by a specific infection peculiar to each, as to those which arise from incidental causes, as cold, intemperance, and the like."[8] Since high predisposition might exist for a long time without blossoming into disease it might be necessary to posit an "exciting" cause (Roberton's "morbific" cause) as an igniter of the fuel of predisposition. Many factors could serve as either exciter or predisposer, depending simply on when, relative to the onset of the disease, they acted.[9]

Well into the 1850s medical textbooks and dictionaries handled "cause" in this way.[10] On one hand, such an agenda reflected the concern of a learned profession with adequate explanation; on the other it fit well a hygiene-centered medical practice because it provided long lists, both of actions people could take to prevent disease and of explanations for why they still sometimes became ill. In most of the physiological models of the period, predispositions, particularly those the poor were likely to suffer from, could be translated readily into a variety of metaphors signifying deficits of energy or vitality. "Causes act primarily on the vital endowment," wrote James Copland in his *Dictionary of Practical Medicine.* Or according to Robert Thomas: "Every thing

state was its most immediate cause. See Parr, *London Dictionary of Medicine,* s.v. "Causa," 381. For a modern discussion see Lester King, *Medical Thinking: A Historical Preface* (Princeton, N.J.: Princeton University Press, 1982), ch. 9–10.

8  John Roberton, *Observations on the Mortality and Physical Management of Children* (London: Longman, Rees, Orme, Brown, 1827), 254fn. His description paraphrases Boerhaave (*Dr Boerhaave's Academical Lectures on the Theory of Physic Being a Genuine Translation of His Institutes and Explanatory Comments Collated and Adjusted to Each Other, as They Were Dictated to His Students at the University of Leyden* [London: W. Innys, 1746], 379–80).

9  Copland, *Dictionary of Medicine,* 559, 562: The analogy is apt because most theorists held that an exciter was not always necessary; something like a spontaneous generation of disease might occur if predisposing forces accumulated to a critical point: "Such is the state of the human frame, that no constitution can ever be pronounced free from predisposition. There is, in every one, some weak organ which requires only an exciting cause to blow the spark into a flame" (Parr, *London Medical Dictionary,* 381, s.v. "Causa"). See also Williams, *Principles of Medicine,* 22; George Wood, *A Treatise on the Practice of Medicine,* 2d ed. (Philadelphia: Grigg, Elliott, and Co., 1849), 126; C. Hamlin, "Predisposing Causes and Public Health in the Early Nineteenth Century Public Health Movement," *Social History of Medicine* 5 (1992): 43–70.

10  Copland, *Dictionary of Practical Medicine,* I, s.v. "Disease," 558; John Elliotson, *The Principles and Practice of Medicine with Notes by Nathaniel Rogers* (London: Butler, 1839), 11–31; J. M. Good, *The Study of Medicine,* 2d ed., 5 vols. (London: Baldwin, Craddock, and Joy, 1825), II, 42; Parr, *London Medical Dictionary,* s.v. "Causa," 381; Thomas Watson, *Lectures on the Principles and Practice of Physic,* 4th ed., 2 vols. (London: Parker, 1857), I, 75–111. By around 1850 these terms were beginning to seem confusing and inutile (see Williams, *Principles of Medicine,* 18–67, esp. 21–23; Wood, *Treatise,* 126–43; *Hooper's Medical Dictionary,* 8th ed, revised, corrected, and improved by Klein Grant, M.D. [London: Longmans, Brown, 1848], s.v. "Aetiologia").

which has a tendency to enervate the body, may be looked upon as a remote cause of fever; and, accordingly, we find it often arising from great bodily fatigue."[11] Because they all acted similarly on the same entity, such causes were interchangeable to a degree.

It should be clear how such a framework made poverty a pathological condition. "It has been determined, by exact observations and calculations," noted Copland, "that those who enjoy easy or comfortable circumstances are much less subject to disease than the poor, the insufficiently clothed, and ill-fed. This arises not only from the former class being less exposed to its exciting causes, but also from the good effects of sufficient nourishment in supporting the energies of life, and thereby warding off the impressions of injurious agents and influences." Joseph Ayre of the Hull Dispensary, writing in 1818, explained that while any individual component of poverty might not harm health noticeably, their combined effect could be strong: "The system, when weakened, is readily affected by agents, which, in a state of vigour, it would have resisted. Thus the cold, to which the children of the poor are subjected by their inadequate clothing, would have much less injurious effects if their food were nutritive and abundant; and for the same reason, the insufficient and watery diet, with which so many of them are fed, would be rendered less hurtful in a climate more temperate and congenial than ours."[12]

It may seem that such explanatory conventions preclude epidemiological investigation. If anything can cause everything and everything can cause anything, it will be impossible to link discrete cause with distinct effect. Indeed, we can be pardoned for regarding all this as the doublespeak of equivocating charlatans.[13] Yet for the hygienist's question of what ways of living are associated with health or disease, these conventions provided an excellent foundation for epidemiology. For example, C. T. Thackrah found dwellers of Lancashire cotton towns to be "small, sickly . . . pallid, thin . . . a degenerate race, – human beings stunted, enfeebled, and depraved." In this holistic medicine it was futile to try to distinguish the effects of "bad habits" and "wretchedness of their habitations" from those of "long confinement in mills, the want of rest, the shameful reduction of the intervals for meals," for all were causes of debility; the way of living in its totality was harmful.[14]

11 Copland, *Dictionary of Practical Medicine*, I, s.v. "Disease," 558; Robert Thomas, *The Modern Practice of Physic, Exhibiting the Characters, Causes, Symptoms, Prognostics, Morbid Appearances, and Improved Method of Treating Diseases of All Climates*, 6th ed. (London: Longman, Hurst, Rees, Orme, Brown, 1819), 27.

12 Copland, *Dictionary of Practical Medicine*, I, s.v. "Disease," 561; Joseph Ayre, *Practical Observations on the Nature and Treatment of Marasmus* (London: Baldwin, Craddock, and Joy, 1818), 155. See also Henry MacCormac, *An Exposition of the Nature, Treatment, and Prevention of Continued Fever* (London: Longman, Rees, Orme, Brown, Green, and Longman, 1835), 40–41.

13 Parr complained of "causes without effects; effects without causes; opposite effects from the same cause; or the same effect from opposite causes" (*London Medical Dictionary*, s.v. "Causa," 381).

14 C. T. Thackrah, *The Effects of the Arts, Trades, and Professions and of the Civic States and Habits of Living, on Health and Longevity: With Suggestions for the Removal of Many of the Agents Which Produce*

This debility might never manifest itself in an increase of any *particular* disease, yet still constitute a significant health problem. Thackrah looked for older workers in a trade. If there were few, he suspected the trade, and the life that accompanied it, were fundamentally destructive, however disease-free the current work force might be.[15] Likewise, diet might best explain the disease experience of laborers in a northern climate. According to J. B. Davis, author of a popular health manual, heavy work in a cold place with too little food resulted in "a want of physical strength, a want of energetic action, and a proneness to all diseases of debility, as well as an especial liability to be affected with all kinds of epidemic diseases." Indeed, lack of good food would be the "prime" factor in disease incidence. Similarly Thomas Bateman, following William Heberden, saw cold as the major factor controlling the London mortality rate.[16]

Not only did such a framework warrant a kind of epidemiology, it implied also that focusing on specific diseases might be counterproductive in obscuring general causes of illness. The very project of distinguishing diseases, which we now see as central to medical progress, might divert the researcher from recognizing the most readily remediable factors. So argued the Manchester dispensary doctor Richard Baron Howard, in *An Inquiry into the Morbid Effects of Deficiency of Food Chiefly with Reference to Their Occurrence amongst the Destitute Poor* (1839). The "starvation" Howard was studying was a combination of chronic malnutrition ("gradual and protracted starvation") coupled with factory work and exacerbated by trade cycles. "Poverty and want exist largely at all times in populous towns," he wrote: "A very large proportion of the mortality amongst the labouring classes is attributable to deficiency of food as a main cause." Yet the postmortem effects of malnutrition were indistinct, for the lives of the malnourished might end in fever, scrofula, dyspepsia, dys-

---

Disease, and Shorten the Duration of Life, 2d ed. (London: Longmans, Rees, Orme, Brown, 1832), 144–46.

15  The idea of premature aging and death is linked to the theory of a quantity or reservoir of vitality that would be prematurely exhausted by those who worked too hard in youth (Thackrah, *Effects*, 35–37, 148–49).

16  J. B. Davis, *A Popular Manual of the Art of Preserving Health* (London: Whittaker, 1836), 144; Thomas Bateman, *Reports on the Diseases of London and the State of the Weather from 1804 to 1816 Including Practical Remarks on the Causes and Treatment of the Former; and Preceded by a Historical View of the State of Health and Disease in the Metropolis in Times Past* (London: Longmans, Hurst, 1819), 52–53, viii; see also William Heberden, *Observations on the Increase and Decrease of Different Diseases* (London: T. Payne, 1801), 46–49, 66–68; John Reid, *The Philosophy of Death, or a General Medical and Statistical Treatise on the Nature and Causes of Human Mortality* (London: S. Highly, 1841), 36. Bateman wrote to correct "a dangerous and fatal impression . . . of the salubrity of cold" (cf. James Johnson, *The Influences of Civic Life, Sedentary Habits, and Intellectual Refinement, on Human Health and Human Happiness, Including an Estimate of the Balance of Enjoyment and Suffering in the Different Conditions of Society* [London: Underwood, 1818], 30–31). There was an issue of class here – Johnson wrote for the wealthy, who didn't get out enough but had the means to get warm; Bateman, as a fever hospital doctor, saw those who could not get warm.

entery, diarrhea, scurvy. So long as starvation was not a recognized diagnosis its extent would be unknown and it would be impossible to provide effective relief. Hence Howard wrote to teach medical men how to recognize starvation by its symptoms: apathy, a low fever, nervousness or inflammation of the brain, coldness, lack of appetite. Because lassitude was so common a symptom, those worst affected complained least.[17]

It may seem that the "physiological" perspective of Collignon and Howard works well enough for chronic illnesses, but what of the acute epidemic diseases that are usually seen as the main business of public health? Some diseases did indeed seem to reflect the specificity of a poison more than the uniqueness of the victim. By the mid-nineteenth century such diseases would become exemplars of a dominant "ontological" conception of disease, in which each disease was a species and for practical purposes the product of a single cause – exposure to its "germ." Because diseases with similar symptoms – say typhoid and typhus fevers – might have different causal agents and routes of transmission and therefore warrant different preventive strategies, accurate diagnosis would be important.

There are striking differences between seeing diseases as imbalances and seeing them as invasions, yet the perspectives are not incompatible, and in the period they were usually complementary.[18] Those studying acute epidemic diseases, like smallpox or typhus, had to explain why not all took the disease, and why it was more serious in some than in others. What distinguished those stricken? It seemed implausible to think exposure to the poison was the answer, for there were always some who must surely have been exposed, yet did not take sick. Strength of constitution (a "physiological" concept) evidently protected them: "Good diet, and good spirits, cleanliness, and fresh air, and proper clothing, and exercise, may all contribute to render the body less

17 Richard Baron Howard, *An Inquiry into the Morbid Effects of Deficiency of Food Chiefly with Reference to Their Occurrence amongst the Destitute Poor* (London: Simpkin, Marshall, and Co., 1839), iii, 1–3, 19–29, 37–40. Howard would write the Manchester report for Chadwick's Sanitary Inquiry; Chadwick, finding Howard's views unacceptable, would virtually ignore it. A few years earlier in Glasgow, Andrew Buchanan, professor of materia medica at the Andersonian University, had raised the same issue even more directly: "In plain language, I am of opinion, that many of the poor in this city *die of starvation*," which in turn was due to policies which "deprive one class of the community of the first necessaries of life, that another class may wallow in affluence." The torpor of the starving was "perhaps, a blessing, as it prevents them from speculating on the causes of their own misery" ("Report of the Diseases Which Prevailed among the Poor of Glasgow, During the Summer of 1830," *Glasgow Medical Journal 3* [1830]: 446–47).

18 For recent discussions of these questions by philosophers of medicine see *Science, Technology, and the Art of Medicine: European–American Dialogues*, Corinna Delkeskamp-Hayes and Mary Ann Gardell Cutter, eds. (Dordrecht: Kluwer Academic, 1993), esp. Dietrich von Engelhardt, "Causality and Conditionality in Medicine Around 1900," 75–104; Anne Fagot-Largeault, "On Medicine's Scientificity – Did Medicine's Accession to Scientific 'Positivity' in the Course of the Nineteenth Century Require Giving Up Causal (Etiological) Explanation?," 105–26; and José Luis Peset, "On the History of Medical Causality," 57–74. See also Riley, *Campaign*, 15.

susceptible of disease; the seeds of which, like those of vegetables, will then only spring up and thrive, when they fall upon a soil convenient for their growth," wrote Heberden.[19]

Often what appear incompatible explanations were answers to different questions. The character of that year's fever (i.e., that it responded to depletative rather than supportive therapy) might be ascribed to the character of the specific poison (contagion, miasm, or unusual state of atmosphere), while remote causes might explain who was stricken and who escaped, and proximate causes might integrate all these into an account of the disease that victims experienced and practitioners treated. While there was a slow shift from physiological to ontological conceptions of disease during the period, medical discussions often employed both, depending on what disease was being explained, what about it was at issue, and what the context of the conversation was: was one talking about unusual cases or urban populations?[20]

The familiar terms "contagion" (the vehicle of person-to-person disease transmission) and "miasm" (a pathogenic emanation dispersed in the atmosphere) belonged to this larger system of causation. Often seen as anticipations of germs, the terms may seem to imply disease specificity. This was not always the case: contagia and miasms might simply be among the many malignant forces that harmed the constitution.[21]

The two terms were variously and vaguely defined and used. To those for whom they were alternative forms of disease-specific poison, they were still often not fully distinct, for both reached their victim through the air, though at greater or lesser distance from their source.[22] But they were not necessarily

19 Heberden, *Increase and Decrease*, 68. Cf. John Haygarth, *A Letter to Dr. Percival on the Prevention of Infectious Fevers and an Address to the College of Physicians in Philadelphia on the Prevention of the American Pestilence* (Bath: R. Cruttwell, 1801), 33–35. Haygarth experimented on susceptibility to typhus, calculating that from 1:23 to 1:33 were not susceptible. "It is not improbable that debility, or indisposition, or fear, or exposure to cold or fatigue, or, as some suppose, a difference of diet, may occasion a greater variety in the quantity of poisonous miasms necessary to produce an infectious fever." See also MacCormac, *Fever*, 40–41.

20 Thus, most of the medical men explaining the Irish fever of 1817–19 gave an anticontagionist (mysterious alteration of atmospheric constitution) explanation of the origin of the epidemic, while appealing to standard contagionism as the primary means of its transmission within Ireland and invoking heavily physiological accounts of debilitation to explain why it struck those it did and affected those it struck differently (J. Barker and J. Cheyne, *An Account of the Rise, Progress, and Decline of the Fever Lately Epidemical in Ireland*, 2 vols. [London: Baldwin, Craddock, and Joy, 1821]). See also A. Tweedie, *Clinical Illustrations of Fever, Comprising a Report of Cases Treated at the London Fever Hospital, 1828–29* (London: Whitaker and Treacher, 1830), 81. These were ancient questions (J. Ferriar, "The Origin of Contagious and New Diseases," in Ferriar's *Medical Histories and Reflections*, 1st American ed., 4 vols. in 1 [Philadelphia: Dobson, 1816], I, 119–20).

21 Nor does "contagion" or "miasm" necessarily translate into "exciting cause" – a contagion might be equally understood as a predisposer, since not all who were exposed to the contagion acquired the disease. "The occurrence of the exciting cause may be, or may not be, accompanied by exposure to contagion" (Hudson, *Fever*, 124–25). See also Williams, *Principles of Medicine*, 36; Copland, *Dictionary*, s.v. "Disease," 565–58.

22 What may seem the most important distinction – that a contagion could only be received from a previous human host, while a miasm could spontaneously generate under proper conditions of

alternatives. Sometimes they were synonyms and sometimes they were answers to different questions. In his 1799 *Medical Dictionary*, Richard Hooper saw no important distinction among "miasma," "contagion" "effluvia," "virus," "lues," "infection."[23] Parr, in 1808, saw "miasm" as a kind of contagion: "Contagion, then, exists in the atmosphere; and we know distinctly but of one kind, viz., marsh miasmata." He suggested also that jail fever arose from miasmata pervading the jail; the "human effluvium" would then be capable of giving "activity to the contagion."[24] John Mason Good would have "miasm" refer to a state of being and "contagion" to the process by which that state of being was applied to a person, as in "contagious miasm."[25] Sometimes "miasm" was used in its restricted sense for an unknown something "arising from stagnant water . . . from vegetable matter in a state of decomposition; from moist absorbent soils exposed to the sun's rays," and similar environments. This was held to cause agues; enlargements of spleen, liver, and glands; rheumatism; and catarrh in cold climates, and remittents, bilious and gastric fevers, dysentery, choleraic diarrhea, and hepatitis in warm climates.[26] Yet some thought this thing from the swamp to be no more than deoxygenated air (resulting from the oxygen demands of decaying organic matter) or conversely to be one of the ordinary products of organic decomposition.[27] "Miasm" often referred simply to air vitiated in some unknown way.

filth – was not completely accepted. Ontologist anticontagionists sometimes did imagine a permanent (i.e., nonlocal, non-spontaneously generated) aerial virus that periodically visited particular places – sometimes they even called it a contagion. See Thomas Mills, *A Comparative View of Fever and Inflammatory Complaints with Essays Illustrative of the Seat, Nature, and Origin of Fever* (Dublin: Cumming and McArthur, 1824), 111–15, 121. The range of contamination was an important issue: How closely could one safely approach a victim? (See Good, *Study of Medicine*, II, 66; Parr, *London Medical Dictionary*, s.v. "Miasm"; Haygarth, *Letter to Dr. Percival*, 6–7, 60).

23 R. Hooper, *Compendious Medical Dictionary* (London: J. Murray, 1799), s.v. "Miasm."
24 Parr, *London Medical Dictionary*, s.v. "Contagio," 482–84. Tweedie similarly held that contagious particles "originate, and spread, in consequence of a peculiar condition of the atmosphere" (*Clinical Illustrations of Fever*, 81–82).
25 Good, *Study of Medicine*, II, 64–65: "No great benefit, however, has resulted from endeavouring to draw a line of distinction between these two terms, and hence it is a distinction that has been very little attended to of late years. *Miasm* is a Greek word, importing pollution, corruption, or defilement generally; and *contagion* a Latin word, importing the application of such miasm or corruption to the body by the medium of touch. There is hence therefore, neither parallelism nor antagonism, in their respective significations: there is nothing that necessarily connects them either disjunctively or conjunctively. Both equally apply to the animal and vegetable worlds – or to any source whatever of defilement and touch; and either may be predicated of the other; for we may speak correctly of the miasm of contagion, or of contagion produced by miasm."
26 Copland, *Dictionary*, s.v. "Disease," 569. Or one could use the new term "malaria": "a peculiar, invisible, and hitherto unexplained exhalation from the ground, supposed to be the consequence of either animal or vegetable putrefaction." With predisposition it was a "powerful agent" (Tweedie, *Clinical Illustrations*, 82–84).
27 Parr, *London Medical Dictionary*, s.v. "Miasm"; Good, *Study of Medicine*, II, 64–65.

## II

Early-nineteenth-century etiological conventions did not imply particular social actions to prevent disease; they did, however, act as a fertile framework
that encouraged medical men to recognize many social factors, more or less
correctable, in their accounts of disease. The social possibilities of this etiology
are especially apparent in two diseases: consumption and continued fever.

Though consumption was a generic term for a wasting disease, pulmonary
consumption was a definite disease entity with recognized links to other "tubercular" phenomena (e.g., scrofula) and to diseases of malnutrition (rickets).
In 1839 consumption was responsible for about a quarter of all deaths and
more than 50 percent of deaths in older children.[28] The authority on consumption in 1839 was the Royal Physician Sir James Clark. Clark held the
ancient view that tuberculosis struck "delicate" persons with a hereditary "cachexia" or "diathesis" for it. Far from taking a "blame-the-victim" stance,
Clark, like many contemporaries, focused on the living and working conditions that determined whether that hereditary disposition ever developed into
full-blown consumption.[29]

The causes Clark identified were those being cited by various critics of
industrializing Britain: poor food, clothing, infant care, ventilation; lack of
light; and overwork. Inadequacy in only one of these might prevent the body's
systems from making use of the others. Thus, impure air impaired digestion
and hence led to malnutrition: "In the confined districts of large and populous
cities . . . food . . . cannot be assimilated even though the supply be unexcep-
tionable." In the country that cachexia might be generated by thin clothes
and lack of meat in the diet. Or it might arise from labor that "exhausts and
debilitates," or uncleanliness, drink, and dashed hopes. At risk was the body's
ability to nourish itself: when predisposers lowered "the power of assimila-
tion" sufficiently, "the tuberculous diathesis will be induced: Whenever . . .
the nutritive functions are vigourously carried on, this disposition will not
manifest itself."[30] Clark found it impossible to distinguish causes which predisposed one to consumption from the exciting causes that initiated the disease. Long exposure to predisposing causes might finally trigger the irreversible

28 William Farr, "Vital Statistics," *A Statistical Account of the British Empire: Exhibiting Its Extent, Physical Capacities, Population, Industry, and Civil and Religious Institutions,* ed. J. R. McCulloch, 2d ed., 2 vols. (London: Charles Knight, 1839), II, 574; Thomas, *The Modern Practice,* 497. Heberden re-ported much the same result in 1801 (*Increase and Decrease,* 42). For recent assessments see F. B. Smith, *The Retreat of Tuberculosis 1850–1950* (London: Croom Helm, 1988); Sumit Guha, "The Importance of Social Intervention in England's Mortality Decline: The Evidence Reviewed," *Social History of Medicine* 7 (1994): 96.

29 Sir James Clark, *A Treatise on Pulmonary Consumption Comprehending an Inquiry into the Causes, Nature, Prevention and Treatment of Tuberculosis and Scrofulous Diseases in General* (London: Sherwood, Gilbert and Piper, 1835), 200–202, 221. Cf. Davis, *Hygiene,* 51–53, 65, 274.

30 Clark, *Treatise,* 239, 12, 219, 230–35. Davis, who followed Clark, held that the "immediate" cause in nine of ten cases was "cold" (Davis, *Hygiene,* 89–95); cf. Thomas, *The Modern Practice,* 498.

decline that constituted the disease, but in a pathology that emphasized the cumulative effect of degrading forces, it was impossible to specify when that event occurred. He acknowledged that consumption might be contagious and that it was unwise to share a bedroom with a consumptive. But it was impossible to say, and pointless: the preventives were social.[31]

Consumption was incurable, Clark believed, but the physician could still help "by convincing the public of the comparative futility of all attempts to cure consumption, and of the signal efficacy of proper measures directed to prevent it." The necessary measures were "simple, and . . . available": airy workshops and apartments, regulation of indoor temperature, exercise, cleanliness, and abstinence from strong drink. Such an attack on predisposition would also "raise the standards of public health, and at the same time advance the moral excellence of man, augment his mental capabilities, and increase the sphere of his usefulness."[32]

It is easy to see how consumption might be linked with deprivation; it is a kind of exhaustion. But it was fever that was the central disease in public health discussions in the half century before 1840. Though it is often suggested that a focus on social and environmental preventives was a product of anti-contagionist (miasmatic) explanations of disease (while contagionist explanations are presumed to limit responses to isolation), most medical men concerned with a social response to fever drew on concepts of contagia.[33]

Typhus fever was not a new disease, but it was becoming increasingly prominent. Its competitors, ague, smallpox, plague, and dysentery, had declined. Moreover it seemed related to life in the new industrial towns: to mo-

---

31 Clark, *Treatise*, 238–40; cf. Thomas, *The Modern Practice*, 498. Occupation was a more central factor in explaining tuberculosis than in explaining most other diseases. Following Thackrah and drawing on the Paris clinicians, Clark saw irritation as the primary pathological process. Workplace atmospheres "loaded with pulverulent bodies or charged with gaseous substances of an irritating quality" were the exciting causes of consumption among stonemasons, miners, coal heavers, flax dressers, polishers of brass and steel, metal grinders, and needle pointers. Also deadly were sedentary occupations, especially those of cobblers, tailors, and dressmakers, because they prevented full expansion of the chest, and thus undermined the constitution (Clark, *Treatise*, 165–69, 186–93; cf. Thackrah, *Effects*, 201; Thomas, *The Modern Practice*, 497).

32 Clark, *Treatise*, iv, xiii–xiv, 202.

33 Cf. Erwin Ackerknecht, "Anticontagionism between 1821 and 1867," *Bulletin of the History of Medicine* 22 (1948): 562–93; Riley, *Campaign*, x. For criticisms see Roger Cooter, "Anticontagionism and History's Medical Record," *The Problem of Medical Knowledge: Examining the Social Construction of Medicine*, eds. P. Wright and A. Treacher, 87–108 (Edinburgh: Edinburgh University Press, 1982); Margaret Pelling, *Cholera, Fever, and English Medicine, 1825–1865* (Oxford: Oxford University Press, 1987), passim; W. Coleman, *Yellow Fever in the North: The Methods of Early Epidemiology* (Madison: University of Wisconsin Press, 1987), ch. 7. Controversies did occur, but as Margaret Pelling has noted, more as concoctions whipped up for immediate political needs than as fundamental antitheses of theoretical medicine. Almost always, the practical response to epidemics included isolating the sick as well as scraping out the drains and hauling off the dung. This eclecticism in explanation was also true in the earlier campaign against plague (see C. Cipolla, *Miasmas and Disease: Public Health and the Environment in the Pre-Industrial Age*, trans. Elizabeth Potter [New Haven: Yale University Press, 1992], 4–5, 45–48, 60).

bility, crowdedness, and periodic unemployment and hunger (though typhus was as bad, if not worse, in the famine-ridden countryside, especially in Ireland).[34] That fever was contagious meant no one was free of risk, a fact reiterated by medical men seeking support for the new fever hospitals or "houses of recovery" they began to establish in the mid-1790s.[35] Fever was a prominent subject of controversy – on therapy (did one deplete or support?), diagnosis (was continued fever one disease or many, or was each outbreak distinct?), and proximate cause (what was happening in a fevered body – debilitation, inflammation, or both?).[36]

The so-called fever contagion was clearly quite different from the smallpox – more volatile, yet weaker (in the sense of being effective only in a concentrated dose). Indeed, it was not clearly distinct from some miasms.[37] Thus there was a premium on one sanitary reform, ventilation. One might safely visit a fever victim so long as the space around the victim was well enough aired to disperse the contagion.[38] A crowded or confined atmosphere, however, would continually generate the poison, as in the Black Hole of Calcutta and many jails.

Because fever was only weakly contagious, predisposition figured centrally in explaining outbreaks. There was broad agreement, based on a large collection of reports of epidemics, that the most important predispositions were unusual deprivation and social crisis. Appealing both to ontological and to physiological conceptions of disease, to predisposing and exciting causes, contagia and miasms, and somatic and psychological factors, Robert Thomas, follower of the eminent Edinburgh professor William Cullen, wrote that ner-

---

34  Reid, *Philosophy of Death*, 88–95; "Epidemic Fever," *Edinburgh Medical and Surgical Journal* 14 (1818): 530, 534; Thomas Bernard, "An Extract from a Further Account of the London Fever Institution," *Report of the Society for Bettering the Condition and Increasing the Comforts of the Poor* 5 (1808): 138.

35  W. F. Bynum, "Cullen and the Study of Fevers in Britain," *Theories of Fever from Antiquity to the Enlightenment*, eds. W. F. Bynum and V. Nutton, Medical History, Supplement, 1 (London: Wellcome Institute for the History of Medicine, 1981), 135–47.

36  Dale C. Smith, "Medical Science, Medical Practice, and the Emerging Concept of Typhus," in Bynum and Nutton, *Theories of Fever*, 121–34; Leonard Wilson, "Fevers and Science in Early Nineteenth Century Medicine," *Journal of the History of Medicine* 33 (1978): 394; Good, *Study of Medicine*, II, 50–63, 240–42; Pelling, *Cholera*, 14–15; W. P. Alison, "Inflammation," *A System of Practical Medicine Comprised in a Series of Original Dissertations*, ed. A. Tweedie, Library of Medicine, 1 (London: J. Whitaker, n.d.), 69–72; Robert Jackson, *A Sketch, (Analytical) of the History and Cure of Contagious Fever* (London: Burgess and Hill, 1819), 150: Robert Thomas, *The Modern Practice*, 4–60; McCormac, *Fever*, 19–21.

37  Henry Clutterbuck, *Observations on the Prevention and Treatment of the Epidemic Fever at Present Prevailing in the Metropolis and Most Parts of the United Kingdom* (London: Longman, Hurst, Rees, Orme, and Brown, 1819), 37, 41; M. C. Buer, *Health, Wealth, and Population in the Early Days of the Industrial Revolution* (London: Routledge, 1926), 166–67; MacCormac, *Fever*, 54–57.

38  Thomas Bateman, *A Succinct Account of the Contagious Fever of This Country Exemplified in the Epidemic Now Prevailing in London* (London: Longman, Hurst, 1818), 14, 144; Haygarth, *Letter to Dr. Percival*, 70–75; cf. William Davidson, "Essay on the Sources and Mode of Propagation of the Continued Fevers of Great Britain and Ireland," in Davidson and Hudson, *Essays on the Sources and Mode of Action of Fever* (Philadelphia: A. Waldie, 1841), 5.

vous fever was "apt to attack those who are weakened from not using a quantity of nutritive food, proportionable to the exercises and fatigue they daily undergo; hence it is very prevalent among the poor." Its "most general cause . . . [was] contagion, communicated through the medium of an impure or vitiated atmosphere, by concentrated effluvia arising from the body of a person labouring under the specific disease; but whatever debilitates the system or depresses the mind, may induce a state of predisposition more readily to be influenced by the operation thereof." A calm and sober person, well fed, clothed, and housed, was less likely to fall into fever though by no means immune.[39] Since crisis, depression, anxiety, or poverty did not always bring on fever or produce contagion, some writers also invoked Thomas Sydenham's concept of an atmospheric "constitution" – a peculiar atmospheric change manifest only in the production of epidemic disease.[40] Indeed, the same atmospheric changes that blighted the crops and led to famine might also produce the fever contagion itself.[41]

Many held that contagion could generate spontaneously, either in a very debilitated body or from exposure to ordinary human effluvia in concentrated form. Wrote Parr: "If many men are confined in a comparatively small place, their health is gradually undermined; their complexions become sallow; their appetite and spirits fail. No real disease may be observable in them; yet, to others, they will some times in this state communicate fever, and fever will appear to arise spontaneously among themselves. . . . When the fever is actually formed, it is well known that it may be communicated by its effluvia."[42] Most believed spontaneous generation to occur rarely, but it explained how fever could arise when there seemed no other apparent contagion. Here the common character of the disease was due to the commonalities of human bodies, which could on occasion produce the same pathological processes usually triggered by exposure to a contagion or miasm.[43] The resulting poisons might be called "contagions," but they were aspecific contagia, simply forms of pathological influence the products of a diseased body could acquire.[44] Such

---

39 Thomas, *The Modern Practice,* 44–46; cf. J. M. Good, *A Dissertation on the Diseases of Prisons and Poor-Houses* (London: C. Dilley, 1795), 25, 67; Wood, *Treatise,* 128–29.

40 Clutterbuck, *Observations,* 30; Jackson, *Sketch,* 148–50. Cf. Wilson, "Fevers and Science," 388.

41 Clutterbuck, *Observations,* 35–36; McCormac, *Fever,* 45.

42 Parr, *London Medical Dictionary,* 645.

43 I.e., "In a great number of instances, the disease has taken place where no *contagion* could be found, or even suspected, to which it might be referred" (Clutterbuck, *Observations,* 30); cf. Davidson, "Fever," 4; Hudson, "Fever," 104–8; MacCormac, *Fever,* 43–44; Haygarth, *Letter to Dr. Percival,* 45, 56, 110; Robert Graham, *Practical Observations on Continued Fever, Especially That Form at Present Existing as an Epidemic with Some Remarks on the Most Efficient Plans for Its Suppression* (Glasgow: J. Smith and Son; 1818). Among those for whom this was an explanation of first resort was Bateman (*Succinct Account,* 11); see also "Epidemic Fever," *Edinburgh Medical and Surgical Journal* 14 (1818): 537.

44 The contagion might be merely "morbid exhalations and secretions . . . constituting a medium of infection capable of generating fever" (Bateman, *Succinct Account,* 13); MacCormac, *Fever,* 44–45; Tweedie, *Clinical Illustrations,* 82–86. This is the case even for Haygarth, a contagionist in a rela-

a view obviated the need to believe that God had created contagia and the need for arbitrary hypothesizing about transmission routes.

In most fever theories the nervous system was central.[45] It followed that the subjective state of the victim could be a cause of the disease. As James Copland explained it, "When mental energies are depressed . . . the powers of life are less able to oppose the debilitating causes of disease." By contrast, with a positive mental state "the depressing causes make little or no impression upon the constitution."[46] Reflection on the loss of liberty was a significant cause of prison fever, wrote Good. John Ferriar included "anxiety and depression of spirits . . . among the efficient causes, because it is not proved that the mere confinement of the effluvia of clean and healthy persons, free from mental uneasiness, can become poisonous; otherwise the close rooms of an elegant house might produce fevers as well as garrets and cellars." Victorious armies were relatively immune to fever; defeated armies susceptible.[47] Terms like "depression" and "anxiety" recur in the literature, referring to a state both somatic and subjective. The sources of depression might be mental events themselves (fear and worry) or physical conditions that produce such outlooks: "low diet, fatigue, previous illness, excessive secretions and discharges, want of sleep, venereal excesses."[48] Ferriar wrote of seeing "patients in agonies of despair on finding themselves overwhelmed by filth, and abandoned by every one who could do them any service; and after such emotions I have seldom found them recover."[49]

### III

Medical theory suggested, then, that the living and working conditions of laboring people shortened life, impaired health, and distressed the soul. Yet that was not necessarily a public problem. Could the poor really expect health and ease of mind? Was not their lot poverty, and were not hardship and some misery concomitants of poverty? One certainly could regard the physical and psychological needs of the poor (and accordingly their justifiable expectations) as different from those of the wealthy (and, conveniently, commensurate with what society was willing to deliver). To adopt a physiological and moral

tively modern sense (*Letter to Dr. Percival*, 129–32). See also Ferriar, "Origin of Contagious and New Diseases," 118; cf. Pelling, *Cholera*, 15.

45  Christopher Lawrence, "The Nervous System and Society in the Scottish Enlightenment," *Natural Order: Historical Studies of Scientific Culture*, eds. Barry Barnes and Steven Shapin, 19–40 (Beverly Hills: Sage, 1979); Gilbert Blane, *Elements of Medical Logick*, 2d ed. (London: Underwood, 1821), 46–47; Davis, *Hygiene*, 96; MacCormac, *Fever*, xi–xii; Reid, *The Philosophy of Death*, 35.

46  Copland, *Dictionary*, s.v. "Disease," 562, cf. Williams, *Principles of Medicine*, 48; MacCormac, *Fever*, 36; Davidson, "Essay," 72–73.

47  Good, *Dissertation*, 81–83; Ferriar, "Origin of Contagious and New Diseases," 125; Thomas, *The Modern Practice*, 44–46.

48  Copland, *Dictionary*, s.v. "Disease," 526; cf. Parr, *London Medical Dictionary*, s.v. "Causa," 381.

49  John Ferriar, "Epidemic Fever of 1789 and 1790," *Medical Histories and Reflections*, I, 78.

universalism (all persons have similar physical and psychological needs), on the other hand was to acknowledge a problem of *public* health.

In Collignon's ancien régime of mutual dependency, physiological universalism did not apply: stations of life were rigid; health and happiness were functions of station. For the poor, security in the necessaries of life – food, shelter, warmth – was enough. It was clearly impossible (and therefore presumably unnecessary) to practice the same fine tuning of constitution that medical men practiced among the rich; the season in Bath or a choice of wine and food was not an option for an agricultural laborer. Accordingly, the keystone of successful social medicine was fulfillment of the duty of charity: Collignon would cultivate responsible landlordism by altering the constitution of those responsible for the poor; he would physick the poor by physicking the rich. There was, indeed, a long tradition that the sufferings of rich and poor were equal but different: the rich suffered from surfeit, the poor from deprivation. James Johnson, editor of the elite *Medico-Chirurgical Journal*, wrote that "the uncultivated boor glides along, unconscious of the pleasures and unacquainted with the sufferings which necessarily grow out of civic society and intellectual refinement." "The *balance* of enjoyment," he held, lay with "the lower classes of society, who have little susceptibility toward intellectual pleasures and pains."[50]

Yet even in Collignon's time, Locke and liberalism were threatening this stable harmony. With educability and liberty came notions of physiological equality: rich or poor, the human "machine" was the same; situations that led inevitably to shorter lives, more disease, and less happiness to poor than rich seemed to violate the possibility of liberty. Medical practice was changing too. In the mideighteenth century the medicine of regimen cultivation had been the stock in trade mainly of an elite of physician gentlemen with exclusive practices. By the end of century, their ranks were being diluted by middle-class doctors, from the new medical schools of Edinburgh and Glasgow. Heirs of Hippocrates by way of Boerhaave, many of these were dissenters, and many had practices among the poor.[51]

A flurry of manuals of health appeared, adapting the ancient art of hygiene to the new middle classes. They told what to eat and drink; how much to

---

50 James Johnson, *The Influences of Civic Life*, 92–93, also 44, 11. See also Davis, *Hygiene*, 90–91. David Roberts finds this argument typical of paternalist social thought (*Paternalism in Early Victorian England* [New Brunswick, N.J.: Rutgers University Press, 1979], 152).

51 Anne Digby, *Making a Medical Living: Doctors and Patients in the English Market for Medicine, 1720–1911* (Cambridge: Cambridge University Press, 1994), 199–233; Anand Chitnis, *The Scottish Enlightenment and Early Victorian English Society* (London: Croom Helm, 1986), 135–46; Robert Kilpatrick, " 'Living in the Light': Dispensaries, Philanthropy and Medical Reform in Late Eighteenth Century London," *The Medical Enlightenment of the Eighteenth Century,* eds. Andrew Cunningham and Roger French, 254–80 (Cambridge: Cambridge University Press, 1990); Andrew Cunningham, "Medicine to Calm the Mind: Boerhaave's Medical System, and Why It Was Adopted in Edinburgh," ibid., 40–66.

sleep and exercise; how to govern one's passions, choose a career, or raise children. Some of these popular hygienic works, like Bernhard Faust's widely translated *Catechism of Health*, were decidedly leveling: according to Faust, the healthy person felt "strong; full of vigour and spirits; he relishes his meals; is not affected by wind and weather; goes through exercise and *labour with ease*, and *feels himself always happy*." The human body, wrote William Farr in 1839, was "framed to continue in healthy action 70 or 80 years." Yet "soon after 40 years of age individuals of the labouring classes begin to suffer from stomach complaints, the consequences of poor diet, poor clothing, exposure to weather, and anxiety; and from these complaints . . . they seldom afterward become wholly free."[52] The historian T. B. Macaulay, earlier a champion of the market, became a ten hours' advocate in 1846: "The great masses of the people shall not live in a way that will abridge life, that will make it wretched and feeble while it lasts, and send them to untimely graves, leaving behind them a more miserable progeny than themselves."[53]

Concepts of liberty were often defined in terms of health: one could only be free to act if one were fit to act. Notions of fair markets in labor presumed physiological parity. Those who were not "able-bodied," political economists generally agreed, were excused from the rigors of competition. But where lay the border between illness and health? And what was one to do if *participation in the market for labor was itself the cause of illness*? Some hoped that however hard their lives, the poor could and would follow the same hygienic rules as the rich. The Manchester fever authority John Ferriar advised the poor to avoid cellar dwellings: "They destroy your constitutions, and shorten your lives. No temptation of low rents can counterbalance their ill effects." They were told, Wash your children "from head to foot with cold water, before you send them to work in the morning. Take care to keep them dry in their feet, and never allow them to go to work without giving them their breakfast, though you should have nothing to offer them but a crust of bread, and a

---

52 Bernhard Faust, *The Catechism of Health, Trans. from the German and Carefully Improved by Dr Gregory of Edenburg [sic]*, 3d American ed. (Raleigh: Thomas Henderson, 1812), questions [qq] 7, 13–14; cf. Q 1: "Dear Children, to breathe, to live in this world, created by God, is it an advantage? Is it to enjoy happiness and pleasure?" A: "Yes. To live is to enjoy happiness and pleasure; for life is a precious gift of the Almighty." In Q 23, we learn from psalm 90 that God promises long life (seventy to eighty years) to those who obey the commandments. It is noted (Q 15) that we have a duty to improve the health of one another, and that parents and schoolmasters do not sufficiently consider that – nothing is said of masters. Nonetheless Faust held most injuries to health to be hereditary (18–19). On Faust see Charles Rosenberg, "Catechisms of Health: The Body in the Prebellum Classroom," *Bulletin of the History of Medicine* 69 (1995): 175–97. Also see Farr, "Vital Statistics," 522, 557; Robert Cowan, "Vital Statistics of Glasgow, Illustrating the Sanatory Condition of the Population," *Journal of the Statistical Society of London* 3 (1840): 270; "Epidemic Fever," *Edinburgh Medical and Surgical Journal* 14 (1818): 529. On physiological equality see E. P. Thompson, *The Making of the English Working Class* (Harmondsworth, U.K.: Penguin, 1968), 90.

53 Quoted in Alfred [George Kydd], *The History of the Factory Movement from the Year 1802, to the Enactment of the Ten Hours' Bill in 1847*, 2 vols. (London: Simpkin, Marshall, 1857), I, 237–38.

little water."[54] Whether it focused on churches, schools, or sewers, such a view was the premise of moral and sanitary reform of the 1830s and 1840s.

Among working people little of this optimism took hold, Thackrah found. Denial was the rule: artisans were unwilling to acknowledge that they led diseased lives. "Health is to most persons a disagreeable subject. . . . It implies a distrust of our sanity . . . most persons . . . will be inclined to admit that our employments are in a considerable degree injurious to health, but they believe, or profess to believe, that the evils cannot be counteracted, and urge that an investigation of such evils can produce only pain and discontent." Lead miners drank heavily, he found, "not with the view of enabling them the better to sustain their unhealthy employment, but confessedly to drown the ever-recurring idea, that they are, from their occupation, doomed to premature disease."[55]

As well as being a precondition of liberty, health was also the readiest yardstick of injustice, and the most unanswerable justification for social change. All this fancy physiology only showed what "any cottager's wife" knew, wrote the surgeon and factory reformer George Kydd: that factory work exhausted and crippled people – "Selfishness and obstinacy could alone require so uncalled-for an exhibition of physiological knowledge – instinct itself . . . proved all that reason, humanity, and science, had contended for."[56]

But medicine held out a physiological as well as a moral rationale for reform. Disease was not just a currency of witness but an instrument of redress. Fever, we have noted, took root in desperate people and became contagious. The belief that subjective outlook affected the generation of fever meant that in a person's *feelings* (and the fragile constitution of her body) lay the power to generate a truly contagious disease. Thomas Bernard of the Society for Bettering the Condition and Increasing the Comforts of the Poor urged "indulgence" of the "prejudices" of the poor against ventilation, for "tho repressed by authority," these "will operate secretly and forcibly on the mind; creating fear, anxiety, and watchfulness" – and possibly disease.[57] In this way fever theory empowered: the *feelings* of the poor person had political signifi-

54 John Ferriar, "Advice to the Poor," *Medical Histories and Reflections*, Appendix 1, 403–6; cf. Ferriar, "Account of the Establishment of Fever-Wards in Manchester," *Medical Histories and Reflections*, III, 337; Ferriar, "Of the Prevention of Fevers in Great Towns," *Medical Histories and Reflections*, II, 233; Clark, *Consumption*, 268–95. Clark admitted, "I am well aware that many of my recommendations will unfortunately be found beyond the attainments of the public at large; but . . . I . . . state them, in order that they may be adopted when circumstances admit."

55 Thackrah, *Effects*, 7, 90.

56 Alfred, *Factory Acts*, 56; see F. Engels, *The Condition of the Working Class in England*, trans. and eds. W. D. Henderson and W. H. Chaloner (Oxford: Blackwell, 1971), 111; MacCormac, *Fever*, 46.

57 Bernard, in Miss Horner, "Extracts from an Account of the Contagious Fever at Kingston-on-Hull," *Report of the Society for Bettering the Condition and Increasing the Comforts of the Poor* 4 (1805): 105. The idea that mental outlook affected physical health was not new: "Passions of the mind" were among Galen's "non-naturals"; the art of physic included producing illusions of hope that might spur recovery.

cance. Fostering a sense and (state) of well-being in others was critical to the success of that least altruistic task of public health, protecting oneself from epidemic disease.

Behind this modern psychophysical science was an ancient moral motif: plague is the oppressor's reward. Warnings of retribution via fever appear often, as medical writers sought support for their endeavors to prevent the disease. Fever was not a natural but an "artificial and accidental" occurrence, wrote MacCormac.[58] Ferriar warned that the "dwellings and persons [of the poor] continually breathe contagion," and it was "hardly possible to prevent the communication of the disease to the families of the rich. . . . The poor are indeed the first sufferers, but . . . by secret avenues it reaches the most opulent, and severely revenges their neglect, or insensibility to the wretchedness surrounding them." The "true danger[s] of luxury" were the "voluptuous habits" that led the rich to withhold charity. Thus "he contributes to the disease and destruction of thousands." The moral: "The safety of the rich is intimately connected with the welfare of the poor . . . minute and constant attention to their wants is not less an act of self-preservation than of virtue."[59] The argument parallels Chartist calls for justice though their retribution would come as revolution. It was also, both for Chartists and for fever doctors, embedded in Christian eschatology and natural theology: God is just; the creation embodies justice; injustice sooner or later triggers retribution.

## IV

Admit that working-class human machines ran by the same laws as upperclass machines, that they required a sense of well-being, and would explode, spewing forth contagion if their "maintenance" were neglected, and you had a political medicine.[60] A medicine that granted everyone a "personhood" is not what one expects of the triumphant years of industrial capitalism and Ricardian economics, and one must ask how far it informed practice. Did

58 MacCormac, *Fever*, 45; cf. "Epidemic Fever," 539; Jackson, *Sketch*, 128.
59 Ferriar, "Origin of Contagious and New Diseases," 125–27. These were central arguments in the campaign for fever hospitals. The tone varies from academic generalization – "wealthy people might get it too unless something is done" – to direct retribution – "the striking down of those who were given the opportunity to act justly, but didn't." The former are more common. Cf. Ferriar, "Epidemic Fever of 1789 and 1790," 77; idem, "Of the Prevention of Fevers in Great Towns," 224–39. See James Kay-Shuttleworth, *The Moral and Physical Condition of the Working Classes Employed in the Cotton Manufacture in Manchester, with a New Preface by W. H. Chaloner*, 2nd ed. (London: Frank Cass, 1970), 7, 11. Cf. Richard Millar, *Statements Relative to the Present Prevalence of Epidemic Fever among the Poorer Classes of Glasgow* (Glasgow: John Smith and Son, 1818), 9–10; Thomas Bernard, "An Extract from a Further Account of the London Fever Institution," 140. The best known version is not Ferriar's but Carlyle's, in *Past and Present*. Carlyle took it from the Edinburgh physician W. P. Alison, and it is at least implicit in nearly every fever writer of the period.
60 Ironically, the view of humans and machines as interchangeable was one of the vehicles of physiological universalism (Thackrah, *Effects*, 220–21).

social causes of disease imply a need for social changes to prevent disease or just for medicines to cure it? What parts of life were changeable? Given that hunger caused fever, was hunger preventable or only an indication of the disparity between population and food? Responses varied. In rural Ireland, where peasants survived by subsistence agriculture, famine and fever were acts of God. One might see the need for soup kitchens during an epidemic yet see no prospect of preventing future famines. Yet for urban workers, food seemed more to depend on the market and the corn laws than on nature. Fever writers of the 1830s and 1840s – Cowan, Davidson, MacCormac, Alison, Hudson – were generally unwilling to see falling wages or rising prices as "natural." Instead, they were errors. Overproduction led periodically to unemployment, and on to hunger and fever. In general medical men did not take on industrial capitalism directly. They did, however, identify some of its features – the division of labor, trade cycles, and wages too low to support life – as medical problems. On occasion they interfered in the market, mitigating rigorous incentives with proclamations that a person or population was in a state of disease and required support.

In part they did so because at a basic level medical ideology was incompatible with political economy. One emphasized dynamism and maximization, the other stability and balance. By definition diseases were contranatural states. Since the human constitution reflected the state of its environment, the social conditions that caused disease must equally be contranatural. In part also they did so as healers. The goal of improving the state of health was independent of the question of why the person was ill. Usually medical men spoke of the economic causes of disease or their interventions in the market not in the charged language of the radical press but in the neutral language of epidemiological generalization or physiological law. One might identify cause and recognize remedy without indulging in blame. Perhaps medical men saw themselves as making medical, not political, statements; perhaps they knew that the best way to be political was to appear apolitical.[61]

A good illustration of this perspective is the Glasgow surgeon Robert Cowan's attribution of the fever of 1836–37 to a textile workers' strike. Unlike many contemporary social analysts, he did not denounce workers' combinations and would say only that the strike was "lamentable." Cowan's problem was the misery of the strikers and their families. A medical problem existed; that the remedy – support for strikers and their families – had political implications, that it might seem to reward the blameworthy and interfere with the systems of incentives that made society work was beside the point.[62]

---

61 Some did wonder why medicine did not have a greater voice in policy (Davis, *Hygiene*, 3–4).
62 Cowan, "Glasgow," 269: "The rapid increase in the amount of the labouring population, without any corresponding amount of accommodation being provided for them; the density, and still increasing density of that population; the state of the districts which it inhabits; the fluctuations of trade and of the prices of provisions, and the lamentable 'strikes' in consequence of combination

A few years earlier, his colleague Andrew Buchanan had explained immorality and crime as physiological effects of desperate poverty.

The moral effect of an actual or apprehended privation of such necessaries, is to rivet [in] the mind the ideas immediately connected with them, and to create a *physical impossibility* of directing it to other subjects, however momentous. The moral condition of the poor, therefore, is in great measure, *the necessary consequence of the privations*, to which they are subject. It can excite no surprise, that, while they are completely and exclusively occupied, from day to day, in a struggle for mere existence, which demands not only their bodily exertions, but engages all their thoughts, they should become indifferent to everything else.[63]

Thus, in highly moralistic Scotland, Cowan and Buchanan saw not evil or righteous persons, but only dangerous epidemiological situations arising from complicated combinations of human errors and natural circumstances.

Fever doctors need not be romantics or humanitarians: Ferriar spoke not of the noble poor, but of their "sullen indolence."[64] But simply to practice effective public medicine, they had to admit that the power to affect the course of an epidemic lay with the poor. The fever hospital had to be much more than a place for isolating diseased bodies; it had to be attractive enough so that people would elect to go to it before the disease had been widely communicated.[65] They had to be persuaded to stay there for a substantial convalescence.[66] There had therefore to be support services for families to

among the workmen, by which the means of subsistence have been suddenly withdrawn from large masses; the recklessness and addiction to the use of ardent spirits, at once the cause and the effect of destitution; the prevalence of epidemic diseases both among the adult and infantile portion of the community, have been the chief causes of the great mortality of the city of Glasgow." Good, writing in 1795, described price inflation as a public health problem. Farmers and manufacturers were doing well, but not laborers: "I have made these observations, because the causes of almost all the diseases I am considering, and consequently the diseases themselves, are to be traced to this general source." He wrote of a typical weaver's family, in which, "if even the strictest economy be made use of," wages "will scarcely suffice to procure the bare necessaries of life." "In such situations, little can be expected from the skill of the surgeon, if he have not influence enough with the chief parishoners to unite their efforts with his own to produce a complete reformation" (Good, *Dissertation*, 44–45, 52).

63 Buchanan, "Report of the Diseases Which Prevailed among the Poor of Glasgow, During the Summer of 1830," *Glasgow Medical Journal 3* (1830): 440. According to Brenda White, Buchanan got himself in trouble with this paper, though probably more for his ad hominem attacks on the patrons of local medical charities than for his political views ("Scottish Doctors and the English Public Health," *The Influence of Scottish Medicine*, ed. Derek Dow, 77–85 [Park Ridge, N.J.: Parthenon, 1988]).

64 Ferriar, "Origin of Contagious and New Diseases," 125.

65 W. F. Bynum, "Hospital, Disease, and Community: The London Fever Hospital, 1801–1850," *Healing and History: Essays for George Rosen*, ed. Charles Rosenberg (New York: Science History, 1979), 102, 109. Cf. Buer, *Health, Wealth, and Population*, 200–201; J. R. Poynter, *Society and Pauperism: English Ideas on Poor Relief, 1795–1834* (London: Routledge and Kegan Paul, 1969), 95. See the comments of Bernard in Miss Horner, "Contagious Fever at Kingston upon Hull," 102, 108.

66 Ferriar, "Epidemic Fever of 1789 and 1790," 77; Bernard, "Extract from a Further Account of the London Fever Institution," 146; idem, "Extract from an Account of the Further Progress of

discourage wage earners from trying to work through a fever or from returning to work too early; and also to maintain the resistance of family members
by providing sufficient food, warmth, and shelter to prevent new cases from
arising. They had to recognize and try to manage perilous stages in the life
course, such as the arrival of a child to a working couple, or the arrival of
jobless newcomers to a manufacturing town, who might "sink under the
pressure of want and despair."[67]

Fever thus became the warrant for a broad program of social welfare. Fever
hospitals orchestrated subscriptions for general relief. A Miss Horner described
the response to an 1803 fever epidemic at Hull:

> Coals were provided for those, who had not the means to buy them. The sick and their
> families were supplied with arrow root, sago, or boiled milk, for their breakfast; and good
> mutton broth was made every day for dinner; each family, according to the number it
> contained, receiving two, three, or more quarts daily. . . . Good wheaten rolls, one day
> old, were distributed at the same time among the families, and in the same proportion;
> rice pudding, a little boiled mutton, or beef steak, with a half a pint of brisk small beer or
> ale, were allowed the convalescents. Milk sago, ale caudle, or arrow root, was prepared
> and given in the evening.[68]

Under Bateman, the London Fever Hospital carried out a program of "whitewashing, cleansing, and fumigating" the homes of their convalescing patients.
Even such programs as these – hospital care, supplies of food, fuel, and clothing – seemed merely "palliative" to Ferriar. Since fever was generated in poor
housing, the "best measure" would be "furnishing the poor with healthy
habitations . . . erecting small houses, at the public expense . . . to be let at
small rents."[69]

Even if an epidemic justified intervening in markets, indiscriminate charity
was surely a brazen invitation to abuse. Surely people would pawn the clothes
they were given, sell the food and fuel to buy drink (ironically, in Cowan's
Glasgow, relief committees allotted funds precisely for "redeeming articles of
clothing from pawn"[70]). Abuses occurred. Ferriar told of a Manchester fever

---

the Fever Institution," *Report of the Society for Bettering the Condition and Increasing the Comforts of
the Poor 6* (1815): 2; Ferriar, "Account of the Establishment of Fever-Wards in Manchester," 323.

67 Ferriar, "Of the Prevention of Fevers in Great Towns," 235, 237–38; idem, "Epidemic Fever of
1789 and 1790," 79.

68 Horner, "Fever at Kingston upon Hull," 100. She gives the ingredients of the broth as 15 pounds
mutton, 3.5 pounds barley, 2 cow heels, 2 sheep's heads, 2 dozen turnips, 1/4 peck onions, 1/2
handful thyme, 1/2 pound salt, to yield 52 quarts broth. Great emphasis is also placed on warm
clothes (Ferriar, "Account of the Establishment of Fever-Wards in Manchester," 321; Bateman,
*Diseases of London,* x). Also see John Pickstone, *Medicine and Industrial Society: A History of Hospital
Development in Manchester and Its Region, 1752–1946* (Manchester: Manchester University Press,
1985), ch. 1–3; Michael Durey, *The Return of the Plague: British Society and Cholera, 1831–2* (Dublin:
Gill and MacMillan, 1979), 84–85.

69 Bernard, "Extract from an Account of the Further Progress of the Fever Institution" (1815), 8;
Ferriar, "Account of the Establishment of Fever-Wards in Manchester," 322.

70 Cowan, "Glasgow," 274.

epidemic in which the usual "beds, clothing, nurses, and food" had been supplied. Yet "great numbers of the poor" had applied "to the Infirmary, under pretence of sickness, for the sole purpose of profiting by the subscription." But the response to the abuse was to meet the request. Since "exposure to hunger and cold had always preceded the fever," the proper response was "to promote subscriptions for the relief of the poor in general."[71]

Actions like these were politically ambiguous. The protracted convalescence that protected the public was also a way to give a laborer rest and a statement that conditions of work were unacceptably exhausting. The provision of food, fuel, and clothing was a real redistribution, but equally a reification of the dependence of one class on another.[72]

## V

It should be plain that at the time of Chadwick there was an essential tension between medicine and political economy. To let the market swing free was to tolerate damage to health; to follow the lead of traditional medicine was to interfere regularly and profoundly in the market. All who were concerned practically or philosophically with the condition of England – philanthropic evangelicals, magistrates, poor law reformers – felt that tension and sought a viable middle ground. The exacerbation of this tension to the point of crisis in the middle to late 1830s is exemplified in the relations of three men who took these questions most seriously: William Pulteney Alison, James Phillips Kay (-Shuttleworth), and Thomas Chalmers.

Alison was from a comfortable Tory Anglican Edinburgh family and was nurtured in the Scottish enlightenment of the late eighteenth century. That Dugald Stewart, his godfather, celebrated his entrance into the world with a gift of a copy of the *Rights of Man* says much.[73] His brother Archibald became a historian and anti-Malthusian political economist of note and, as Lanark sheriff, Scotland's most important social administrator. W. P. held several chairs at Edinburgh, culminating in the prestigious "theory and practice of medicine," and was an exemplary dispensary doctor, visiting the sick poor in their homes. In the early 1840s he led the campaign for reform of the Scottish poor law.

Kay, beneficiary of the new wealth of Lancashire cotton, had been one of Alison's prize pupils. Returning to Manchester, he sought a career in dispensary medicine and then medical journalism, as coeditor of the *North of England Medical and Surgical Journal* (1831–32). He would go on to become an assistant

71 Ferriar, "Of the Prevention of Fevers in Great Towns," 228.
72 Ibid., 235. Roberts (*Paternalism*, 42) notes the centrality of this welfare of dependency among paternalist writers. Cf. R. A. Lewis, *Edwin Chadwick and the Public Health Movement, 1832–1854* (London: Longmans, Green, 1952), 115–16; and Kilpatrick, " 'Living in the Light.' "
73 Chitnis, *The Scottish Enlightenment*, 23.

poor law commissioner and then secretary to the Privy Council's Education Committee.[74] Kay's pamphlet, *The Moral and Physical Condition of the Working Classes Employed in the Cotton Manufacture in Manchester,* was a product of his work during the cholera of 1832 for the quasi-official Manchester Board of Health. It is the apologia of a medical liberal and a decade later was a key source for Engels to defend views opposite Kay's.

Both Alison and Kay were responding to the optimistic Malthusianism of the Reverend Thomas Chalmers, political economist, mathematician, natural theologian, leader of the evangelical party in the Scottish church and of the breakaway Free Kirk in 1843. A charismatic minister, Chalmers held that demoralization, destitution, and disease could be overcome not by impersonal institutions of state but by a morally united parish community, through a mix of exhortation, market incentives, pervasive moral oversight, and, at last resort, minimal and carefully targeted relief in kind. With a cadre of deacons, Chalmers carried out his experiment in Glasgow's St. John's parish in the late teens and early twenties. What the St. John's approach accomplished was debatable – had pauperism really dropped or was relief simply being denied? Yet in the years prior to the 1834 new poor law, this Scottish approach was enormously popular in England. Chalmers seemed to represent a Christian political economy that merged the call to help the needy with a faith in the market. Indeed, the founders of University College, that "Godless College on Gower Street," tried their best to persuade him to take their chair of moral philosophy (Chalmers took the Edinburgh divinity chair instead; an accomplished mathematician, he had earlier run second for the chair of natural philosophy).[75] Kay dedicated *The Moral and Physical Condition* (second edition) to Chalmers rather than to his teacher Alison; in September 1840 (with Chadwick in the audience) Alison, in glorious forensic combat with Chalmers at the Glasgow meeting of the British Association, overthrew the Chalmersian paradigm of social policy.[76] Yet he did so within Chalmers's terms, only adding medicine to the mix of Malthus, the market, and moral duty. Kay and Alison are both representative and immensely influential figures. They show us "public health" at the time Chadwick began his work and the cultural framework in which solutions were conceived and assessed.

---

74 Frank Smith, *The Life and Work of Sir James Kay-Shuttleworth* (London: John Murray, 1923); R.J.W. Selleck, *James Kay-Shuttleworth: Journey of an Outsider* (Ilford, Essex: Woburn Press, 1994). Kay was the son of a Rochdale cotton manufacturer. He was Alison's principal clerk, practiced briefly in Dublin (1826), and by 1828 was senior physician at the Ardwick and Ancoats Dispensary.

75 Stewart J. Brown, *Thomas Chalmers and the Godly Commonwealth in Scotland* (Oxford: Oxford University Press, 1982), 156, 177. See also Anthony Brundage, *The Making of the New Poor Law: The Politics of Inquiry, Enactment, and Implementation, 1832–1839* (New Brunswick, N.J.: Rutgers University Press, 1978), 70; Audrey Peterson, "The Poor Law in Nineteenth Century Scotland," *The New Poor Law in the Nineteenth Century,* ed. Derek Fraser, 171–93 (London: Macmillan, 1976).

76 W. Hanna, *Memoirs of the Life and Writings of Thomas Chalmers D.D.,* 4 vols. (Edinburgh: Constable, 1852), IV, 196–216; Brown, *Chalmers,* 288–96. Kay, *Moral and Physical,* 3, explains that he dedicated the second edition of the pamphlet to Chalmers after Chalmers had praised the first.

Kay had become interested in political economy through his experience as Alison's assistant, during which he realized that the causes of disease were social. He gained "insight," he later wrote, "into the grave questions affecting the relations of capital and labour, and the distribution of wealth, as well as the inseparable connection between the mental and moral condition of the people and their physical well-being." His shift to Chalmers began after his return to Manchester.[77] In 1830 Alison was an established medical authority and a paragon of the quiet duty of charity, but not yet a social reformer. By contrast Chalmers led a noisy army of moral regeneration based equally in godliness and science. It is not hard to see the attraction for the dissenter, Whig, and evangelical Kay, himself inflamed with a religiosity so intense that it would lead to nervous exhaustion on several occasions.

Both Kay and Alison were unusual in their empathy for the poor about whom they wrote and whose outlook on the world they tried to imagine and explain. Their writings are thus difficult to categorize or dismiss: Kay, for example, was probably cited more often by supporters of factory legislation than opponents, though he opposed such interference.[78]

Kay's pamphlet is often taken to typify early Victorian social discovery. Exploring the unknown land of the slum, Kay is aghast at what he finds: not just filth and poverty, but the self-destructive (and irrational) defiance of moral standards. In large part his response is typical too: to preach virtue, religion, education, and the free flow of capital. What makes the analysis unusually forceful is the extent to which it reflects a medical view of society. For Kay, as for most contemporary medical men, predisposing causes – "every thing which depresses the physical energies" – were central. These included "imperfect nutrition; exposure to cold and moisture . . . uncleanliness of the person, the street, and the abode; an atmosphere contaminated . . . extreme labour, and consequent physical exhaustion; intemperance; fear; anxiety; diarrhea, and other diseases."[79] Because these were pathological *forces*, they necessarily caused harm, even if acute disease never arose. Because the nervous system was the medium of pathological action, they also had moral effects. "It is utterly impossible," Kay wrote, "to separate any event which is witnessed by human intelligence, from a certain inevitable moral sequence; or that they who know that to drop a pebble on the surface of the world disturbs the planet, *should not perceive how, of equal necessity, events acting on the human*

77  Smith, *Kay-Shuttleworth*, 13–14, 20, 26–30; Selleck, *Kay-Shuttleworth*, 56–61.
78  Nicholas Coles, "Sinners in the Hands of an Angry Utilitarian: J. P. Kay (-Shuttleworth), *The Moral and Physical Condition of the Working Classes in Manchester (1832),*" *Bulletin of Research in the Humanities* 86 (1985): 455, 462; Frank Mort, *Dangerous Sexualities: Medico–Moral Politics in England since 1830* (London: Routledge and Kegan Paul, 1987), 22–23; Mary Poovey, "Curing the Social Body in 1832: James Phillips Kay and the Irish in Manchester," *Making a Social Body: British Cultural Formation, 1830–1864* (Chicago: University of Chicago Press, 1995), 55–72.
79  Kay, *Moral and Physical*, 27–28. I quote from the second edition; on the changes from the first see Selleck, *Kay-Shuttleworth*, 66–77.

*spirit, in proportion to their novelty and power, disturb, for good or ill, the constitution of society.*[80] That, explained Kay, was why cholera was coextensive with vice.

As the pebble analogy makes clear, Newtonian images of complex fields of force and delicate equilibria provided the master metaphor. The interacting physical, social, and moral forces of factory work, along with the rest of the Manchester environment, produced an accelerating degradation nearly irresistible to the soul of the mill hand.

> Prolonged and exhausting labour, continued from day to day, and from year to year, is not calculated to develop the intellectual or moral faculties of man. The dull routine of a ceaseless drudgery, in which the same mechanical process is incessantly repeated, resembles the torment of Sisyphus. . . . The mind gathers neither stores nor strength from the constant exertion and retraction of the same muscles. The intellect slumbers in supine inertness; but the grosser parts of our nature attain a rank development. To condemn man to such severity of toil is, in some measure, to cultivate in him the habits of an animal.[81]

In a similar manner, brief mealtimes and poor food prevented adequate digestion; this, combined with dampness and other predisposing conditions, induced a form of bowel disturbance which exacerbated (and was exacerbated by) a "deep mental depression" that led directly to the gin shop. "The exhausted artisan, driven by ennui and discomfort from his squalid home . . . [strives], in the delirious dreams of a continued debauch, to forget the remembrance of his reckless improvidence, of the destitution, hunger, and uninterrupted toil."[82] It led also to crime, illicit sex, sedition, violence.

Kay's language leaves no room for acts of will. Manchester workers are victims of a social, moral, and physical disease which they no more choose than we choose the flu. Seeing disease as a consequence of environment might seem to absolve the victim of blame.[83] It did not for Kay. Though the interplay of forces led to an unfortunate result, yet it still did not constitute an error in a cosmic sense. For Kay as for Chalmers, natural events were not arbitrary, but the outcome of natural laws, which were the laws of God's Providence; one no more blamed Providence for the degradation of the operative than for the fall of heavy objects. Providence (not Malthus) was author of the principles of population and political economy. The actions a society took must not oppose Providence, but they could complement it. Poor laws, factory acts, revolution, or interference with markets would worsen matters. That these were the preferred solutions of the working classes did not matter. One

80 Kay, *Moral and Physical*, 4 (italics mine). Chalmers's holding of such views verged on the unorthodox inasmuch as they seemed to threaten the doctrines of predestination and grace central to the Westminster Confession (Brown, *Chalmers*, 14).

81 Kay, *Moral and Physical*, 22.

82 Ibid., 23, 25, 43–44. See also James Phillips Kay, "Physical Condition of the Poor. I. Diet. Gastralgia and Enteralgia, or Morbid Sensibility of the Stomach and Bowels," *North of England Medical and Surgical Journal* 1 (1830): 220–30.

83 But see Coles, "Sinners," 475.

could understand sympathetically why working-class people might be attracted to such solutions (just as one understands why two-year-olds throw tantrums), but since dehumanizing conditions had already deprived them of their full claim to humanity, their own analysis was no more credible than that of any ill person who cries out for something the doctor knows must be withheld.[84]

Thus, the very attempt to take working-class experience seriously led Kay to discredit it. While dehumanized factory hands could not be blamed for their situation (on the grounds that they were not full moral agents), they, and not the conditions in which they lived, might still be the proper site of remediation – through countervailing forces, such as "spiritual discipline," education, police, and sewers.[85]

For Alison the need for medically informed social policy arose from the failure of Chalmers's effort to revitalize Scottish poor relief. Unlike the English poor law, the Scottish law denied public relief to the ablebodied. There was no official recognition of unemployment, increasingly common as a result of the fluctuations of an industrial economy. Even those with a right to relief, the disabled and the elderly, did not have a right to much. In most parishes there were no legal assessments for support of the poor and contributed funds were often too little. In St. Andrews the allowance was often a few pence per week and a bit of coal: a "*system of protracted starvation,*" wrote Alison.[86] There were many charities in Scottish towns, and also many beggars. Alison protested that medicine was being made to substitute for a proper poor law in a way that was both ineffective – by the time the indigent came to the attention of a medical charity or benevolent doctor little could be done – and unfair: displaced people, from Highland clearances or from Ireland, overloaded the medical charities in the larger towns or appealed to individual medical men, who often supplied them with the "necessaries" without hope of reimbursement. His solution was a Scottish version of the English poor law: it would recognize a right to relief, perhaps in conjunction with some needs test; would

84  Kay, *Moral and Physical*, 9; [Kay], "Review of M. T. Sadler's Law of Population," *North of England Medical Journal* 1 (1830): 105–26.

85  Kay, *Moral and Physical*, 6–7; see also 42–43, 45, 48–53, 78, 91–93, 94–97, 105–11; Smith, *Kay-Shuttleworth*, 46. In some sense Providence determined these social responses too, quite as much as it had originally determined the problems. That the solutions had not yet come was due to the slow action of the societal sensorium, or nervous system (Kay spoke of the need for a "natural faculty" to recognize the state of society). It was in this sense that the cholera epidemic was welcome – an indication of both divine "mercy" and divine "judgment" – as a pain stimulus strong enough to provoke preventive action. The task of the therapist Kay was then to invigorate the dulled nerves of society with the tonic of social statistics (Kay, *Moral and Physical*, 27–30, cf. Coles, "Sinners," 465, 483, 486).

86  Alison, "Illustrations of the Practical Operation of the Scottish System of Management of the Poor," *Journal of the Statistical Society of London* 3 (1840): 229. Cf. Ian Leavitt and Christopher Smout, *The State of the Scottish Working-Class in 1843: A Statistical and Spatial Inquiry Based on the Data from the Poor Law Commission Report of 1844* (Edinburgh: Scottish Academic Press, 1979), 161, 220–21.

be administered by a professional staff, including a paid medical staff; and would be supported by rates.

*Observations on the Management of the Poor in Scotland, and Its Effects on the Health of Great Towns*, Alison's first and chief work on the subject, appeared in spring 1840, a response to a report on the Scottish Poor Law by the General Assembly of the Scottish Church. The church seemed unlikely to solve the problem. Unpopular ministers "intruded" by patrons into parishes were unlikely candidates to revitalize those parishes à la Chalmers; nor, in many places, did the public seem likely to endorse taxes to support the poor. Seizing on the opportunity provided by Chadwick's great Sanitary Inquiry, Alison quickly organized The Association for Obtaining an Official Inquiry into the Poor Laws of Scotland, preponderantly made up of medical men, which would try to broaden Chadwick's inquiry into a general investigation of the Scottish poor law.

For years, Alison explained, he had been "applying remedies to diseases which have obviously been the result of privations . . . [and] known that they could be only temporarily useful, simply because he had no remedy for the privations from which they originated." He would undertake an epidemiology of the "grand evil of Poverty itself, and endeavour to apply to it the same principles of investigation, by which physicians are guided in determining the immediate causes and remedies of disease."[87] The medical police tradition warranted this trespass of the usual bounds of medicine. Contagious fever was a far greater problem in Scotland than in England, Alison argued.[88] While destitution was rarely its direct cause, it was most common and most dangerous among destitute people.[89] Thus "a poor family wandering in search of employment, and infected with fever, who were driven from one part of the town to another . . . introduced the disease into three different districts, all inhabited by very poor people." Fifty cases were traced to them; all could have been prevented by an effective poor law.[90] In practical terms, destitution

87 W. P. Alison, *Observations on the Management of the Poor in Scotland, and Its Effects on the Health of Great Towns,* 2d ed. (Edinburgh: Blackwood, 1840), x.

88 Ibid., 14; W. P. Alison, *Reply to Dr Chalmers' Objections to an Improvement of the Legal Provision for the Poor in Scotland* (Edinburgh: Blackwood, 1841), v. Thus fever accounted for 20 percent of mortality in Glasgow in 1837, 15 percent in Dundee in 1836, but no more than 8 percent in any English town during the century.

89 "It is not asserted that destitution is a cause adequate to the *production* of fever (although in some circumstances I believe it may become such); nor that it is the *sole* cause of its extension. What we are sure of is, that it is a cause of the *rapid diffusion* of contagious fever, and one of such peculiar power and efficacy, that its existence may always be presumed, when we see fever prevailing in a large community to an unusual extent. The manner in which deficient nourishment, want of employment, and privations of all kinds, and the consequent mental depression favour the diffusion of fever, may be matter of dispute; but that they have that effect in a much greater degree than any cause external to the human body itself, is a fact confirmed by the experience of all physicians who have seen much of the disease" (Alison, *Observations,* 10–11).

90 Alison, "Illustrations," 240–41.

was *the* public health problem. So strong was this relation that Alison would treat fever incidence as the "test to the legislator" of the adequacy of provision for the poor: " '*As the botanist can tell the quality of the soil from the flowers that spontaneously arise upon it, the physician knows the state of a people from the epidemics that mow it down.*' "[91]

While medicine warranted Alison's involvement, he was equally adept making the case on theological and economic grounds. In *Observations*, Alison accused Chalmers of exegetical error, arguing that the command to charity was unqualified. All humans were a mix of good and bad; thus none was fully undeserving, and to punish sinful parents was also to punish innocent children. Yet behind the moral argument was the medical: those most in need (regardless of desert) were those "among whom fever and other epidemics are most apt to break out and to extend; and that this result can only be prevented by some improvement of their condition and comforts. . . . For the sake of the morals, but quite certainly for the sake of the health of the community, it is most important, that the wants (well ascertained by inquiry) of the vicious poor should be promptly relieved."[92] Alison rejected the prominent view that poverty implied sin, that, for example, a high mortality rate was the just reward of drink. Infant deaths were the chief component of higher than normal mortality rates, he noted; furthermore, the poor were too poor to drink themselves to death. And granting that intemperance was a problem, how was one to stop very depressed people from drinking heavily?[93]

While *Observations* spoke to the Scottish church, "Illustrations of the Practical Operation of the Scottish System of Management of the Poor," his address to the Statistical Section of the British Association in September 1840, targeted political economists. Alison accepted Malthus's views of the problems of poor relief, but argued that Malthusian policies were inconsistent, ineffective, and, by generating disease, dangerous. The Malthus–Chalmers approach was illogical because it presumed a clear demarcation between problems that stemmed from moral error (indigence, irresponsible reproduction, intemperance) and those resulting from "a visitation of Providence."

Malthus and Chalmers had held medical relief to the sick pauper to be acceptable because it did not tempt one to become ill. Alison found this distinction illusory. How could it be right to assist when incurable disease disabled the able-bodied worker but wrong to assist those "disabled by that visitation of Providence which the mere advance of years brings upon all"? Admittedly destitution sometimes resulted from moral failing, yet many became destitute as a result of causes "over which they have had as little control

91  Alison, *Observations*, 18; idem, *Reply to the Pamphlet Entitled "Proposed Alteration of the Scottish Poor Law Considered and Commented on," by David Monypenny, Esq. of Pitmilly* (Edinburgh: Blackwood, 1841), 46.
92  Alison, *Observations*, 80–83.
93  Ibid., xi–xii.

as over the dispensations of Providence . . . the failure of any particular line of industry in consequence of improvement in art, the glut of markets, commercial embarrassments from failure of banks or other establishments, or the general increase of population." Chalmers's error was the assumption that whoever was not a pauper was, in a meaningful sense, independent. Yet few were; the welfare of almost all was tied directly to the whims of landowners or the speculations of capitalists.[94]

Either the Chalmersites had to be more rigid in their enforcement of social responsibility or one must disentangle public morality from public health, leaving the former to the church, treating the latter by the most effective means.[95] On empirical grounds Alison denied that either deterrent social policies or a fatalistic response to epidemics did anything to slow population growth. On the contrary, they exacerbated the problem: "In a country advanced in civilization, population makes the most rapid progress where least is done for the poor; . . . its tendency . . . to outstrip the means of subsistence, is most effectually restrained where a fixed and uniform provision, securing them against destitution and degradation, is known to exist." Ireland, with (until recently) no legal provision for the poor, was the exemplar of Malthusian misery and regularly swept by epidemics.[96]

Alison's writings in the early 1840s mark the epitome of a medical critique of industrialism and capitalism the like of which did not reappear until the twentieth century. He went further than others in exploring the possibilities of a supportive social policy. In his hands the deterrent workhouse of Chadwick became a hostel for the destitute and a fever-prevention institution. The invisible poor of Edinburgh, deserted elderly women who silently starved or froze in lodging houses, might live there "in comparative comfort, and, if they should take fever, would be prevented from communicating the infection."[97] His critique was rooted, on the one hand, in eighteenth-century sentiment, on the other in practical experience. He realized that fever hospitals were ineffective if fever victims did not trust them and that the economists' theories of rational behavior did not describe the actions of the desperate people with whom he worked. Among the most eloquent of his observations was of three young mothers in Edinburgh:

94 Alison, "Illustrations," 246; idem, Reply to Dr. Chalmers, 17–20.
95 Alison, "Illustrations," 212, 253–55.
96 Among many contemporary political economists the carrot of "artificial wants" that might be acquired through prudence was coming to seem a better motivator than the stick of misery, the punishment for imprudence (Alison, Observations, v–vi; "Illustrations," 244–45; Alison, "Further Illustrations of the Practical Operation of the Scotch System of Management of the Poor," Journal of the Statistical Society of London 4 [1841]: 290–93).
97 "Illustrations," 243; Observations, 109. In general, Alison favored outdoor relief, arguing that "it never can be wise or useful, to break down those habits of comfort and cleanliness, and those artificial wants, which at present characterise the great body of the labouring poor, and even of the aged and disabled poor in England or to outrage the feelings of family affection" (Reply to Monypenny, 38).

During the inclement weather of spring 1838, I saw three young women with natural children on the breast, who were out of work, in a miserable state of destitution, and who were refused admission into the workhouses, and were very scantily relieved by the other charities here. After some weeks of severe suffering, the children all died, certainly of the effects of cold and imperfect nourishment. If anyone supposes, that the effect of this sacrifice of innocent life was to improve the morals of these women or their associates, I can only say, that he knows nothing of the effect of real destitution on human character and conduct.[98]

What then of Kay, schooled in the same traditions of physiology and medical practice, likewise concerned with the condition of the people and adept in the scholasticism of political economy? Kay had gone far in wrestling with the question of what must be the effect on a person of a life in Manchester's mills. Yet his conclusion – that such a life bred monsters – only reinforced his belief in the need for invisible chains that would control them. He endorsed Chalmers. Unlike Alison, who held, in effect, that if destitution, fever, and overpopulation were consequences of the creation of the industrial proletariat, then there must be something wrong with that system, the providentialist Kay found himself trapped by what he, Chalmers, and many others saw as God's laws for the conduct of economic, moral, and social relations. One can of course attribute their differences to their upbringings, and the cultural climates they worked in. It is also well to remember that Edinburgh's problem (immigration of displaced people into a nonindustrial town) was not Manchester's (management of an "angry and alien" proletariat during a period of fluctuating trade and technological change). Would each have thought the same had he practiced in the other's town?[99]

Their divergent analyses of the relations of public health to social policy are of great importance, however. For the early Christians the great question was "Athens or Jerusalem?" In public health it was "Manchester or Edinburgh?" Kay's approach led to the public health of Chadwick (according to Kay, he dumped the "sanitary idea" in Chadwick's lap when he took the post of secretary to the Privy Council's Education Committee). Outside Scotland the Alison approach disappeared, surfacing only briefly in the early 1860s, the first years of John Simon's reign over British public health. As we shall see in later chapters, Chadwick virtually ignored Alison; the reader of the *Sanitary Report* will not know of the *Observations* nor of the fireworks in Glasgow in September 1840, though both dealt centrally with the relation of fever to

98 Alison, *Observations*, 83fn.
99 Cf. Alison, *Reply to Monypenny*, 42–43. Alison emphasized the differences between Manchester and Edinburgh to highlight the contrast between a society with legal relief for the poor (England) and one without (Scotland). Accordingly he made working-class life in Manchester appear positively bucolic. For the handling of similar issues in America see Charles Rosenberg, *The Cholera Years: The United States in 1832, 1849, and 1866* (Chicago: University of Chicago Press, 1962), esp. 40–64, 133–50.

poverty, ostensibly the subject of the inquiry. Throughout the decade – which, after all, produced the massive fevers of the great Irish famine – Alison continued to produce analyses of the economic causes of disease, yet he was unable to halt the juggernaut of sanitarianism.[100] For Chadwick had conceived a policy far more innocuous than the redistributionism of a food–work conception of health, and one with a real treat for the dutiful middle classes: new porcelain water closets and ready water, for cooking, cleaning, even drinking.

100 Brenda White, "Scottish Doctors and the English Public Health," 77–85. On the Irish famine fever see Joseph Robins, *The Miasma: Epidemic and Panic in Nineteenth Century Ireland* (Dublin: Institute of Public Administration, 1995).

# 3

## Prelude to the *Sanitary Report*, 1833–1838

Let us set this drama in motion. The social crises of the 1830s exposed the tension between new political economy and old medicine; by the middle of the next decade the sanitary movement would emerge as the anodyne to soothe the raw wound of contradiction.

Food, work, and money: the decade began with rick burning in the countryside and in the towns a new crusade against the "Yorkshire slavery" of debilitating factory work. In 1831–32 the Lords' efforts to derail parliamentary reform led to the brink of revolution. In 1834 came the hated and violently resisted new poor law, stigmatizing the pauper. By 1837 a deep depression had developed in agriculture and manufacturing, leading to the Chartist movement, founded in early 1838, as a demand for social justice through suffrage. In 1839 riots and rebellion followed Parliament's dismissal of the first Chartist petition, bearing more than a million signatures (the second, in 1842, would bear more than three million). By the end of the decade the plight of several hundred thousand hand loom weavers was desperate. Bidding for work against one another and the new power loom, they were finding it nearly impossible to keep body and soul together.

At the center of this strife was the ordinary lower-class Man. It was his collective soul, body, behavior, character that Carlyle dubbed the "condition-of-England" question. One could have talked of a Scotland, Wales, or Ireland question, each equally serious. Responding to these questions were reformers of many stripes – followers of Bentham, or Robert Owen, or the young Englanders. Often they justified their missions with social investigations. The sweeping philosophies of the Godwins, Paleys, Smiths, and Malthuses were giving way to surveys, case studies, social experiments, and stacks of facts. Everywhere the investigators found problems; usually disclosing them was held to be the only important requisite to implementing whatever solution the investigator was promoting. Reality was full of directions for reform; every fact had its message, to be unloaded by these burly investigators. In fact, as David Roberts wryly notes, these reports were really "essays" – "on the social, moral, and physical condition of the labouring classes . . . scarcely ever was 'moral' omitted from the formula, and scarcely ever did it include 'economic.' " And "social conditions" were usually but a stalking horse for "moral condition," which in turn meant something like "matters pertaining to whether society as we know it will fall apart and/or a revolution will occur."[1]

One of the most effective of these writers of moral essays was Edwin Chadwick, secretary of the Poor Law Commission (PLC), whose 1842 *Report on the Sanitary Condition of the Labouring Population of Great Britain* is often seen as the foundational text of modern public health. It is usually considered the outcome of considerations that began in the winter of 1837–38, when a severe fever epidemic had struck the poor East End of London. Faced with the growing costs of supporting fever victims, the Whitechapel guardians had asked Chadwick for advice and had in fact drained a foul pond, which they believed was causing the fever. When such use of poor relief funds was disallowed by auditors, Chadwick asked three physician–friends to look into the causes of fever in London. Two, Southwood Smith and Neil Arnott, were old friends from Bentham's inner circle. The third, James Phillips Kay, was on the staff as an assistant commissioner. Reporting in early May 1838, the three confirmed that foul ponds and like conditions caused fever, thus vindicating the union.[2] To strengthen the case for bringing preventive medicine within the domain of the poor law, at the end of 1839 Chadwick convinced the bishop of London to request an analogous study of fever in England and Wales. Against the wishes of his Poor Law Commission bosses, who feared antagonizing powerful interests, Chadwick published the study in July 1842.[3] So strong were its claims, so vivid its details, that the Royal Commission on the Health of Towns and Populous Districts was quickly convened. Reporting

1 David Roberts, *Victorian Origins of the British Welfare State* (1960, reprint; Hamden, Conn.: Archon Books, 1969), 211–12. Cf. Nicholas Coles, "Sinners in the Hands of an Angry Utilitarian: J. P. Kay (-Shuttleworth), *The Moral and Physical Condition of the Working Classes in Manchester (1832),*" *Bulletin of Research in the Humanities 86* (1985): 477. In general see Gertrude Himmelfarb, *The Idea of Poverty: England in the Early Industrial Age* (New York: Random House, 1985).

2 B. W. Richardson, "Edwin Chadwick C.B., A Biographical Dissertation," *The Health of Nations: A Review of the Works of Edwin Chadwick, with a Biographical Dissertation,* 2 vols. (1887, reprint, London: Dawson, 1965), I, xlii: "So sudden and severe was the attack, that the parochial authorities were at their wits' end to know what to do or whom to consult. In their distress they thought of the active and resolute Secretary of the Poor Law Board, and to him they applied." See also Maurice Marston, *Sir Edwin Chadwick (1800–1890)* (London: Leonard Parsons, 1925), 93; John Simon, *English Sanitary Institutions, Reviewed in Their Course of Development, and in Some of Their Political and Social Relations* (London: Cassell and Co., 1890), 178, 182–85; S. E. Finer, *The Life and Times of Sir Edwin Chadwick* (London: Methuen, 1952), 150, 155–57; Edward H. Gibson, "The Public Health Agitation in England, 1838–1848: A Newspaper and Parliamentary History" (Ph.D. diss., University of North Carolina, Chapel Hill, 1955), 22.

3 The standard account of the report is M. W. Flinn, "Introduction," Edwin Chadwick, *Report on the Sanitary Condition of the Labouring Population of Great Britain,* ed. M. W. Flinn (Edinburgh: Edinburgh University Press, 1965), 43–58.

in the mid-1840s, it confirmed Chadwick's findings. In 1848, despite the apathy of Tory and Whig governments alike, the Public Health Act passed, and modern public health began.

The legend unites virtue and discovery. It is persuasive because it is simple. But it leaves out much. We are never invited to ask whether other explorers had perceived differently, whether all the important facts were there, whether they led so inexorably to Chadwick's conclusions, and whether the good Chadwick offered was the most important good that one in his place, with his stated intentions, should have offered.

## I

Let us then join three doughty social investigators as they tour the East End of London in the 1830s. They find "great ravages" from fever: "unpaved yards, and filthy courts, and the want of drainage and cleansing rendered their houses hotbeds of disease." "In whole streets," they find "nothing worthy of the name of bed, bedding, or furniture; a little straw, a few shavings, a few rags in a corner formed their beds – a broken chair, stool, or old butter-barrel their seats." They find one man in the act of suicide.

But wait. These are not Chadwick's trio of Smith, Kay, and Arnott, but another team of investigators, studying the same area in 1831. One is Thomas Wakley, *Lancet* editor and later radical M.P.; another is William Lovett, later leader of the "moral force" Chartists. Theirs was a very different political medicine than that of Chadwick's investigators, as we learn when we read that it was "fever *combined with hunger* [that] was committing great ravages among them" and when we find that the suicidal man (he had only a fork to do the deed) had been "reduced to a miserable state of despondency from the want of food." In March 1832, when Bishop Blomfield had called a penitential fast to save the country from cholera, Lovett held a feast. He and his fellow trade unionists were sure "that the ravages made by that dreadful disease were chiefly to be attributed to the want and wretchedness." Such causes "were greatly within the power of Government to remove," insisted Lovett.[4]

Discovery is central in the Chadwick legend, the idea that no one who counted had ever before bothered to look into the alleys and courts. "Discovery" talk made what was in fact a contentious matter – rethinking "public health" – seem the simple opening of one's eyes. In fact, the picture of squalor and disease in the Chadwick reports is not so different from that in reports of others in the previous half century. But the revelations of Lovett, Wakley,

4 William Lovett, *Life and Struggles of William Lovett in His Pursuit of Bread, Knowledge, and Freedom with Some Account of the Different Associations He Belonged To and of the Opinions He Entertained*, 2 vols. (New York: Knopf, 1920), I, 71–72, 80 (italics mine). See also Michael Durey, *The Return of the Plague: British Society and Cholera, 1831–2* (Dublin: Gill and MacMillan, 1979), 197–200.

and others had to be suppressed. Not only did they challenge the fiction that no one had known, but, in treating disease as an element of misery, they forced on society the unwelcome truth that you could not just skim "public health" from the great social questions of the day. The *Sanitary Report* did its work well; it enhanced the credibility of the new poor law and of Chadwick. In part because of the great public health movement it led to, and in part because of the paper trail Chadwick left, historians, even while recognizing Chadwick's biases, have accepted that the report was about exactly what he said it was: improving the lives and health of the poor, because they needed improving.

To understand the *Sanitary Report* we must see it not as the foundation of what would come after 1848 but in light of the problems of administering the new poor law of 1834. In 1839, at the outset of the Sanitary Inquiry, Edwin Chadwick was thirty-nine. Caricatured as the "briefless barrister," he had a double legal qualification as barrister and attorney. Though in government service for only five years, he was already well known, indispensable in some circles, infamous in others.

Almost always he is labeled "Benthamite." Chadwick had been Bentham's secretary, yet calling him a Benthamite is as unhelpful as calling Aristotle a Platonist. There are common themes, but other influences and concerns were often more important. He was much less concerned with maximizing happiness or expanding democracy than with ensuring discipline and order.[5] He shared his mentor's passion for micromanagement and complex organizational plans. Any system that required serious trade-offs or seemed a zero-sum game was surely wrong – a mark of correct organization was a cascade of collateral benefits. Sewage farming, for example, was simultaneously a means of sewage disposal, an endlessly expandable source of food, a source of jobs, and a source of capital needed for other beneficent undertakings. He made no pretense at serious philosophical utilitarianism; in contrast with the usual theorists, he would be the empirical political economist.[6] He differed from many political economists in his optimism for industrial growth. For Chadwick, there was no "surplus population," no limited fund of wages, but an economy that could always absorb workers provided they were released from the bondage of antiquated paternalism.[7]

Chadwick's public career had three phases – first, the period of designing the new poor law, 1832–34, in which he had some hope of seeing passage of

---

5 On Bentham, Chadwick, and democracy see Finer, *Chadwick,* 31; Roberts, *Victorian Origins,* 149; Michael Ignatieff, *A Just Measure of Pain: The Penitentiary in the Industrial Revolution* (New York: Pantheon, 1978), 212. On Chadwick's centrality see Oliver MacDonagh, *Early Victorian Government, 1830–1870* (London: Weidenfeld and Nicolson, 1977), 34, 53–54.

6 R. A. Lewis, *Edwin Chadwick and the Public Health Movement, 1832–1854* (London: Longmans, Green, 1952), 13.

7 Chadwick was not the Malthusian he was often labeled (Lewis, *Chadwick,* 17–18).

a program shaped by science rather than political expediency. Here the hand of Bentham was strong. Others felt it too and could provide support, from Lord Brougham in the Whig cabinet to Francis Place in the London vestries. Beginning with his leadership of the Factory Commission in 1833 and throughout his service as secretary to the commission administering the poor law (until 1847) Chadwick was a pragmatist, fighting for the survival of the new law and for his own career. Though Chadwick felt more comfortable with the Whigs, who were his first patrons, his politics were often closer to those of Peel and Sir James Graham: maintaining order took priority.[8] A third phase (1847–54) began with Chadwick's rise to power at the end of 1847. As chief member of the investigatory Metropolitan Sanitary Commission (1847–48), the administrative General Board of Health (1848–54), and the legislative and executive consolidated Metropolitan Sewers Commission (1847–49), he was in a position to shape policy. The agendas of all three were at least loosely Benthamite, but political crises overwhelmed their activities. Nor, by 1850, did there remain a cadre of reliable Benthamite allies. Indeed, the Benthamites Joseph Hume and Sir William Molesworth were among those who scuttled the General Board of Health and drove Chadwick out of office.

In person Chadwick was humorless, domineering, single-minded, with no sense of proportion. He was hard to work with, or for, or to have as a subordinate. Much taken with Bentham's systems of checks and balances, he leapt easily to dogma and accordingly would not countenance partial or compromise approaches. Hence he was no politician. Nor was he suited to be the sort of administrator he dearly wished to become. Poor law commissioners, like colonial governors, needed a justice-of-the-peace style: equal parts of humanity, gentility, severity, and not knowing too much about anything. Chadwick, on the other hand, sought authority through dogma and detail. He found it hard to see those he differed with as other than enemies and easy to imagine the conspiracies they were surely hatching. Sadly this outlook generated self-fulfilling prophecies: his failures to win favor did reflect others' assessments; the harder he tried the more he failed; and the more he failed the more self-righteous he became. Under the command of that self-righteousness, his lawyer's training only confirmed to him the unanswerability of his own case. Some of his letters reflect a search for friendship, but for him friendship was discipleship, and the relationships did not prosper.[9] These factors are important: Chadwick's personality probably affected the course of the sanitary revolution even more than his ideas.

The commission of which Chadwick was secretary had been created in 1834 to administer the act passed in response to the report of the investigative

---

8 He had this in common with a number of the philosophical radicals (see R. K. Webb, *Harriet Martineau: A Radical Victorian* [London: Heinemann, 1960], 363–64).

9 Finer, *Chadwick*, 2–6, 195; Lewis, *Chadwick*, 14; Maurice Marston, *Chadwick*, 62.

Poor Law Commission of 1832. Chadwick, who was elevated from assistant to full royal commissioner during the inquiry, was, with Nassau Senior, the main author of that commission's report. That report would be marked by what would become characteristic Chadwickianisms: strings of quotations chosen to support predetermined answers.[10] Chadwick had been led to expect that he would be one of the three commissioners appointed to administer the new act, and when that did not occur, that the secretary would effectively be a fourth commissioner. The commissioners, however, tended to see him as an office manager. And rather than conducting most business as a board, which would have allowed Chadwick significant autonomy, they divided the country among themselves, each keeping in close touch with several of the nine to eighteen regional assistant commissioners. The assistant commissioners were quite literally the front line of the new poor law. Their unpleasant and even dangerous job was to form vestries into unions and to teach the elected guardians and their officers how to manage.

In 1839 the commissioners were Thomas Frankland Lewis, George Nicholls, and J. G. Shaw-Lefevre. Lewis's son, George Cornewall Lewis, would replace his father in 1840. They have been seen as shallow creatures of patronage. "It is not difficult," writes Marston, "to imagine the disgust" of these commissioners at "Chadwick's exuberant energy, sincerity and horror of inefficiency. How they must have hated this man who worked so abominably hard and was so keen, this worker among the drones!" In fact each appears to have taken his post seriously, thought deeply about poor law principles, and spent much time advising field staff.[11] Had they been so blasé, Chadwick would surely have had an easier time. Though several of the staff were more Malthusian and pessimistic than Chadwick, the chief source of friction was his principle versus their pragmatism. They accepted government by muddle: some opposition could not be kicked away; it could be compromised with, bypassed, or even temporarily surrendered to.[12]

It is sometimes suggested that Chadwick took up sanitation either to pursue his true métier or to distance himself from the hated poor law. The move is

10 Raymond Cowherd *(Political Economists and the English Poor Laws: A Historical Study of the Influence of Classical Economics on the Formation of Social Welfare Policy* [Athens: Ohio University Press, 1977], 224–25) notes that the recognition by several assistant commissioners of the economic bases of destitution was ignored. See also Ursula R. Q. Henriques, *Before the Welfare State: Social Administration in Early Industrial Britain* (London: Longman, 1979), 26.

11 Marston, *Chadwick,* 52–53; Finer, *Chadwick,* 3, 108–9. Roberts, *Victorian Origins,* 142–43; historians of the poor law have generally been more respectful. See also William C. Lubenow, *The Politics of Government Growth: Early Victorian Attitudes toward State Intervention, 1833–1848* (Newton Abbott: David and Charles, 1971), 26.

12 Finer, *Chadwick,* 82, 281–91. The reports of friction between Chadwick and the commissioners at the time of the *Sanitary Report* date from the Andover hearings of 1847, in which secretary and commissioners brought the commission down in a flurry of blame laying. This evidence warrants about the same credibility as the retrospections of spouses in a messy divorce. Poor Law Commission [PLC] archives do not suggest such a polarized situation.

seen as precipitated by his growing disenchantment with the commission. Passed over for promotion, ignored by superiors who were mismanaging the system he had designed, he was ready for fresh pastures. His superiors, it is suggested, acquiesced in this hobby as a way to prevent him from meddling in things that mattered.[13] The explanations are inadequate. Chadwick's forte was public administration; the domain was less important. It is true that urban living conditions were an early interest, but so too were roads, police, and education.[14] As for being hated, Chadwick was not one to dodge criticism. Knowing himself right, he saw criticisms as the work of fools or interested parties. He was sure that after the rough patch of adjustment the newly freed labor force would generate unparalleled prosperity. One role of the commission and its secretary was to draw wrath to itself, making it easier for local unions to act.[15] Finally, whatever anger Chadwick harbored at the Whig politicians who had failed to come up with a promised commissionership, and however difficult his daily dealings with the commissioners and staff, in 1838–39 he was still active in forming and executing poor law policy and wholly dedicated to the principles of the act. Even in the summer of 1842, after Chadwick had been again humiliated and relations with the commissioners had deteriorated even further, the sanitary initiative remained much more than a diversion for a troublesome secretary.

## II

The sanitary initiative was so important to the commission because it was an alternative to the claim that destitution caused disease. That claim was fundamentally incompatible with the new poor law. The poor law was intended automatically to deflect potential claimants of relief back to the labor market to accept the prevailing wage. It did so by imposing the workhouse test. "Outdoor relief" (aid to maintain a poor family within its own dwelling and community) was to be banned; relief was to go only to those willing to enter a workhouse and elect the despised status of pauper. But while the law sought to balance access with disincentive, a balance was hard to strike. The presence of any destitution was an embarrassment; it showed that the balance had not been found, that the terror of the workhouse was too successful. Worse, if virtuous laborers were starving themselves into disease to avoid the workhouse, then the deterrent system was "morally indefensible" and might even

13 Lewis, *Chadwick* 34; Margaret Pelling, *Cholera, Fever, and English Medicine, 1825–1865* (Oxford: Oxford University Press, 1978), 11.
14 In 1841 Chadwick was asked what sort of position he might occupy within the Home Office. Sanitary administration was not on his list (Chadwick to Lord Normanby, 12 May 1841, University College London [to be cited as UCL], Chadwick Papers, #1578).
15 Anthony Brundage, *The Making of the New Poor Law: The Politics of Inquiry, Enactment, and Implementation, 1832–1839* (New Brunswick, N.J.: Rutgers University Press, 1978), 50; Lewis, *Chadwick*, 22; Finer, *Chadwick*, 93.

be augmenting pauperization and poor law costs by indirectly increasing disease.[16] If those diseases were contagious, then forcing people into privation would spread contamination throughout the population. The whole deterrent edifice would appear penny-wise, pound-foolish, not to mention immoral, and even, in a broad sense, criminal.

Beyond these concerns, to admit that destitution could cause disease was incompatible with the liberal principles of staying out of markets and fostering independence. Providing food, medical care, education, or support for the aged was no way to foster responsibility. One could not have dependency *and* liberty. Such relief had hampered the freedom of the labor market, forcing wages either too high (since workers had an alternative to work) or too low, as when farmers relied on the parish to subsidize their laborers.[17]

Chadwick in particular was uncomfortable with the Malthusian implications of the destitution–disease view. If one held that preventable lethal disease was a public problem, one had to argue that it led to the loss of something valuable. Yet Malthus had presented humans as demanders of finite resources and many still saw high mortality among a residuum as a corrective. To Chadwick, however, humans (or at least adult males) were the stuff of industrial growth and their premature deaths could be reckoned as so much lost profit. It was important, then, to see disease as a product of ill-considered arrangements, not, as the Malthusians would, as proof of an industrial society's tendency to create an imbalance between population and food.[18]

These were not abstract considerations. The "medical problem" was central in poor law administration and raised the deepest moral conundrums for the administrators. The 1832 Royal Commission had neglected the subject of disease, ignoring the tradition (and felt obligation) of providing public medical care.[19] Its automatic machinery could not accommodate disease very well. Clearly it made no sense, morally or financially, to install an entire family in a workhouse whenever illness led to temporary inability to work. In such cases it made sense to provide both medical care for the ill breadwinner and

---

16 Rumsey observed that the PLC seemed to regard medical care as a commodity or even a luxury, "a sort of personal gratification . . . of doubtful if not of dangerous tendencies" ("Medical Care of the Poor in England, with Notices Relating to Ireland – Part I. Historical," *Essays on State Medicine* [London: Churchill, 1856], 157, 169, 173). See also Henriques, *Before the Welfare State*, 126; Roberts, *Victorian Origins*, 258.

17 Chadwick did think wages were too high in manufacturing districts (Finer, *Chadwick*, 83; Lewis, *Chadwick*, 64, 66).

18 Cowherd, *Political Economists*, 228, 231; Pelling, *Cholera*, 11; Finer, *Chadwick*, 23; Lewis, *Chadwick*, 17–18, 45, 62–65.

19 Neglected in the report despite substantial attention to it in the evidence, noted Henry Rumsey ("The Medical Care of the Poor in England, I," 154). Rumsey claimed four fifths of Englishmen in places where there were no charitable institutions received parish medical care; with passage of the act this proportion decreased by about half (ibid, 164, 168). For the importance of regular public care in Bristol see Mary Fissell, *Patients, Power, and the Poor in Eighteenth-Century Bristol* (Cambridge: Cambridge University Press, 1991), esp. ch. 5.

"necessaries" for the family until money was again coming in. And if it were prudent to provide medical care to return the wage earner to work, could one withhold it from nonearning family members? One could permit only the ill family members into the workhouse, but Chadwick opposed that as simply another form of outdoor allowance.[20] If one withheld medical care, one risked violating a principal tenet of the law: that in an emergency people had a right to relief. The PLC tried to solve the problem by inventing a bureaucrat. The union relieving officer was to assess requests for medical care and send on only those judged worthy, who might then receive relief without taking on the pauper stigma. On the grounds that relieving officers were unqualified to diagnose, medical officers often bypassed them, using the excuse that emergency care was needed.[21]

Even more worrisome was the possibility that the deterrent system might itself cause disease. Chadwick had argued that elimination of the various pre-1834 allowances in aid of wages would ultimately raise wages since employers would be competing for the services of free laborers. In some notorious cases the reverse happened. The law left the labor force less mobile than Chadwick had hoped, and guardians, who in rural areas were often also employers, found they could bargain down wages, always making sure that the comforts of the workhouse were lower than that available outside. The resulting wage levels (five shillings/week for agricultural laborers in Andover) seemed below subsistence. If it were true, as most medical men held, that the predisposing causes of low diet, cold, poor clothing, and misery could themselves cause disease, then the poor law caused disease among cold, ill-fed people in the workhouses or among those scraping along on almost nothing in trying to stay out of them.[22]

Accordingly, for Chadwick and the commission disease among the poor was a touchy subject. At times he would insist that disease victims were never innocent, that all disease reflected moral error and could be avoided. The commission would suggest also that for the poor demand for medical care was

---

20  Finer, *Chadwick*, 188.

21  Rumsey, "Medical Care of the Poor in England, I," 188–89; idem, "The Medical Care of the Poor in England, with Notices Relating to Ireland – Part II. Its Present Condition and Requirements; Its Relations to Political Economy and Sanitary Management," *Essays on State Medicine*, 248; Ruth G. Hodgkinson, *The Origins of the National Health Service: The Medical Services of the New Poor Law, 1834–1871* (London: Wellcome Historical Medical Library, 1967), 20–21, 23, 25, 38–39.

22  Henry Rumsey, paragon of mid-Victorian medical politicians, would speak of "the injury deliberately inflicted on the cause of public health by . . . the influence of one [Chadwick], who has been held up by his partisans as the chief sanitary reformer of the age" ("Medical Care of the Poor in England, I," 171). On wages see Finer, *Chadwick*, 94, 257. Additionally a workhouse might facilitate the spread of contagious disease; Farr estimated the mortality rate to be 50 percent greater there. Farr, "Vital Statistics," *A Statistical Account of the British Empire: Exhibiting Its Extent, Physical Capacities, Population, Industry, and Civil and Religious Institutions*, ed. J. R. McCulloch, 2d ed., 2 vols. (London: Charles Knight, 1839), II, 545. See also Hodgkinson, *Medical Services of the New Poor Law*, 8–9, 15, 60, 150–52.

a function of supply. Do away with public care and you would find that illness disappeared.[23] While mutterings like these reflect class hostility more than serious policy options, it was still politically and morally imperative that the commission offer some solution. Ideally, argued Chadwick, families should save for medical emergencies, perhaps through medical clubs. But that didn't work. The clubs usually went bankrupt and most people simply didn't (or thought they didn't) have extra income to save. Chadwick urged unions to offer medical relief as a loan, but it was a loan rarely repaid.[24]

If this were not enough, the medical profession, which could unite on little else, was united in opposition to the reorganization of public medical practice under the new poor law. The act of 1834 established union medical officers to replace the old system of parish surgeons. By amalgamating parishes into unions, Chadwick and the commissioners hoped to improve care and cut costs. Each union would be split into a few medical districts, each with an officer. With larger patient loads, practitioners could become expert in the medical problems of the poor. At the same time, competition for fewer posts would force down salaries.[25]

Costs fell, but care did not improve. Districts became unmanageably large. Appointments (renewable yearly) were often made on lowest tender, frequently to outsiders who knew nothing of the district or their patients. Often the small stipends had to recompense both the practitioner's time and the medications used – the best way, thought Chadwick, to combat over-prescribing. Those taking the posts cut corners elsewhere: some were novices willing to live on a pittance while starting a practice. Others used union appointments to attract apprentices, who actually did the union work. Still others, as we shall see, altered prescriptions to avoid costly medication.[26] Care deteriorated; some felt that the humanity essential to medical practice would erode in such conditions of practice.[27]

General practitioners began to organize almost immediately after passage of the poor law act. Both the Provincial Medical Association (mainly rural practitioners) and the first British Medical Association (mainly metropolitan) were

23 Hodgkinson, *Medical Services of the New Poor Law,* 2–3, 5, 93.

24 Ibid., 249; Finer, *Chadwick,* 243; Rumsey, "Medical Care of the Poor in England, II, Present," 255–59; M. W. Flinn, "Medical Services under the New Poor Law," *The New Poor Law in the Nineteenth Century,* ed. Derek Fraser, 58–59 (London: Macmillan, 1976).

25 Finer, *Chadwick,* 158.

26 R. D. Thomson noted that wholesale druggists offered inferior lines of medications for use in poor law practice. "Select Committee on the Poor Law Amendment Act, 44th–46th Reports (Medical Inquiry)," *Parliamentary Papers [P.P.],* 1837–38, *18 pt. 3,* (518.), questions [qq] 15590–91; Edward Evans of Southwark noted (q 15763) that about half of his salary went to drugs.

27 Wakley questioning H. W. Rumsey and William Farr, "Select Committee on the Poor Law Amendment Act," qq 14907–13; 15382–84; John Yelloly, *Observations on the Arrangements Connected with the Relief of the Sick Poor; Addressed in a Letter to the Rt. Hon. the Lord John Russell, Secretary of State for the Home Department* (London: Longman, Rees, Orme, Brown, Green, and Longman, 1837), 20.

founded to press for improvements in poor law appointments. They were supported by both the Royal Colleges and Thomas Wakley's furious *Lancet* editorials. In 1838, Wakley (M.P. as well as *Lancet* editor and crusading coroner) managed to get a Commons select committee packed with supporters of the act to hold four days of hearings on the medical provisions of the law.[28] An 1844 select committee would focus exclusively on poor law medical practice and such issues would be at the heart of the Andover scandal, which in 1846–47 would bring down the PLC.

Medical men claimed the right to pronounce on the determinants of disease and health and claimed that given freedom to practice, they could eliminate much pauperism and lower the cost of relief.[29] The grand threat they held was moral – that the principles and administration of the new poor law were inhumane and caused much illness. They seemed immune to the truths of political economy, taking the view that care for the poor was a public duty, and that free care did not pauperize.[30] William Farr, recently appointed (with Chadwick's help) as statistician to the Register General, argued that medical provision could not "lead to the same abuse as relief in aid of wages . . . no one will break his leg willingly, or take physick as an amusement; medical relief has no tendency to increase." But even if it did, that made no difference: Farr and his colleagues recognized a duty to heal, refused to make medicine a commodity, and expected the parish to reimburse them. Farr went on: "No one, with a human heart can deny relief to the sick, medical men cannot. If a poor man came to a medical man, and he was conscious that the poor man could never pay him, the medical man must go to him, if it were a case of emergency; such being the case . . . the public should provide that man with medical relief . . . he should not be thrown entirely on the charity of the medical profession."[31] Many seemed willing to grant relief to all applicants. Perhaps for some this was a way to popularity, yet in a profession whose central institutions included dispensaries and voluntary hospitals, such charity held a central place in professional identity. Others insisted for reasons of social

28  Rumsey, "Medical Care of the Poor in England, I," 172; Finer, *Chadwick*, 130.

29  In light of Chadwick's depictions of selfish medical men it is interesting to note that several leaders of the general practitioners, including William Farr and Robert Ceely, saw the medical officer as having a key role in prevention ("Select Committee on the Poor Law Amendment Act," q 15832 [Farr], 15239 [Ceely]). J. P. Kay suggested that such an enlargement of the role of the medical officer was exactly the goal of the sanitary investigations he had just completed (ibid., qq 16074, 16078). See also Hodgkinson, *Medical Services of the New Poor Law*, 140.

30  But see Rumsey's views in "Select Committee on the Poor Law Amendment Act," qq 14930–33, 15011–12; Henry Rumsey, "The Medical Care of the Poor in England, II, Present," 243–46, 252, 256–57, 292–94. The solution to the problem of the pauperizing tendencies of medical care, suggested by both Rumsey and Kay, was simply to withdraw medical care from the domain of commodities and offer free care without stigma of pauperism (Hodgkinson, *Medical Services of the New Poor Law*, 61–62; MacDonagh, *Early Victorian Government*, 116–19).

31  "Select Committee on the Poor Law Amendment Act," q 15787; R. Ceely in ibid., q 15442.

stability that it was essential that poor and gentry be attended by the same practitioner, just as they were by the same clergyman.[32]

Still worse, poor law medical men had discovered a loophole that extended their stipends at the expense of the rigor of the law. While medical officers had to supply their own medicines, the parish supplied food for the convalescent. Thus it paid to medicate with food rather than pharmaceuticals. At the cost of the parish they ordered ample doses of mutton, ham, wine. To Chadwick this was tantamount to malpractice and fraud. These doctors were prescribing mutton only because someone else was paying. This was hardly "less eligibility": those getting public medical care were better off – in medical care narrowly construed and in the "necessaries of life" – than the independent poor.[33] Medical men denied the insinuation. One can clearly see how, working within a framework in which disease was debility and practicing among those who, by Chadwick's own admission, were managing on a smaller diet than prisoners received, such treatment could be justified.[34]

Yet Chadwick and his friends could not wring a confession or condemnation out of the medical brotherhood – even from Assistant Commissioner James Phillips Kay, who was, after all, one of their own as well as being a doctor. Asked by the committee whether food was the best medicine, and how it could be right that one practitioner prescribed far more necessaries than another in an adjacent district, Kay refused to second guess a colleague's management of a particular case. Instead, the guardians must "show great respect [for] . . . the opinions of the medical man on a subject on which his opinion must have greater weight than the opinion of the Board." The most he would say was that if an officer habitually prescribed large amounts of

---

32 Hodgkinson, *Medical Services of the New Poor Law,* 38–41; Robert Ceely, Rumsey in "Select Committee on the Poor Law Amendment Act," qq 15397–99, 15011–12; Rumsey, "Medical Care of the Poor in England, I," 155; idem, "Medical Care of the Poor in England, II, Present," 282. Indeed Rumsey envisioned a distinctly pastoral role for the state doctor, a "Missionary of Health . . . practically proving to the helpless and the debased, the disheartened and disaffected, that the State cares for them."

33 In their 7th Annual Report (1841), the commissioners would write: " 'If the pauper is always promptly attended by a skillful and well qualified medical practitioner; . . . if the patient be furnished with all the cordials and stimulants which may promote his recovery; it cannot be denied that his condition, in these respects, is better than that of the needy but industrious ratepayer who has neither the money nor the influence to secure equally prompt and careful attendance, nor any means to provide himself or his family with the more expensive kind of nutriment which his medical superintendent may recommend. This superiority of the condition of the pauper over that of the independent labourer as regards medical aid will, on the one hand, encourage a resort to the poor rates for medical relief, so far as it is given out of the workhouse, and will thus tempt the industrious labourer into pauperism; and on the other hand, it will discourage sick clubs and friendly societies' " (quoted in Hodgkinson, *Medical Services of the New Poor Law,* 60).

34 Hodgkinson, *Medical Services of the New Poor Law,* 38–41, 120; Rumsey, "Medical Care of the Poor in England, I," 214; idem, "Medical Care of the Poor in England, II, Present," 259–61; Finer, *Chadwick* 159, 189–90.

necessaries, the guardians might query this practice at reappointment.[35] Asked whether doctors were substituting food for "expensive" stimulants, Kay refused to say.[36]

Given the power of the guardians over the fates of young practitioners in an overcrowded profession, the boldness of these medical men is remarkable. Most really were cowed, Henry Rumsey insisted. Yet those who were not were mounting the most serious challenge to the new poor law and the rule of political economy, one more serious, because more respectable, than that of O'Connor, Stephens, and the northern Chartists.[37] They recognized, at least implicitly, a right to health that was being jeopardized by industrialization, urbanization, liberalism; indeed one critic of poor law medical men sniffed at these "petits amis de droits de l'homme."[38] Still, we should not regard these practitioners as purposefully political. The diagnostic power of French hospital medicine with its ambivalence toward its subjects had done much to displace the sympathetic sensibility taught in Edinburgh.[39] Nor were medical men necessarily happy as Tory radicals.

Still, a threat existed, one which Chadwick felt more strongly than his colleagues. Because of the way medical men insisted on practicing their profession there was an incentive to be ill; it was the route to relief without stigma. "Teething, bruises, even measles [were being taken] to validate claims for relief," he fumed. "Considering the facility with which medical certificates are obtained, especially where the medical man get popularity both with the labourer and the employer, this rule would procure permanent out-door relief, during the whole period of breeding up a family."[40]

Thus so very much depended on that most basic question of medical phi-

35  Kay, "Select Committee on the Poor Law Amendment Act," qq 5135–45, 5154.

36  Surely no practitioner could acquire popularity with the poor by prescribing inferior medicines? the committee insisted. Rumsey painted a picture of medical men compensating for their failure to use the proper medications with long chats and acquiring popularity thereby ("Select Committee on the Poor Law Amendment Act," qq 14942–48).

37  Hodgkinson, *Medical Services of the New Poor Law*, 16, 59, 118; Rumsey in "Select Committee on the Poor Law Amendment Act," qq 14748–49.

38  "Review of Report of a Committee on the New Poor-Law Act Appointed by the Provincial Medical and Surgical Association," *Medico–Chirurgical Review* 25 (1836): 326. On such social rights see Peter Mandler, "The Making of the New Poor Law *Redivivus*," *Past and Present*, 117 (1987): 131–57.

39  Dale Smith, "Afterword: The Study of Continued Fever in Victorian Britain," William Budd, *On the Causes of Fevers*, ed. Dale Smith (Baltimore: Johns Hopkins University Press, 1984), 130.

40  Quoted in Finer, *Chadwick*, 189–90; see also 188, 204; Chadwick to Lord Normanby, 7 March 1840, UCL Chadwick Papers, #1578. Rumsey agreed but drew the opposite conclusion: Because it could not discriminate between the pauper and the working poor, any program for preempting debilitating disease and "quickly restoring the sufferer to his previous condition of capacity for work – was . . . wholly irreconcilable with the Poor-Law principle of withholding relief, except in cases of destitution, lest the 'industrious labourer or needy rate-payer be tempted into pauperism.'" Rumsey, "Medical Care of the Poor in England, I," 190; also 182. On Chadwick's attitude toward doctors see Pelling, *Cholera*, 12; Finer, *Chadwick*, 158; Lewis, *Chadwick*, 47, 75–77; Marston, *Chadwick*, 152.

losophy: what disease was. The medical officers' approach assumed a contin-uum between health and disease; it assumed that people living in poverty slid into disease and that relief in the form of food, clothes, warmth, and good air pulled them out. If disease remained debility, if medical men persisted in seeing economic liberty as a disease requiring their intervention, then society would never achieve its potential. The only way to fight theory was with a different theory, one with vastly different implications for the relations of environment to disease, one in which disease was not a continuum but a binary phenomenon, either present or absent. Its presence would be random with regard to economic conditions and occupations, dependent instead on structures and behavior.

## III

The theoretical tenet that disease was not a function of poverty was essential for Chadwick to defend the claim that prolonged existence on a marginal diet, whether within or without the workhouse, did not adversely affect health. Among his first investigations as a poor law administrator was a study of prison diets. He claimed to find that prisoners on a "low" or minimal diet were actually healthier than those on a "high" diet.[41]

Chadwick's sensitivity to this issue is clear already in the 1833 Reports of the Royal Commission on the Employment of Children in Factories. The Whig government had established the commission to neutralize the incendiary testimony given to Michael Sadler's 1832 select committee. Although Sadler had convened the committee to make a case to limit the workday of factory children (and, necessarily, of their adult co-workers) to ten hours, witnesses represented factories as sites of wholesale deformation and destruction of hu-man beings. Sadler's exposés seemed to allow no equivocation and the com-mission was required to report quickly. It consisted of three Benthamites as central commissioners, Chadwick, Southwood Smith, and Thomas Tooke; several local investigators, and three medical commissioners: Charles Loudon, F. Bisset Hawkins, and Sir David Barry.[42] Effectively the chairman, Chadwick wrote its report. Its chief recommendation, which quickly became law, was to restrict the workday of children under thirteen more than the Sadlerites called for, to nine hours, and to require that factory children also spend four hours in school. This, however, allowed the working of two shifts of children, making for an even longer day for adults (i.e., those over thirteen). The ten

---

41 Finer, *Chadwick*, 83; Wakley and Farr would show this conclusion to result from statistical slop-piness (Lewis, *Chadwick,* 32; Henry Rumsey, "On Sanitary Inquiry: Its Methods and Defects in England – The Directions in Which It Needs Extension under State Authority," *Essays on State Medicine,* 92–94, 114).

42 Finer, *Chadwick*, 53. Chadwick had no choice of assistants and was particularly uncomfortable with Loudon.

hours' movement saw this as a cynical attempt to split its support. Others have seen Chadwick's policy as an ingenious compromise.[43]

Here it is important to focus on the tension between the commission's conclusions and the separate conclusions of the medical commissioners, for these same tensions would give rise to the Sanitary Inquiry – medicine had to be kept out of economics. Chadwick's tactics too were the same he would use nine years later: to select only facts that agreed with his views; to reject the burden of proof; to divert attention to safer matters – "sanitary conditions"; and, finally, to discredit medical men. Any residue of pathological effects that could not thus be explained away was to be ascribed to factors incidental to the work itself: high temperature, poor ventilation, dustiness, or even smelly privies – all of which were being eliminated in newer factories.

Pressure to legislate prevented thorough inquiry. The commission made its recommendations in a first report in early June, then issued a second in mid-July, when the evidence, particularly the medical reports, was all in. Thus there was a need to make the medical findings compatible with recommendations already issued. The first report had admitted that fatigue and lack of sleep did produce physical symptoms, such as aches and swollen ankles, and sometimes "serious, permanent, and incurable diseases." It found the case proved for amended legislation, yet opposed the ten hours' bill on the grounds that its real purpose was to regulate adults, not aid children.[44] Despite the medical reports appended to it, the second report was even more dismissive of health concerns. To a degree, the medical commissioners had left themselves open to misrepresentation. They had been given far too much to do: they were to examine the factories, the workers, their houses, their streets, and especially women (some Sadler witnesses had claimed that factory work inflamed female sexual desire yet interfered with puberty, conception, and parturition, so there was to be a grand study of this matter).

Each of the medical commissioners had approached his task differently. Barry, a Paris-educated physiologist and former army surgeon, toured Scottish factories, taking special interest in the stature of women, chatting with local medical men, and following up leads suggested by local workers' committees. His reports were disorderly, and Chadwick took them to show that there was no evidence of factory-induced deformity. He ignored most of Barry's conclusions.[45] In fact, Barry had damned factory work in general. Despite good

43 Finer, *Chadwick*, 56; MacDonagh, *Early Victorian Government*, 42–43; Charles Wing, *Evils of the Factory System Demonstrated by Parliamentary Evidence* (London: Saunders and Otley, 1837), xxxviii.
44 "First Report of the Royal Commission on the Employment of Children in Factories," *P.P.*, 1833, *20*, (450.), 28–29, 33–35, 45–47.
45 "Second Report of the Royal Commission on the Employment of Children in Factories," *P.P.*, 1833, *21*, (519.), 3. On Barry see *Dictionary of National Biography* [DNB]. Barry had found some skeletal deformities in factory workers, though he could not prove factory work caused them, as well as a number of persons who had lost limbs to machinery, a significant amount of consumption, and a good deal of local medical opinion that disease and deformity were attributable to very long

wages and better food and clothing, factory workers were no healthier than their unemployed neighbors. Factory work harmed children's health, first by "the undeviating necessity of forcing both their mental and bodily exertions to keep exact pace with the motions of machinery propelled by an unceasing, unvarying power"; second, by requiring long periods of standing; third, by depriving them of sleep. Other harmful factors were dust, damp, heat, and the absence of time for play. Male spinners typically suffered from "capricious appetite and dyspepsia," Barry found, and as few were "tall, athletic men," it was "fair to conclude, that their mode of life is not favourable to the development of the manly form." Women seemed "less deteriorated." Many were asthmatic.[46]

F. Bisset Hawkins, society doctor and pioneer statistician, simply summarized medical opinion in Greater Manchester, Preston, and Derby. Thus his report was full of "conflicting statements," noted Chadwick, and dismissed it.[47] Most troublesome was Loudon's Yorkshire report. A Leamington practitioner and population theorist, Loudon confirmed the Sadler witnesses. The state of one youth who had sometimes worked forty hour shifts was "a case of injury to the limbs from pure labour."[48] A ten hour day should be the maximum for adults as well as children, Loudon advised. In giving this advice, however, Loudon was "speaking merely 'as a physician'," Chadwick explained. This "purely medical point of view" might be accepted "without weakening the . . . moral and social considerations which discountenance all legislative interference with the disposal of labour extending beyond the age of childhood." And since Loudon's conclusion was not "exclusive . . . to labour in factories," it ought to be applicable to all labor. Thus there were no grounds for singling out textile workers and no basis for legislation.[49] Rarely was Chadwick's scorn for medicine so sweeping – at issue were not just doctors' ideas or practices but medicine itself, repudiated as a ground for social action. Medical men might perhaps ply their art in some ideal world when "moral" and "social" (i.e., economic) criteria were finally met, but to rethink the moral or the economic in terms of health seemed absurd.

Especially important in the factory reports are two stratagems Chadwick would use to attack medicine in the *Sanitary Report*. The first was the appeal to statistical rigor. The medical commissioners were to do a controlled study: "Whatever number of answers are obtained from the factories, the same number must be obtained from the population living in the same place, but not

hours of labor (Sir David Barry, "Northern Districts," in "Second Report of the Royal Commission on the Employment of Children in Factories," Appendix A-3, 1–4, 11–12, 16, 30, 33).

46 Barry, "Northern Districts," 72–73. Ultimately Barry backed off from the implications of these comments and would urge only some restriction of hours of child labor.

47 "Second Report of the Royal Commission on the Employment of Children in Factories," 6.

48 Dr. Charles Loudon, "North-eastern District," in "Second Report of the Royal Commission on the Employment of Children in Factories," Appendix C-3, 7–8.

49 "Second Report of the Royal Commission on the Employment of Children in Factories," 5.

engaged in factories." Only in this way could one distinguish the effects of factories from those of town life or of work in general. For the reproduction study all married women not factory-employed living on the same street as women employed in factories were to be interviewed – "omitting none, that no exception may be taken to the results obtained."[50] Several times in his career Chadwick would argue that medical men were misled about causes of disease because they practiced in one place only. Seeing many cases of a disease (e.g., skeletal deformity), they would infer a local cause (factory work) without asking whether the local incidence was typical of its incidence generally.[51]

Sound concerns, surely, but impossible to address in the time available. Still, the dazzling prospect of statistical certainty could neutralize claims founded in medical theory or clinical experience. Those who alleged the harmfulness of factory work bore the burden of proof, Chadwick held. Since he would accept only a statistical proof, which was in practice, impossible, he could conclude that the case against factories was not proved: there were no grounds for interference with adult labor.[52]

The second tactic was to exploit the richness of medical theory. Because any case of disease could be seen as the product of many causes, one was free to focus on plausible causes that diverted attention from a threatened activity. The commission's regional investigators were

to investigate minutely the *concurrent* causes . . . the state of the drains in and about the factory, the state of the neighbourhood of the factory as to dryness or dampness, cleanliness or filthiness; the state of the houses and neighbourhood in which the children and adult workpeople take their meals and exercise . . . and where they sleep; the state of the air within the factory . . . whether it be fresh or whether it be not fresh, owing to deficient

50  Chadwick advised that local medical students be recruited to carry out this inquiry, a suggestion of appalling insensitivity in the wake of the cholera riots of the previous year and in light of contemporary views of medical students ("Supplementary Instructions to the Medical Commissioners," in "First Report of the Royal Commission on the Employment of Children in Factories," 82): "It is only medical men who can be safely entrusted with several of the inquiries to which it is of the greatest importance to obtain correct answers; and a few medical pupils each, or what perhaps would be better, two by two, taking a street, and making the inquiries from house to house, would speedily and effectually accomplish the task. In hope that this suggestion will be carried into effect, the tables of inquiries to be made of married women have been made up into books of fifty each, which may be distributed to each medical man or medical student."

51  "Instructions to the Medical Commissioners," in "First Report of the Royal Commission on the Employment of Children in Factories," 80–81. This was part of a general argument against the authority of professions. Cf. [Thomas Southwood Smith], "Contagion and Sanitary Laws," *Westminster Review* (1825): 135, 137; Cowherd, *Political Economists*, 210–11.

52  He accepted interference with child labor without statistical demonstration. There was great disagreement as to the age at which the body developed the ability to work an adult day. Most attention focused on puberty as a time after which the skeleton was no longer in jeopardy. But as to the age of puberty, there was much disagreement, with the commissioners using the figure of eleven to twelve years in girls and fourteen in boys, while much of the medical testimony showed it to be later (in the late teens for females), "Second Report of the Royal Commission on the Employment of Children in Factories," 1.

ventilation; whether it be pure or whether it be rendered impure by effluvia floating in it, and if so, what the effluvia are.[53]

Thus the causes of harm might be either independent of, or at worst only incidental to, the factory. The implicit and unfounded assumption was that but for these causes, factory work was safe, however long the workday might be.

It was in this way that the "sanitary" problems Chadwick would take up a few years later crept into an investigation of the effects of work on health. Indeed, one Leeds factory apologist, Dr. James Williamson, offered Chadwick what was virtually the charge for the Sanitary Inquiry. It was not work but housing that had a "most pernicious . . . influence on health," Williamson wrote to the commission: "The greater proportion of cottage streets formed within the last fifteen years in most of the manufacturing towns are unpaved, or very partially paved and sewered; the houses are undrained; and these situations are the most frequent haunts of pestilential disease; besides contributing by their noxious exhalations to depress the health and to induce chronic disease." Williamson saw "the only adequate remedy" as a law requiring builders "to provide . . . sufficient drainage, and to pave the streets."[54]

The greatest gift Chadwick took from the factory inquiry was the word "sanitary" itself. Sir David Barry headed sections of his report "Sanitary Differences between Wet and Dry Flax Spinning" and "Sanitary State of Hand-Loom Weavers."[55] The roots of this neologism were clear enough: "cordon sanitaire" was familiar as a way to exclude epidemic disease; the adjective "sanitary" (or "sanatory" as Chadwick would spell it) could be readily coined to refer to factors affecting health or, collectively, "sanitary conditions" or "sanitary condition."[56] In the *Sanitary Report* Chadwick would become master

---

53 "Instructions to the Medical Commissioners," 81; "First Report of the Royal Commission on the Employment of Children in Factories," 15–16.

54 James Williamson, in Loudon, "North-eastern District," 12. Williamson, physician to the Leeds Infirmary, General Dispensary, and House of Recovery, uses precisely the arguments Chadwick uses, invoking all causes of disease other than long hours (i.e., diet, irregular habits, anxiety, as well as physical causes), highlighting the failings of statistical demonstrations, asserting that only workers with hereditary susceptibility were adversely affected by factory work. He denied that dusty workplaces were the cause of pulmonary ailments; instead these were caused by "improper or innutritious diet, or . . . inebriety. The internal membranes of the stomach being morbidly excited, sympathetic irritation is often propagated to the lungs, which *then* become more susceptible to the noxious influence of a dusty atmosphere" (ibid., 9). Williamson was recruited to write the local report on Leeds for the Sanitary Inquiry, but declined on the grounds that Henry Baker had also been asked (Williamson to Chadwick, *Leeds–Poor Law Commission [PLC] Correspondence,* 29 December 1840, Public Record Office [PRO] MH 12/15225).

55 Whether Barry himself coined the term is not clear; certainly it was not common, and I have found no earlier use. Barry, "Northern Districts," Appendix A–3, table of contents, and p.1. Cf. Pelling, *Cholera,* 31.

56 Chadwick used "sanatory" throughout the inquiry, yet "Sanitary" appears on the title. As was pointed out in letters to the *Times* in 1847, "sanitary" and "sanatory" have different origins (Gib-

of this word and would give it the close association it still has with structures that affect health, and particularly with water, wastes, sewers, and so forth. He did this not by an act of definition, but through use – as the label for subjects he wished to include in the report and as the grounds for excluding matters he wished to avoid. Even if diet and work affected health, they were not parts of "sanitary condition."

Barry had not used the term for such purposes, but simply as shorthand for "factors tending toward health or disease." He had even outlined what an inventory of "sanitary circumstances" might include. Only a few of his twelve items, quality of air and temperature, for example, overlapped with Chadwick's "sanitary conditions." Barry's list gave much attention to social and economic determinants: wages, education, inculcation of standards of behavior, family structure, as well as working and living conditions. Item 12, "sources of unhealthfulness," included "hard labor" and "poor living" in the case of the weavers, and "constant upright position," "wet feet and person," "personal labour only source of support," and "attention obliged to be as unremitting as the motion of a steam engine" for mill workers.[57]

## IV

Chadwick's turn to sanitation in the spring of 1838 is best understood as part of the PLC's attempt to deal with the "medical problem" within the framework of this sort of inquiry-as-apologetic. Ostensibly, the reports by Arnott, Kay, and Smith on the causes of fever in the East End of London were to make the case for investing poor law funds in nuisance removal. This would lower disease, and ultimately lower poor law costs. The idea of investing poor funds in capital projects to prevent pauperism was not new. Under the old poor law, vestries had been more or less at liberty to use the poor rate as they saw fit. The 1835 Royal Commission on Municipal Corporations found instances of its being used for general municipal purposes and for particular projects such as harbor improvements. That "sanitary" structures should be the sole focus is odd, however, for the argument that preventing disease prevented destitution could equally have sanctioned expenditure on soup kitchens, dispensaries, workplace regulation, provision of churches or schools, or other economic development.[58]

What evidence would warrant such an investment? Who needed convinc-

son, *The Public Health Agitation*, 47). Thomas Southwood Smith had referred to "sanitary laws" in his "Contagion and Sanitary Laws," *Westminster Review* (1825): 134–57, 499–530.

57  Barry, "Northern Districts," 9–10.

58  In a general form the argument was a fundamental premise of medical police. See William Farr, "Vital Statistics," 522–23; Miss Horner, "Extract from an Account of a Contagious Fever at Kingston upon Hull," *Report of the Society for Bettering the Condition and Increasing the Comforts of the Poor* 4 (1805): 103–4. On the use of poor rates for other purposes see "First Report of the Royal Commission on Municipal Corporations," *P.P.*, 1835, *23*, (116.), Appendix, 672, 836.

ing? In fact, Chadwick did not claim that fighting fever was the best invest-ment, or that the best way to fight it was by removing filth, nor did he try to calculate the costs and benefits of such a program. He was not in fact suggesting anything like the vast systems of water and sewers that he would be promoting by 1842, but only sanction for the small charges "irregularly incurred by parish officers" in removing nuisances.[59] The reports simply doc-umented removable filth, which was held to contribute to fever, other disease, and other social problems. As Chadwick's reporters recognized, few medical men would have denied the harmfulness of "filth" or the benefits of sewers, wider streets, and so on, though they might not have agreed on how "nui-sances" harmed health or on the priority of sanitation.[60]

The reports, I believe, were undertaken less to facilitate some public actions than to undermine others. While it is clear why Chadwick might wish to show that filth caused fever and thus destitution, the inquiry was also an occasion to pretend that destitution didn't cause disease. Hardly anyone would have denied that disease, through either the death or the disablement of wage earners, led to destitution. Yet, while admitting this, most would have ac-knowledged also that destitution typically indicated exposure to a host of constitution-weakening "predisposing causes" that led sooner or later to acute disease. That disease struck the susceptible seemed obvious; accordingly they recognized a feedback loop of destitution leading to disease, and to further destitution and further disease.[61] Only comprehensive improvement of living standards would break that loop. Chadwick would deny half that feedback. That denial, implicit in the 1838–39 reports, is explicit in the *Sanitary Report* and would remain a central tenet of sanitarianism through the 1840s.

In 1838 the need to reclaim authority from medical men had become crit-ical. In February, Wakley had made a frontal attack on the food issue, sneering at Chadwick's claims from prison studies that less food was better.[62] The new poor law was more unpopular than ever. As the depression worsened, the PLC kept pushing the act on the industrial North. Even liberal manufacturers,

---

59 Lewis, *Chadwick*, 34; "Report of the Poor Law Commissioners Relative to Certain Charges Which Have Been Disallowed by Auditors of Unions in England and Wales," *P.P.*, 1838, *38*, (539.), 4. But see Rumsey, "Medical Care of the Poor in England, I," 185.

60 "This connexion [between fever and exhalations] has been long known" (Thomas Southwood Smith, "Account of a Personal Inspection of Bethnal Green and Whitechapel in May 1838," *Fourth Annual Report of the Poor Law Commissioners, Supplement, P.P.*, 1837–38, *28*, [147.], 92). "The want of proper attention to these things . . . has often been complained of by medical men, and is evident to any attentive observer" (Neil Arnott and J. P. Kay, "Report on the Prevalence of Certain Physical Causes of Fever in the Metropolis Which Might Be Removed by Proper Sanatory Mea-sures," in ibid., 69).

61 Lewis, *Chadwick*, 45. For example, Rumsey ("Select Committee on the Poor Law Amendment Act," qq 15216–20) argued that medicine ought to receive a definite proportion of a union budget. This would take into account that medical costs must rise when conditions worsen and fall when they improve. Rumsey took as axiomatic that "distress invariably produces pauper disease."

62 "The Poor Law Amendment Act," *Lancet*, 1838, i, 777–84.

his usual allies, could see no grounds for enforcing a workhouse test when there was no work going, yet Chadwick kept up the call for strict enforcement. In parts of Lancashire, the West Riding, and the Northeast collieries, assistant commissioners were encountering an absolute unwillingness to cooperate. They (and Chadwick) were harassed and threatened. The ten hours' campaign had evolved into an anti-poor law crusade, which in turn gave the loftier goals of Chartism an immediacy and militancy they lacked in the South. As instigator and chief member of a Royal Constabulary Commission, Chadwick was building a case for a national police force. One could hardly rely on vapid and vacillating magistrates to uphold order; they were the very ones overturning the guardians' attempts at discipline. Throughout the year he and the Home Office were considering when to arrest the rabble rousers; they moved only in late December, when Chadwick led a team to Ashton to arrest the Reverend Joseph Rayner Stephens for fomenting riot. That two companies of dragoons accompanied them indicates the tension.[63]

The commission faced heavy weather in Parliament too. The PLC's mission was temporary: to group parishes into unions, oversee elections and workhouse construction, and settle other start-up problems. In 1839 the law would be up for renewal. Chadwick and the commissioners were having trouble merely implementing the act. Union formation was slow. Besides outright disobedience, unimagined legal and financial problems had arisen, and a much larger staff had been required. It was by no means clear that the commission would survive. Its chief survival strategy, observed the *Times*, was inventing busy work, like sanitary investigation and its (ultimately successful) campaign to control vaccination.[64]

But sanitation was also a counterattack, a way to scotch both doctors and Chartists. As in the factory investigation, here too a cesspool or foul privy was a scapegoat. Political concerns are apparent also in the site of the main case study: the East End of London, particularly Whitechapel and Bethnal Green, including Spitalfields. To be sure, the area was poor, disease-prone, and familiar to Southwood Smith, the investigator, but more importantly it was home to many militant artisans and a key battleground in the social policy wars. The first Spitalfields Act of 1773 established a mechanism for fixing piece rates in the cottage silk industry, and Spitalfields became (so it seemed

63 Nicholas C. Edsall, *The Anti–Poor Law Movement, 1833–44* (Manchester: Manchester University Press, 1971), 56–57; Finer, *Chadwick*, 141, 182–83. Chadwick had written to Russell in February 1838 that the *Northern Liberator* was calling for the assassination of Sir John Walsham, the assistant commissioner for the Northeast, and for Chadwick's liquidation. Others had been chased, assaulted, and shot at. See also J. T. Ward, *Chartism* (New York: Barnes & Noble, 1973), 120.

64 "[Poor Law Commission and Public Health]," *Times*, 25 November 1840, 4b–c; *Provincial Medical and Surgical Journal* 1 (1840): 199. Cf. Lewis (*Chadwick*, 37), who treats this expansion in "revolution-in-government" terms, as a product of social investigation. See also Finer, *Chadwick* 181; Marston, *Chadwick*, 91.

in retrospect) a paradise of educated and pious artisans with advanced views on politics and labor.

When the acts were repealed in 1824 Spitalfields was in decline, trade having moved north. Many locals blamed the Whigs with their free trade fancies and argued that Spitalfields-like acts were necessary for the weaving trade in general. They fought the new poor law, offering "medical" relief (including food) to those who asked for it, and argued that the government was starving and humiliating those whose only faults were self-education and democracy. All the while Smith and his colleagues were investigating, Spitalfields was being investigated by the Royal Commission on Hand-Loom Weavers (chaired by the Benthamite Nassau Senior, Chadwick's coauthor on the great poor law report). That commission's local investigator, Chadwick's friend the actuary Dr. James Mitchell, would attribute conditions in Spitalfields to moral failings and artificial wages, which had led too many people into weaving. To find that the East Enders were not being starved, but instead falling victim to their own filth, resonated in a way it would not have elsewhere.[65]

The 1838–39 London reports are in fact five studies published as four titles. Three are by Southwood Smith, one by Arnott, and one by Kay (those of Arnott and Kay were published as a coauthored report). Four kinds of studies were done. First were the theoretical claims of Arnott and Smith that among the many factors that harmed health, filth was the cause for real concern. Second were reports of tours led by local medical officers of "fever" hotspots (Smith went to Bethnal Green and Whitechapel; Arnott and Kay to the Wapping–Stepney area). From these tours they hoped to generalize about the *places* where fever was common. Third was a survey of metropolitan medical officers

---

65 William Hale, *An Appeal to the Public in Defence of the Spitalfields Act: With Remarks on the Causes Which Have Led to the Miseries and Moral Deterioration of the Poor* (London: Justines, 1822), 43, 45. Cf. Dr. James Mitchell, "On the East of England," *Royal Commission on Handloom Weavers. Reports of the Assistant Handloom Weavers' Commissioners*, Pt II, *P.P.*, 1840, *23*, [43-I.], 379–81. On the political debate see Duncan Bythell, *The Handloom Weavers: A Study in the English Cotton Industry During the Industrial Revolution* (Cambridge: Cambridge University Press, 1969), 139–75; Paul Richards, "The State and Early Industrial Capitalism: The Case of the Handloom Weavers," *Past and Present* 83 (1979): 110–15; Lovett, *Life and Struggles*, 77; Thompson, *Making of the English Working Class*, 332. On economic aspects see D. C. Coleman, *Courtaulds: An Economic and Social History*, 3 vols. I, *The Nineteenth Century, Silk and Crepe* (Oxford: Clarendon Press, 1969), 7–8, 20–21. On medical services see Hodgkinson, *Medical Services of the New Poor Law*, 23, 41–43, 135; Thomas Mackay, *A History of the English Poor Law*, vol. III, *From 1834 to the Present Time* (New York: Putnam, 1900), 244–46. Chadwick had met Mitchell about 1829 when Chadwick was becoming interested in sanitary matters (B. W. Richardson, "Edwin Chadwick C.B., A Biographical Dissertation," xxvii) and had used Mitchell's talents on the Factory Commission (Wing, *History of the Factory Acts*, xli). Mitchell, in turn, would use Smith's report in the Handloom Commission report (see Arthur Helps, *The Claims of Labour: An Essay on the Duties of Employers to the Employed*, 2d ed. [London: Pickering, 1845], 99); Chadwick himself had earlier praised the rigor with which Reverend Stone of Spitalfields denied charity to the local Irish (Cowherd, *Political Economists*, 233).

on the "physical" causes of fever in their districts. This made up the bulk of Kay's report. Last, and published a year later, was Smith's analysis of the geography of fever in the metropolis.[66]

These reports are the medical foundation of Chadwickian sanitarianism. Their authors gave Chadwick the gift of medical authority. He would represent them as identifying the causes of fever in London; the mission of the great Sanitary Inquiry was to confirm that these were the causes of fever in general. While they would be circulated as reflecting the state of the art in public health, they were in fact defining that field. One finds them cited often, but aspecifically – the evidence was not reviewed, the conclusions never questioned or compared with others' investigations of fever. Smith and Arnott would contribute with greater or lesser friction to Chadwick's sanitary projects during the next sixteen years, reiterating their 1838 views or applying them in particular cases, but none of their later works displaced these short reports.

The reports do not warrant the use Chadwick made of them. Their empirical arguments are careless and inconclusive, their theory dated and arbitrary. And though they were presented as independent studies, Chadwick had much to do with their shaping. Let us start with the Arnott–Kay report, which is effectively a condensed version of the *Sanitary Report* to come. Its title, "Report on the Prevalence of Certain Physical Causes of Fever in the Metropolis, Which Might Be Removed by Proper Sanatory Measures," is a clue to the reorienting character of the project. It orients "public health" in three ways, in focusing on fever, on "physical causes," and on remediability through "proper sanatory measures."

The first focus was unambiguous. Effectively, however, it marginalized occupational disease, tuberculosis, and infant mortality as public health problems. Less clear was the realm of "physical causes" remediable by "proper sanatory measures." Neither author defined "physical causes"; under it Kay included not only structures that might be built or repaired, like sewers and houses, but also behavior – yet he excluded occupational and economic causes. Chadwick would sometimes imply that "physical causes" exhausted the realm of cause and other times use the phrase to exclude causes he wished to avoid.

---

66 The reports are Neil Arnott and J. P. Kay, "Report on the Prevalence of Certain Physical Causes of Fever in the Metropolis, Which Might Be Removed by Proper Sanatory Measures," *Fourth Annual Report of the Poor Law Commissioners, Supplement, P.P.,* 1837–38, *28,* (147.), 67–83 (the contributions of each author are evident in the Mss report in the *PLC–Kay Correspondence,* PRO MH 32/50); Thomas Southwood Smith, "Report on the Physical Causes of Sickness and Mortality of Which the Poor Are Particularly Exposed; and Which Are Capable of Removal by Sanitary Regulations, Exemplified in the Present Condition of the Bethnal Green and Whitechapel Districts," in ibid., 83–88; idem, "Account of a Personal Inspection of Bethnal Green and Whitechapel in May 1838, with a Supplement," in ibid., 88–98; "Report on the Prevalence of Fever in Twenty Metropolitan Unions or Parishes During the Year Ended March 1838," *Fifth Annual Report of the Poor Law Commission, P.P.,* 1839, *20,* (239.), Appendix C–2, 100–106.

"Proper sanatory measures" meant measures acceptable within "Recognised Principles of Legislation," but the bounds of appropriate public action, too, were assumed rather than addressed. They did not include action against economic causes of illness: thus Smith would focus on causes of disease "incident to the condition of poverty," which made poverty part of the background within which the problem had to be solved, rather than a health problem in its own right.[67] In fact, early-nineteenth-century parliaments frequently went beyond Chadwick's "recognised principles of legislation," regulating the workplace and the supply of food and fuel. "Proper sanatory measures" were, like "physical causes," devices to deflect inquiry from the great social issues of prices, wages, hours, liberty.[68]

The most valuable part of the reports was the survey of medical officers, which would warrant Chadwick's claim to be representing the views of practitioners. The work of digesting the responses into generalizations fell to James Phillips Kay. In 1838 Kay was on the way out of medicine to a brief if successful career as a reformer of primary education. After his famous pamphlet *The Moral and Physical Condition of the Working Classes Employed in the Cotton Manufacture in Manchester* Kay had left practice and been appointed assistant poor law commissioner, posted first in East Anglia, and then in mid-1838, in London. Kay would later claim credit for the "sanitary idea." "Ambitious, impatient and vain," he has also been called the "most skilled, articulate, and intelligent" of the assistant commissioners.[69]

The survey itself was the work of Chadwick, not Kay, and it was neither an instrument for determining which factors most strongly correlated with

---

67 Smith, "Physical Causes," 83. In practice "physical causes" and "proper sanatory measures" defined each other: "physical causes" were what proper sanitary measures removed; "proper" sanitary measures were what was indicated to remove physical causes.

68 Roberts (*Victorian Origins*, 214) claims the PLC reports introduced this concept of "Physical."

69 R. J. W. Selleck, *James Kay-Shuttleworth: Journey of an Outsider* (Ilford, Essex: Woburn Press, 1994), 128; Brundage, *Poor Law*, 91; Edsall, *Anti–Poor Law*, 35; see also Coles, "Sinners," 459. In 1877 Kay wrote that when his health broke down, he was "at a critical period of my inquiries, for I had turned from the examination of the defects of municipal arrangements to an examination of the best existing examples of the arterial drainage of towns, however partial, and of the sources whence they derived any supply of water, however inadequate, and the means by which it was conveyed and distributed. These questions had not then become the familiar problems of scientific engineers. I had to grope my way from one imperfect example to another. . . . At that time there would have been no hope that any municipality, though clothed with sufficient powers, would expend the vast sums which have been most wisely applied in many great cities to their drainage and water supply. Nor would engineers probably have then been ready with well-devised schemes for a sufficient supply of pure water and for carrying away the sewage." He had been considering a foreign journey to investigate these matters. Yet "after I found myself likely to be absorbed in the efforts of the Government to establish a system of national education, I recommended to Mr. Edwin Chadwick to undertake the prosecution of this investigation into town drainage and water supply, and other connected questions of sanitary improvement" (Smith, *Kay-Shuttleworth*, 33). Dating this interest is problematic. If Kay was really the source of Chadwick's involvement, it must come from c. 1838–39; but Kay did not become involved in education until 1842.

fever nor a means for determining practitioners' views on the causes of fever. Instead, the questionnaire, which Kay did not include in his report, asked something quite different:

> The Poor Law Commission have been informed that within many districts chiefly inhabited by the labouring classes fever and other diseases occur at regular intervals or are never absent.
>
> It has also been stated that such diseases arise in places where there is no drainage; where filth is allowed to accumulate, or where there are other physical causes of disease which are removable if steps be taken.
>
> It is further stated that where such causes exist the suffering of disease, often fatal, is extensively inflicted on the inhabitants, mostly of the labouring classes, and very heavy burthens are cast upon the ratepayers. – Instances have been given to the commissioners where setting aside the higher consideration, even regarding only the expenditure of the rates, it would be good economy to remove the causes in question at public expense if there were no other means for their removal.
>
> You will . . . describe to them the nature of any such places it may have been your duty to visit, and specify the number of cases of illness ascribable to such causes, which have become chargeable to the parish.[70]

The survey assumed what it would be held to demonstrate, that filth caused fever. Medical men were only asked how much filth-caused fever there was, and few answered. The view that filth or bad drains harmed health was neither new nor controversial, and the government's interest welcome. But it did not follow that filth was the *primary cause* or its removal the most effective remedy. And though asked only about "drainage," "filth," and "other physical causes," respondents ranged far more widely in explaining fever.

Kay divided their views into causes "independent of habits" – insufficient sewers and drains, uncovered or stagnant drains, open stagnant pools, undrained marshes, accumulation of refuse, inadequate ventilation, and exhalations from cesspools, noxious trades, and overcrowded burial grounds – and causes "originating in habits": the state of lodging houses (for vagrants and for "a certain class of the Irish poor"); crowded houses; uncleanliness in dress, person, and house; intemperance; inappropriate dwellings (in squats and cellars or near to pigs); unwillingness to be hospitalized or vaccinated.[71] Typically fever writers did not classify causes according to whether they were acts of will (or habit); halting contagion was more important than blaming people. But such distinctions were central in discussions of poor relief and crime.[72] If

---

70 Circular to Greater London vestries, 27 April 1838, PRO MH 3/1.
71 Arnott and Kay, "Physical Causes," 70–71.
72 For example, the early nineteenth-century police reformer Patrick Colquhoun distinguished "culpable indigence" from "innocent indigence." He recognized twenty-six forms of the former and twenty-nine of the latter (J. R. Poynter, *Society and Pauperism: English Ideas on Poor Relief, 1795–1834* [London: Routledge and Kegan Paul, 1969], 202). Chadwick was emphasizing this distinction at the time with regard to the causes of pauperism (Finer, *Chadwick*, 147–48).

"fever" were to be abducted from medicine and made part of the great questions of morality, a concept of the bounds of personal responsibility was essential. For surely some elements of one's world (drains) were conditions of moral action, while others (drinking alcohol) were moral acts for which one was responsible. Deciding which were which was another matter. Is crowdedness a habit, as Kay will have it – either an insensibility to decent living conditions or a horrid enjoyment of life en mob? Or is it simply a mark of a disparity between supply and demand in housing? And if so, does that disparity reflect a failure of builders and landowners or the bad "habit" of irresponsible procreation? Was dirtiness a "habit" or a product of lack of water? And why was living near "poor Irish" more a habit than living near undrained ponds? And what of *being* poor and Irish, for surely at some level Kay knew that the "poor and Irish" were victims of fever too. Perhaps for Kay, seeking a convenient way to classify responses, all this didn't matter; for Chadwick, seeking a mechanism of social stability, it did.

The factors Kay identified (save unwillingness to be vaccinated, which had to do with smallpox) do figure in contemporary explanations of fever. As we have seen, medical men recognized many kinds of causes, existing at varying temporal distance from the event and acting in various ways. Cesspool exhalations might contain an exotic fever poison or ordinary gases that undermined the constitution. Intemperance led to fever by causing one to live in the dreadful conditions where fever thrived. The "Irish poor" might cause disease economically, by diluting the fund of wages, or morally, by setting an example of squalid living. Or they might be held responsible for miasma-generating filth or seen as a reservoir of contagion. But Kay offered none of the usual careful distinctions of how the causes worked. And missing from his list were the destitution factors usually included as predisposers: hunger, fatigue, cold, and damp. In fact, several respondents had mentioned these. Jordan Lynch (whose letter Kay used to illustrate slaughterhouse nuisance as a cause of fever) observed that the majority of fever victims were those "unable to procure adequate nutriment from want of employment during the past inclement winter, which predisposed them to the attack of the contagion, and deprived them of the power to resist its ravages." James Appleton (bad drains) included as a cause of fever "privation . . . with respect to food."[73] For Kay as for Chadwick, *some* social conditions, but not others, might be admitted as

---

73 Appleton's multicausalism is typical: "Considering the filthy habits of the people dwelling in this particular locality; considering the privation that many of them undergo with respect to food, and their intemperate use of ardent spirits; that they are huddled together in ill-ventilated rooms, and that this place is the rest of Irish lodgers . . . it is exceedingly difficult to give an opinion how far these cases of fever have had their origin in such causes; how far they have had their origin in states of atmosphere equally affecting the crowded parts of this metropolis; and how far they have originated in the local causes above named." See also Hatfall, Evans, Byles, and Mitchell in Arnott and Kay, "Physical Causes of Fever," 73, 75–80.

causes of disease. Willing to include so many "causes," Kay excluded destitution.


## V

For Chadwick, the most important items on the list were the cesspools, piles of filth, puddles, and stagnant drains, the producers of the supposed miasm which would increasingly be seen as the only significant cause of fever. This would be the dogma of Arnott and Smith. Both in their early fifties, each had a claim to relevant expertise, Smith as physician to the London Fever Hospital, Arnott as a ventilation authority. Each fancied himself a philosopher and had a penchant for grand theories of health. Neither was in the mainstream of medicine. They were "the authorities" only within the Benthamite circle so dominant in social inquiry.[74]

Neil Arnott would serve as Chadwick's "bulldog" in an 1840 controversy with W. P. Alison on the social causes of fever. In 1853, he would disappoint Chadwick by finding that Chadwick's new sewers were responsible for a fever epidemic in Croydon. After brief study of medicine and surgery at Aberdeen and at St George's Hospital, Arnott had been appointed surgeon in the East India Company. After two voyages he left that service for a career as a scientific lecturer and fashionable London practitioner, including among his patients Chadwick's nemesis Thomas Wakley. As a Catholic fluent in languages, he found a large practice among diplomats and exiles from Continental politics. In 1837 he was made physician extraordinary to the new queen. He was a popularizer of science, the author of a popular physics text, and an inventor (of a water bed for invalids and a fuel-efficient stove) but (with the exception of ventilation) not a research scientist. A founder of the University of London, he became a major benefactor of higher education, particularly for women.[75]

Arnott's contribution comprises the first two pages of the Arnott–Kay report. He began by representing fever as a poisoning. Just as a contagion was the smallpox poison, a malaria from decaying filth was the fever poison. Though typically found in the "uncultivated" tropics, this malaria must exist wherever there was decomposing matter. Even if there were no apparent filth, the very fact of disease indicated hidden filth nearby.[76] This malarial poison

---

74 Cf. Marston, *Chadwick*, 94; Pelling, *Cholera*, 7, 25.

75 DNB; Neil Arnott, *On Warming and Ventilating; with Directions for Making and Using the Thermometer–Stove or Self-Regulating Fire* (London: Longman, Orme, Brown, Green, and Longmans, 1838); Chadwick to Lord Morpeth, 20 September 1848, UCL Chadwick Papers, #1855.

76 Significantly, in his ventilation book, Arnott attributes most disease to "deficiency, excess, or other misgovernment" of the four great necessaries of life: food, warmth, air, and exercise. He speaks, for example, of "diseases from deficiency arising during famines, as putrid fevers, scurvy, dropsies, etc." Arnott recognizes a category of poisons, which includes malaria from filth but does not emphasize it (Arnott, *On Warming and Ventilating*, 4–6).

was not distinctly different from a contagion. In typhus there might be generated a "contagious malaria, often more quickly operative on other persons than the original cause."[77] Crowdedness was problematic not by concentrating decomposition but by preventing separation of the fevered from the healthy.

Offered as proof of the malarial hypothesis were "illustrative facts which have occurred to Dr. Arnott in the course of his professional engagements." First was a girls' school in an area of cowsheds, ditches, and sewers. Every year the girls were ill with something, convulsions, or typhoid, or ophthalmia, or constipation. Then there were the grave robbers struck down by a putrid corpse, or cesspool cleaners meeting a similar fate. Three families successively occupying a house on Baker Street were struck with fever, from foul drains, Arnott claimed. Arnott wrote of his tour with Kay of Wapping and Stepney that "we found as we were prepared to find wherever the fever had appeared, one or more of the causes now to be active": houses without privies or covered drains, or with stagnant drains, or large open ditches, or "houses dirty beyond description as if never washed or swept and extremely crowded," or pig sties and "half-putrid pig food" and "heaps of refuse rubbish." Surely prevention would cost less than care for the sick and support "for the helpless widows and orphans of those who die," Arnott concluded.

Arnott's brief report illustrates how utterly arbitrary was the reasoning on which the sanitary movement was founded. His malaria is an ad hoc hypothesis to account for any disease he chooses to assign to it. Its plausibility relies on a correlation argument, but the malaria with which fever is to be correlated is so imprecisely defined and its presumed effect modified by so many variables that the correlation can never be tested. The girls' school case is to indicate the range of effects of the poison. While it was plausible enough at the time to think of a single cause having varied effects, a succession of epidemics might at least as plausibly have suggested a succession of different causes. The occasional asphyxiation of otherwise healthy gravediggers or sewer workers was well known and usually attributed to carbonic acid.[78] As for the Baker Street case, Arnott had to admit that his knowledge was secondhand: it had occurred long before and been reported by Armstrong. Yet Arnott would present this as sophisticated induction. "Malaria being invisible and intangible, men in

---

77  In his 1838 report Smith admitted that prior to the arrival of a fever victim, even poor sanitary conditions in a workhouse would not trigger an outbreak (Smith, "Physical Causes," 87); cf. Pelling, *Cholera,* 44.

78  Arnott is ambiguous on the sewer workers, referring to the "mephitic air from putrid animal and vegetable matters, etc." (Arnott and Kay, "Physical Causes," 69). But see John Ferriar, "Origin of Contagious and New Diseases," *Medical Histories and Reflections,* 1st American ed., 4 vols. in 1 (Philadelphia: Dobson, 1816), I, 121–22, or the more recent authority, Robert Christison, *Treatise on Poisons in Relation to Medical Jurisprudence, Physiology, and the Practice of Physic,* 1st American ed. from the 4th Edinburgh ed. (Philadelphia: Barrington and Haswell, 1845). On Baker Street see "Sanitary Report – Sewers and Water Supply," UCL Chadwick Papers #45.

rude states of society [were still] totally ignorant of its existence," he soberly observed.[79] With malaria "invisible and intangible," having many sources, acting at distance, and productive of many effects, one could hardly fail to find what one was "prepared to find."

The physician and Unitarian minister Thomas Southwood Smith – like Kay and Alison, an Edinburgh graduate – made much the same arguments, but in a more sophisticated way. Smith, through no desire of his own, would be Chadwick's rival for leadership of the sanitary movement in the next two decades. Arguably he was the more indispensable in transforming public health: one can imagine others drafting legislation and administering a board of health, but Smith offered the counterweight to Alisonian medicine. His persona was important too: many in the Health of Towns Association in the mid-1840s found the gentle Smith a refreshing change from the rigid and aggressive Chadwick.[80] As members of Bentham's inner circle, Smith and Chadwick shared a faith in progress and liberalism.[81] But they came to it from different directions. At heart Chadwick was a social engineer who would rationalize systems to rationalize people, while Smith was a liberal theologian and a compassionate doctor. Chadwick thought of populations, Smith of individuals. If, as Benthamites, both were concerned with happiness, Chadwick's happiness was a condition delivered by (and defined by) a scientific state, while Smith's was felt by real people.

If Smith was so moved at the plight of the individuals caught by the Moloch of industrialism we may wonder why he did not adopt the radical politics of Cobbett, Oastler, or Wakley, or the evangelical humanitarianism of Lord Ashley. While he shared much with these men, he was deeply uncomfortable with the stifling paternalism of Tory radicalism. Yes, the industrial revolution had placed people in unacceptable situations, but the answer was not some mythical organic village past in which the parish bountiful endlessly ladled soup to a peasantry of vile incompetents. That seemed too much like the slavery one was fighting so vigorously. Instead, Smith, like Kay, Thomas Chalmers, and a great band of liberal reformers, was searching for a mechanism that would foster independence and competence. For many it was education or temperance. It was churches for Chalmers, sanitation for Smith.

Smith's searchings took place within a necessarian theology that emphasized God's goodness and absolute responsibility for the world. In this view, the evils of industrialism and the rest of the "condition-of-England" problem were

79 Arnott and Kay, "Physical Causes," 68.
80 In the title page of Smith's *The Common Nature of Epidemics, and Their Relation to Climate and Civilization. Also Remarks on Contagion and Quarantine,* ed. T. Baker (London: Trübner, 1866), Smith is called "the father of sanitary reform." See also Lewis, *Chadwick,* 35.
81 Webb, *Martineau,* 88–90, argues that necessarians like Smith were not utilitarian, though the two movements ran "parallel."

to be seen as a stage in human progress, necessary but temporary; the result of ignorance more than of evil. By discovering and implementing scientific truths, humans would ultimately come to run the world as God had intended.[82] These views appeared in Smith's first book, *Illustrations of Divine Government* (1818). There he argued that disease was not God's fault: putrefaction, though a cause of disease, "could not in the nature of things have been avoided" since there could be no chemical combination without repulsion between particles. The great evil was not poverty but "dependence and servitude." Inequality was God's prod, Smith argued; equality would diminish happiness. "The difficulty, yet absolute necessity of procuring food, puts all the faculties of the mind on the stretch, to invent expedients for increasing its quantity, and for abridging the labour necessary to raise it. . . . There is not, indeed, among the inestimable blessings of civilisation, a single good for which man is not indebted, directly or remotely, to this stimulus."[83]

When Smith moved to London in 1820 he was already a significant Unitarian theologian. In 1824 he obtained positions at the London Fever Hospital, the Jews' Hospital, and the Eastern Dispensary, remarkable for an outsider and a mark of the clout of both the London Unitarians and Bentham. In the controversy between those for whom fever was debilitation (to be treated with supportive therapies) and those for whom it was inflammation (warranting depletive therapies like bleeding) Smith, like John Armstrong, his senior at the London Fever Hospital (also a dissenter), was an inflammationist.[84]

Smith's first contribution to "public health" was a long article, "Contagion" – principally of plague – for the Benthamite *Westminster Review* during the quarantine controversy of the mid-1820s. As Erwin Ackerknecht noted long ago, this controversy was over burden of proof. On discovering a case of plague, should one hypothesize contact with an unknown plague carrier or a mysterious pathogenic state of atmosphere? The assumptions were equally gratuitous. Smith decided the atmosphere caused plague; hence quarantine was futile. That view reflects his liberalism, his necessarianism, and probably also his jealousy of the old guard Anglican monopolists of the Royal College of Physicians.[85] On the grounds that it is actually plague modified by the English climate, he gave much space to typhus, arguing that what was often

82 Ibid., 71–83.
83 Thomas Southwood Smith, *Illustrations of Divine Government;* 1st American from the last London ed. (Boston: B. Mussey, 1831), 89–90, 109, 111–14.
84 Pelling, *Cholera*, 9, 21.
85 [Thomas Southwood Smith], "Contagion and Sanitary Laws," *Westminster Review* (1825): 134–67, 499–530; E. H. Ackerknecht, "Anticontagionism Between 1821 and 1867," *Bulletin of the History of Medicine* 22 (1948): 562–93. See also James C. Riley, *The Eighteenth Century Campaign to Avoid Disease* (London: Macmillan, 1987), xi, xv; Pelling, *Cholera*, 27–29. In attacking Blane, Faulkner, and Granville ("Contagion," 501, 505, 514), Smith makes clear he is attacking the Royal College of Physicians.

called "contagious fever" was not contagious. He made the claim less by challenging well accepted observations and inferences than by redefining concepts and by abusing those who did not use his definitions.[86]

In the article are many arguments that would later appear only as assumptions. Central were a new, narrow definition of "contagion" and a distinction between "contagious" and "epidemic" diseases. Smith held that contagious diseases properly so called were specific diseases. The "specific animal poison" that produced a disease must produce it in any exposed person who had not previously had it. An outbreak would end only when there were no new victims.[87] Most important, he saw no room in the concept of contagion for predisposing causes. A case of contagious disease required only the placing of "a *healthy* person within a certain distance of the diseased." The old Cullen–Bateman–Alison view that fever could "arise from cold, from wet, from a peculiar constitution of the atmosphere, or from any of the common causes of fever, and become contagious," was "as great an absurdity as the spontaneous generation of an animal." Even assuming animals and diseases were analogous, the statement went well beyond contemporary opinion.[88]

That older view had explained how it was that typhus sometimes developed in those with no apparent contact with previous victims. To explain such events, Smith would appeal to a new concept of "epidemic" diseases, which

86 Smith, "Contagion," 135–38, 514: "The physicians of the London Fever Hospital, and all other physicians who are extensively acquainted with the typhus fever of the metropolis, know that the plague constantly exists in London; that is they know that cases constantly occur in this city with symptoms *exactly similar* to those of plague: . . . with bubo, with swelling, and suppuration of the glands of the axilla, and with carbuncle superadded to all the other symptoms of malignant fever." The idea did not originate with Smith; see William Heberden, *Observations on the Increase and Decrease of Different Diseases* (London: T. Payne, 1801), 87; Dale Smith, "Afterword," 130; Pelling, *Cholera*, 7, 35.

87 Smith, "Contagion and Sanitary Laws," 145, 147; Pelling, *Cholera*, 18, 22–25.

88 Smith, "Contagion and Sanitary Laws," 135, 139–41, 145, 147: "Contagious matter being applied to the unaffected, the disease it produces would as readily arise in the rich as in the poor; in the well-fed as in the ill-fed; in the well-clothed as in the ill-clothed; in the well-lodged as in the ill-lodged; in the idle as in the laborious; in those who dwell in a pure, as in those who dwell in an impure atmosphere, and in the natives of a country, as in strangers." While many held something like this view with regard to smallpox, they certainly did not with regard to fever (145). Henry Clutterbuck argued the opposite, that contagion explained the susceptibility of the impoverished: "Supposing the disease to be capable of being propagated by *contagion*, . . . it is obvious that the poor are peculiarly obnoxious to every circumstance favourable to the operation of this cause. The close and crowded state of their dwellings; their general disregard of cleanliness, increased as it is by that indifference to the common decencies of life, which poverty is so apt to generate; and the depression of mind with which this state is necessarily accompanied; are all circumstances favourable to the operation and spreading of contagion, and from which the higher orders are exempt" (*Observations on the Prevention and Treatment of the Epidemic Fever at Present Prevailing in the Metropolis and Most Parts of the United Kingdom* [London: Longmans, Hurst, Rees, Orme, and Brown, 1819], 34). For contemporary opinion on the specificity question see William Henry's commissioned review: "Report on the State of Our Knowledge of the Laws of Contagion," *4th Report of the British Association for the Advancement of Science* (1834): 67–72. One of the few to agree with Smith is William Budd, "On the Causes and Mode of Propagation of the Common Continued Fevers of Great Britain and Ireland," in Budd, *On the Causes of Fever*, 72–73.

resulted from a "condition of the air." He could not say what mix of aerial qualities was responsible; moisture and warmth appeared important, but mainly one attributed epidemics to an indefinable state of the air simply because their variability excluded all other determinants.[89]

This "condition of the air" included at least five hypothetical pathogenic processes, in three classes. First was the transitory "epidemic constitution," which when combined with local weather produced major epidemic waves. In cold, wet Britain it produced true typhus; in warmer places it appeared as plague or tropical fevers. Second, a generic "common" fever, as well as a range of other diseases, might arise from a local "corruption" of air. But "corruption" itself referred to three quite different things. It meant in the first place a concentration of "the healthy exhalations of the human body" (e.g., carbonic acid), in the second "the morbid exhalations of the human body" (i.e., exhalations from a body suffering from some indefinite disease), and in the third "exhalations arising from the putrefaction of dead animal and vegetable matter." The effects of these several corruptions were indistinguishable; they varied "from the head-ache, produced by a crowded theatre, to the mortal fever . . . as occurred in the blackhole of Calcutta."

Finally, a true typhus was *"capable, under certain circumstances, of generating [typhus] fever.* It is a fact established by frequent observation, that if the apartment of a person labouring under typhus fever be small, close and dirty; if it be unventilated, and if the effluvia from the body be allowed to accumulate in it, the air will become so contaminated, as to produce fever in those who breathe it." There were the many cases of medical men visiting typhus patients who remained unharmed so long as they stayed near windows or doors, but when they turned "to receive both the effluvia and the breath in the most concentrated state . . . felt a sudden disagreeable sensation [and] . . . immediately became affected with fever." This sort of transmission process had been the raison d'être of the fever hospital movement. Allowed to follow its course in clean and airy conditions, a fever would lose its contagiousness and thus pose no threat to house staff or to the surrounding neighborhood. But where ventilation was poor, "animal steams from foul and diseased bodies" might become so thick as to bring on fever in anyone who came through the door.[90]

Familiar with the spread of typhus in crowded and ill-ventilated military hospitals, Sir John Pringle, the eighteenth-century authority on the diseases of armies and longtime Royal Society president, had inferred its contagiousness. Yet Smith insisted that these were "contaminative" not "contagious"

---

89 Smith, "Contagion and Sanitary Laws," 135, 141–42.
90 Ibid., 150, 519–20; cf. Clutterbuck, *Observations,* 39. Smith himself had suffered from this kind of fever from visiting a patient in a tiny unventilated room: "I could not breathe the air of that room. I could not remain in it long enough to write a prescription for the poor patients. As I was writing it at the street-door I shivered and felt sick. I knew that I had taken fever. I passed through a very severe form of it" (*Common Nature of Epidemics,* 53).

fevers, because *"no fever produced by contamination of the air can be communicated to others in a pure air,"* while a true contagion must be "equally communicable in every possible state of the atmosphere." An epidemic disease, he concluded, could not *become* contagious simply because it could not *become* specific.[91]

On one level the controversy, as Smith admitted, was "a mere dispute about words." In treating the diffusible "something" as not a contagion, Smith would make "contagion" a more precise term, but at the cost of loading "conditions of the atmosphere" with a bewildering array of pathological processes with indistinguishable effects.[92] Nonetheless, this rearrangement of central medical concepts did have implications. Predisposition was severed from a constitutional medicine in which persons either succumbed directly to debility or were left susceptible to contagia, and appended to the new category of "condition of the air" diseases. There it was superfluous and gradually faded, taking with it the possibility of mounting any general social critique from the ground of medical theory.

In 1825 Smith still acknowledged the traditional range of predispositions, even if they no longer figured in contagious diseases. He agreed with his predecessor Thomas Bateman that fever was "sure to be generated, to prevail extensively and to prove highly mortal wherever there is a scarcity of provisions."[93] Yet "atmosphere" had already begun to displace social conditions. True, in towns, epidemics struck in low and damp places, places "inhabited . . . by the poor." But their poverty was incidental: the key factor was their "crowded . . . ill ventilated and dirty" houses. "The most certain and the first victims of epidemic diseases are those who, from their poverty or their occupations, *are most exposed to the air.*"[94] Where the chroniclers of London mortality for the previous century, William Heberden, Robert Willan, and Bateman, had taken the winter mortality peak as evidence of the deadly effect of cold and damp on a poor, hungry, and overcrowded population, Smith argued that such seasonal changes in diseases were exactly what one would expect from an atmospheric cause.[95]

91 This argument that a contagion was a "gratuitous" assumption unless one could show that it could also be transmitted in good air didn't help, since there was no way to define or measure what "goodness" meant (Smith, "Contagion," 151, 520).

92 Ibid., 519–21; cf. Thomas Bateman, *A Succinct Account of the Contagious Fever of This Country Exemplified in the Epidemic Now Prevailing in London* (London: Longman, Hurst, 1818), 142. Smith's reasons were probably a mix of theological and practical. To Smith the providentialist it was more fitting to think that God had left a world in which intelligent and responsible humans could produce health than one in which humans were fated always to be the victims of manifold species of hostile entities. Smith the fever hospital doctor faced the problem of reassuring neighbors that the hospital was safe and that they possessed means to combat the disease. He wrote that when the words were finally properly used people would no longer be scared ("Contagion," 516, 522–23). Yet while many fever hospital doctors wrote about the same problem, none that I know of saw the rejection of the term "contagion" as an appropriate solution.

93 Smith, "Contagion," 515.

94 Ibid., 135, 144 (italics mine). This is with the exception of unacclimated newcomers.

95 Ibid., 143.

Smith drew on this "condition of the air" model in his 1838 report to Chadwick. Yet there were three key differences, reflecting the context of the report, developments in science, and a new concept of predisposition. First, in 1838 he would be concerned only with one atmospheric agency, emanations of decay. This reflected a shift of focus from fever generation and transmission to prevention. Chadwick was not interested in epidemic constitution, and the other forms of aerial poison were relevant mainly to fever hospitals and medical practice.[96] But Smith was also beginning to think that emanations of decay explained all fever, and most other diseases. In his 1830 *Treatise on Fever*, he had held the exciting cause of fever to be "a poison formed by the corruption or the decomposition of organic matter." At that point it was still to be known only by its effects, though the effects of animal decay differed from those of rotting vegetation.[97] By 1838 that had changed. Hitherto "ascertainable only by its mortal influence," now the poison had been isolated by "modern science." He reported experiments in which mice and dogs had been injected with or exposed to a condensate of putrefactive emanations. In high concentration this killed instantly, and Smith noted that "by varying the intensity and dose of the poison . . . it is possible to produce fever of almost any type, endowed with almost any degree of mortal power." Ten to twelve drops, for example, produced in a dog the black vomit of yellow fever.[98]

Most dramatic was the even more marginal status of predisposition. At best, debility now only determined how quickly one succumbed to the malarial poison. "Wretched" people "with enfeebled constitutions" – like Bethnal Green weavers – would succumb quickly, but even those "in robust health" would "sooner or later, by the mere residence in these places, either fall into fever, or suffer from some other of the diseases indirectly produced by the febrile poison." No "constitution, no conservative power in wealth," could resist "constant exposure to the exhalations which are always arising from these collections of filth."[99] Smith also reinterpreted the mode by which predisposing causes acted. They might be seen not as cumulative assaults on the

96  Smith had not given up his notions of a quasi-contagious process of fever transmission. He noted that fever outbreaks typically showed a pattern of succession of cases rather than the simultaneous outbreak that one would expect from a massive dose of an environmental poison: "When fever breaks out and becomes prevalent . . . the evil is frightfully increased by the extension of the infection to neighbouring houses and districts. The exhalations given off from the living bodies of those who are affected with fever, especially when such exhalations are pent up in a close and confined apartment, constitute by far the most potent poison derived from an animal origin." So powerful were these exhalations that admitting a fever case into a clean workhouse would still spread fever among the inmates (Smith, "Physical Causes," 84, 87).

97  Thomas Southwood Smith, *A Treatise on Fever* (Philadelphia: Carey and Lea , 1830), 360–61, 372, 376–77, 381–82.

98  Smith, "Physical Causes," 88. The argument was circular since Smith could not independently measure the malaria in the environment. He claimed to be interested in correlating fever with "the presence and intensity of malaria," yet fever was the only measure of malaria.

99  Ibid., 84–85.

constitution, but as part of a train of causes triggered by a single factor. For example, breathing an atmosphere of decay could lead to indigestion, which left one poorly nourished, susceptible to temperature changes and accordingly to inflammation of the lungs or consumption. Therefore, to the total of fever deaths (half of all world deaths, Smith claimed) one had to add all deaths due indirectly to the poison.[100] The factors Kay had drawn from the medical officers' responses – damp, intemperance, crowdedness, or any of the destitution indices – might be seen as consequences of the malaria (or as facilitators of its action). Without them, the poison would still eventually have its effect; without the poison, they would never lead to fever.

Nearly a year later Smith supplemented the report with a statistical analysis of the relations of population, percentage of paupers, and fever incidence among paupers in several metropolitan districts. The data came from a survey of medical officers. In a loose sense this was to be a test of whether fever was more closely linked to place or to economic status, a test of whether filth or destitution was the more important determinant. He found no correlation of fever to percentage of paupers and concluded that the presence of the malarial poison, not the lack of necessaries of life, caused the disease. But there had been no attempt to map cases within large areas, or to relate fever to economic conditions, or to discover how much unreported fever or unrelieved (transient) destitution existed in those areas. While casting doubt on the claim that fever reflected want, the results were equally incompatible with the claim that fever caused pauperization: were that so, one would find a high correlation between fever and paupers.[101]

By this time the malaria was no longer an hypothesis to explain puzzling effects but an axiom. One need not even provide bad smells or tangible rot; its presence could be seen in its effect; indeed, one no more asked for proof of its existence than one asked for proof of gravity.[102] Grant Smith this hypothetical morbid force, and he can explain everything. Since all *must* succumb to it, all symptoms can be explained by it. Science was superfluous; the malaria was as unfalsifiable as any political or religious dogma.

There are several implications of Smith's new perspective. First, it trivializes health by focusing on a single cause of deadly disease. The important fact is that all *must* succumb to the malaria; that some, who happen to be ill fed and ill clothed, succumb more quickly is a matter of accident. The causes of that

100  Ibid., 83–85.
101  Smith, "Report on the Prevalence of Fever." Although the results were not compiled until late April 1839 they were to refer to the year ending 25 March 1838, and therefore to the same period as the 1838 reports. Although all districts were asked to reply, there were only 20 respondents, representing a population of 850,000.
102  The image is Smith's: "Though we are unacquainted with the physical form or chemical properties of this body, this is no reason why we should not understand its force as a special agent in the production of disease, just as we know the forces of other physical bodies, though not their nature" (*Common Nature of Epidemics*, 24).

accident, such as economic conditions, do not really count as causes of disease, since the malaria must ultimately have its effect. Taken to an extreme, Smith's argument can be construed that since all die (as a result of a law of mortality as inexorable as a mysterious malaria), the circumstances of the event are relatively unimportant.

The converse of denying the medical importance of social differences is a model that unites society. The malarial disease, like death itself, is universal-izing. All of us in a particular locale belong to a brotherhood of breathers. Smith tells us how the poison will spread from Bethnal Green to "the most remote streets and the great squares" of London. And if it can spread this far, it can in theory spread anywhere (being unable to isolate it, we can hardly limit its range).[103] He has thrown down a challenge to the middle and upper classes, indeed, to everybody: "Sewer or die!"

But the cost of this universalizing is that we must grant Smith authority to define our disease. This was, of course, a period of great change in relations between doctors and sick people, and Smith is part of that. Constitutional medicine had been centered in the subjectivity of illness. It had inferred the multiple causes of illness by taking seriously the uniqueness of each case. In Smith's poison-centered view of disease, we lose that subjective authority. No longer is the ill person a self, cultivating a constitution with the advice of a helpful healer, but only a sort of barograph displaying contact with decom-posing matter. Those matters relating to the victim as a self, unique in social relations, work, and environment are so much noise masking the signal of bad air. Because the poison is hypothetical, Smith, the expert, can tell us when we are sick. He and Chadwick can also tell us what about us is sick. Once they know where we live, then any part of our behavior – our moral life, say, or our political participation – can be attributed to the poison. There is no room for complaint. Cold and hungry people will no longer be allowed to *say* they are made ill by cold and hunger. Cold and hunger return to their proper significations as incentives to get back to work. Far from being an expression of self, the locus of disease was now only incidentally in humans; it became a matter of "places, not persons," as Smith put it.[104] Disease lay in house design, street width, or sewer slope, and therefore in houses, streets, and sewers. Occasionally humans wander into these pathological force fields with the sorry result that they, or their surviving dependents, become social problems, needers of "care."

A most powerful political medicine, this.[105] But what Smith would do with it was not what Chadwick would do. The two saw different problems: Smith's

---

103 Smith, "Prevalence of Fever," 106.
104 Smith, *Common Nature of Epidemics*, 32.
105 Pelling, *Cholera*, 20–22; cf. Coles, "Sinners," 473–74. Smith's arguments were used by several medical witnesses to the 1834 Select Committee on Metropolis Sewers, *P.P.*, 1834, *15*, (584.), qq 874–78, 941–43, 954.

was theological; Chadwick's, policing. For Smith it was why humans, essentially good and responsible beings, did not act thus. The reason was *environment*: it prevented the expression of their goodness and responsibility. In explaining difference, environment had leveling implications; his faith in sanitation was part of his faith in Providence. In time the world would be perfected, made normal, through a "principle of kindness" exemplified in sanitation: "We . . . neglect body and mind, and then the disorders and vices which necessarily follow we endeavour to repress by punishments that harden but never reform."[106]

Even if he might agree in principle with Smith's "there but for a good sewer go I," Chadwick lacked Smith's charity. He had faith in progress, but not in the innate goodness of humans. Throughout his career he would focus on greed, sloth, lust, intemperance, hypocrisy, even if he did not talk of "sin" explicitly. The need was less to return the world to some hypothetical normality where the good folk would wash regularly, speak modestly, and act decently than to build a machine to instill those "habits." Hence Chadwick would go further than simply removing impediments to health and good citizenship; he would urge automatic systems of discipline.[107]

---

106  Smith, *Common Nature of Epidemics*, 59.
107  As would Kay; see Coles, "Sinners," 473, 486; Roberts, *Victorian Origins*, 179; Finer, *Chadwick*, 180. Smith, by contrast, was much more comfortable with moral force Chartism (Pelling, *Cholera*, 7).

# 4

# The Making of the *Sanitary Report,*
# 1839–1842

Legend has it that the reports of Smith, Arnott, and Kay on sanitary conditions in the East End of London were "the passing novelty of the time." They were quickly "so much in demand that as many as seven thousand were distributed amongst the people."[1] In fact, there was little interest initially because there was little new – just "the wonted inflation of matter-of-fact which characterize the lucubrations of the Poor-law organs," as one writer later characterized it.[2] Their great distribution occurred mainly because, in connection with the Sanitary Inquiry, Edwin Chadwick sent three copies to every poor law union.

The Sanitary Inquiry was only launched in August 1839, over a year after the reports, when the queen ordered the poor law commissioners to determine "the extent to which the causes of disease" identified in the Smith–Kay–Arnott inquiries "prevail also amongst the Labouring classes in other parts of England and Wales." The request came from the House of Lords, and in particular from Benjamin Blomfield, bishop of London, former Royal Poor Law commissioner, initiator of the call for a fast during the 1832 cholera.[3]

Why resurrect these brief and obscure reports that had lain dormant more than a year?[4] Not, as sometimes suggested, to make work for Chadwick:

1 B. W. Richardson, "Edwin Chadwick C.B., A Biographical Dissertation," *The Health of Nations: A Review of the Works of Edwin Chadwick, with a Biographical Dissertation,* 2 vols. (1887; reprint, London: Dawson, 1965), xiii; S. E. Finer, *The Life and Times of Sir Edwin Chadwick* (London: Methuen, 1952), 162; Maurice Marston, *Sir Edwin Chadwick (1800–1890)* (London: Leonard Parsons, 1925), 99–100: "As he anticipated, the effect was instantaneous. The report came before Parliament and greatly disturbed statesmen, politicians and influential public men."
2 "[Fever in London – Arnott, Kay, and Smith Reports]," *Lancet,* 1838, ii, 630–33; see also 691–94; "Report on the Sanitary Condition of the Labouring Poor," *The Spectator* 15 (1842): 760–61.
3 Lord John Russell to Poor Law Commissioners, 21 August 1839, *Report to Her Majesty's Principal Secretary of State for the Home Department on an Inquiry into the Sanitary Condition of the Labouring Population* (London: Clowes, 1842), iv (this front matter is not included in the modern edition of the *Sanitary Report* edited by Flinn). On Blomfield's involvement see Edward H. Gibson, "The Public Health Agitation in England, 1838–1848: A Newspaper and Parliamentary History" (Ph.D. diss., University of North Carolina, Chapel Hill, 1955), passim.
4 The request does closely follow the Poor Law Commission's Fifth Annual Report, which included Smith's compilation of the London medical officers' returns on pauper fever. Smith, however, was

having finished the first report of the Constabulary Commission in March, he was fighting to get its recommendations into law and beginning a second report – sanitation was an interruption.[5]

A Sanitary Inquiry seemed suddenly imperative for many reasons. Revolution, for one: the first Chartist petition had just been delivered and rejected; in November there would be an armed rising in South Wales. Then, too, the hated Poor Law Commission was in deep trouble, on the first of several one-year reprieves.[6] A great study might help justify its existence. Finally, there was William Farr, whose first letter analyzing causes of death in England and Wales had just appeared in the first report of the Registrar General. As we shall see, Chadwick saw Farr as a serious threat to the commission.

The form is odd too.[7] Despite the royal warrant, this was not a royal commission, only a command to the Poor Law Commission, which often undertook its own investigations without supplemental authorization and published them in its reports. It has been suggested that the royal warrant reflected Chadwick's attempt to bypass his uninterested superiors. Yet at the outset it was not clear that this would be his special project: LeFevre and Lewis recruited informants; as we will see, the full commission did take responsibility for the report.[8]

Requests for information went out in early November 1839. One set went to the nine assistant poor law commissioners, another to clerks of boards of guardians, who were to transmit a third to union medical officers. The latter were to supply "returns of . . . contagious or infectious disease, the spread of which . . . has been promoted by the circumstances referred to . . . [with] observations thereon." In Chadwick's summary, these "circumstances" shifted further from person to structure and geography: medical officers were to note the commission's focus on "the *visible and removable* agencies promoting the prevalence of such diseases as are commonly found connected with the defects in the situation and structure or internal economy of the residences of the labouring classes."[9] Assistant commissioners were also to solicit a report from

merely supplementing his earlier report; the returns were over a year old (for the year ending 31 March 1838).

5 Stanley H. Palmer, *Police and Protest in England and Ireland* (Cambridge: Cambridge University Press, 1988), 427; Anthony Brundage, *England's "Prussian Minister": Edwin Chadwick and the Politics of Government Growth, 1832–1854* (University Park: Pennsylvania State University Press, 1988), 57–77.

6 Thomas Mackay, *A History of the English Poor Law*, vol. III, *From 1834 to the Present Time* (New York: Putnam, 1900), 265.

7 Its legality would be questioned ("Vaccination Extension Bill," *Lancet*, 1840, ii, 579).

8 This was a natural way of proceeding, since assistant commissioners recruited local medical men and each assistant commissioner was paired with one commissioner. See the *Poor Law Commission [PLC]-Twistleton Correspondence*, November 1839–November 1840, Public Record Office [PRO] MH 32/72. The third commissioner, Nicholls, was on assignment in Ireland. More likely the seeking of a royal instruction reflects a recognition of the need for cooperation of people far outside the commission, such as prominent urban medical practitioners.

9 Chadwick to Medical Officers, 12 November 1839, *Report to Her Majesty's Principal Secretary of State*, xiv. How many medical officers responded is not clear. Chadwick boasted of sixteen hundred

an "eminent" medical man in each large town who would be familiar with dispensary or infirmary practice. The idea here was to find prominent practitioners who, like Kay, Smith, and Arnott, could digest the raw returns of poor law medical officers.

Although the Arnott–Kay–Smith reports were central, other matters appeared inexplicably on the agenda: rents, household income, building costs, and model cottage projects. Chadwick wanted to know whether cottage occupants paid rates; waiving rates invited deterioration of cottages, he believed.[10] This might seem to lie outside the charge, he admitted, but drafty and leaky cottages led to disease and harmed morals. Rural housing had long been an important poor law issue, and some informants focused mainly on it (a few did not even address effluvia–fever issues). Cottages, morals, and rate-paying would, however, become part of the sanitarian agenda. All this was to be done in a few months, yet the *Sanitary Report* appeared only in early August 1842, followed a few weeks later by two volumes of local reports by the assistant commissioners and by "eminent" medical men. Periodically in those three years Chadwick chastened tardy informants, yet he himself was still opening new lines of inquiry as late as April 1842.[11]

In those three years this "fever inquiry" would evolve from a topic of sociomedical exploration into a paradigm of social analysis, with its own vocabulary, assumptions, and forms of argument. The long gestation reflected neither the tardiness of contributors nor Chadwick's "care and thoroughness" so much as the adaptation of the project to changing circumstances.[12] Here we examine five sources of change: "medical criticism of sanitarian principles," "Scotland," "starvation," "Slaney and sewers," and "Graham and revolution."

I

The main reason for lack of interest in the London fever reports was that they appeared to say nothing new. The political moral Chadwick would draw, that the most important causes of fever were *incidental* rather than *essential* to poverty, was nowhere stated. On the other hand the value to health of drainage,

returns, which seems a very high rate (Edwin Chadwick, "Mr. Chadwick's *Sanitary Report,*" *The Spectator* 15 [1842]: 1001); few of these survive. See A. Power to Chadwick, 1 February 1840, *PLC–Power Correspondence,* PRO MH 32/64.

10 Despite their faith in market forces, there was some feeling among PLC staff that cottage rents were unconscionable (Mott to Chadwick, 20 November 1839, University College London [UCL] Chadwick Papers #1449).

11 Sir John Walsham to PLC, 2 March, 8 April 1840, *PLC–Walsham Correspondence,* PRO MH 32/79; PLC to Assistant Commissioners," *PLC Appendices to Minutes,* 23 November 1840, PRO MH 3/2; Charles Mott to Chadwick, 4 February 1841, UCL Chadwick Papers #1449.

12 Gibson, "The Public Health Agitation," 114.

water, ventilation, effective "police" of the streets, and less crowded housing was well accepted.[13]

Georgian medical men knew well that large towns were mortality sinks. Whether acting as a miasm, transmitting contagion, or in some other way, town air seemed an obvious cause. It was a fearsome solvent of smells, wrote John Roberton, the Manchester obstetrician, in 1827: "The offensive vapours of a thousand manufactures, odours arising from the preparation of food, from animal bodies in health and disease, from offal, and from common sewers – are dissolved or suspended in the air. Added to this is the want of ventilation, or agitation of the atmosphere . . . it is probable that these effluvia, when not dispersed, undergo fresh [changes] that render them more injurious to living animals." In crowded and unventilated cellars and "houses in deep narrow lanes," air became "so charged with effluvia, as to be unfit for the maintenance of health."[14] In 1818 interior air in Edinburgh slums was held to be "literally incapable of serving the purposes of healthy respiration to so many individuals as exist upon it, besides being contaminated by the accumulation of all their effluvia, and abundance of other filth."[15]

This "other filth," the emanations of decomposition, would become for the Chadwickians chief of the sins to which air was heir, "the all pervading cause." The idea that decomposition was pathological was at least as old as the Ebers Papyrus and similarly well accepted among British medical men. John Haygarth of Chester, writing in 1801, called for street cleaning on the grounds that street "*dirt . . . is always in a putrid or putrescent state.*"[16] Ferriar of Manchester wrote that "fever prevailed most, in streets which were not drained, or in which dunghills were suffered to accumulate, or where the blood and garbage from slaughter-houses were allowed to stagnate." Whether or not such "nuisances" caused disease, they "assist its progress, and . . . operate as remote causes of fever, in whatever manner pathologists may choose to explain their action."[17]

Still, these writers did not see a "sanitary crisis," but instead an ongoing process of improvement – much had been done; there was much yet to do.[18]

---

13 "It would be possible to quote pages of extracts from eighteenth century doctors preaching the efficacy of soap and water and fresh air" (M. C. Buer, *Health, Wealth, and Population in the Early Days of the Industrial Revolution* [London: Routledge, 1926], 138).

14 John Roberton, *Observations on the Mortality and Physical Management of Children* (London: Longman, Rees, Orme, Brown, 1827), 207–8.

15 "Epidemic Fever," *Edinburgh Medical and Surgical Journal* 14 (1818): 540.

16 John Haygarth, *A Letter to Dr. Percival on the Prevention of Infectious Fevers and an Address to the College of Physicians in Philadelphia on the Prevention of the American Pestilence* (Bath: R. Cruttwell, 1801), 114.

17 John Ferriar, "Of the Prevention of Fevers in Great Towns," *Medical Histories and Reflections*, 1st American ed., 4 vols. in 1 (Philadelphia: Dobson, 1816), II, 226.

18 William Heberden, *Observations on the Increase and Decrease of Different Diseases* (London: T. Payne, 1801), 96. See also William Moss, *A Familiar Medical Survey of Liverpool* (Liverpool: Hodgson, 1784), 18–19.

Admitting the danger of rot, they yet remained skeptical of the existence of an all-powerful putrefactive poison à la Southwood Smith. Ferriar criticized the ancient belief (which Chadwick would resurrect) "that pestilential disorders are occasioned by the effluvia of dead bodies." Fever did not "rage more severely in houses surrounding church-yards . . . though the stench of the putrid bodies, over-heaped in such receptacles, is often insufferably offensive."[19] Misery remained more important than those physical causes of disease that Chadwick would make the domain of "sanitary condition" because it was the more fundamental cause. William Moss of Liverpool explained that "manner of living" superseded other causes since station in life determined the geographic (and economic) causes to which one was exposed. One could, perhaps, never eliminate misery, but one could mitigate it: London's improved health reflected an "absence of dearth for several years," noted Thomas Bateman in 1819. Yet "dirt, closeness, and starvation" remained "as fully adequate as ever to produce and nurture the contagion of fever."[20]

Given these views it is no surprise that fever writers often anticipated Chadwick's program of sanitary improvement. Writing in 1818, the Glaswegian Robert Graham called on the police to remove dung heaps, pave surfaces, renew "closes" so they ran downhill, improve street cleanliness. From Belfast Henry MacCormac urged construction of "roomy and capacious sewers" – and also housing regulations, daily scavenging, ventilation, and provision of the necessaries of life. When fever hit Hull in 1803, the "street was paved anew, the drains, which were defective, repaired, and a proper descent given to carry off the foul water." Thomas Bernard of the Society for Bettering the Condition and Increasing the Comforts of the Poor observed that "too much attention cannot be paid in large populous towns to prevent the air from being contaminated by noxious effluvia exhaling from corrupt and putrid substances, arising from the neglect of the cleansing of the streets, lanes, and sewers sufficiently and frequently, and of suffering soil carts to stand in the streets at improper hours, and heaps of manure to remain in a town."[21]

Henry Clutterbuck of the General Dispensary described London's sanitary failings and needs at length in 1825: "Houses . . . in long and narrow alleys,

---

19 Ferriar, "Origin of Contagious and New Diseases," *Medical Histories and Reflections*, I, 121–22; MacCormac was making exactly the same arguments in the late 1830s (Henry MacCormac, *An Exposition of the Nature, Treatment, and Prevention of Continued Fever* [London: Longman, Rees, Orme, Brown, Green, and Longman, 1835], 50).

20 Moss, *Medical Survey of Liverpool*, 18–19; Thomas Bateman, *Reports on the Diseases of London and the State of the Weather from 1804 to 1816 Including Practical Remarks on the Causes and Treatment of the Former; and Preceded by a Historical View of the State of Health and Disease in the Metropolis in Times Past* (London: Longmans, Hurst, 1819), 257–58.

21 Robert Graham, *Practical Observations on Continued Fever, Especially That Form at Present Existing as an Epidemic with Some Remarks on the Most Efficient Plans for Its Suppression* (Glasgow: J. Smith and Son, 1818), 63–65; MacCormac, *Fever*, 193–94; Bernard, in comments on Miss Horner, "Extract From an Account of a Contagious Fever at Kingston-on-Hull," *Report of the Society for Bettering the Condition and Increasing the Comforts of the Poor 4* (1805): 98.

with lofty buildings on each side; or in a small and confined court. . . . These places are at the same time the receptacles of all kinds of filth, which is only removed . . . at distant and uncertain intervals; and always so imperfectly, as to leave the place highly offensive and disgusting." He outlined a program for inspection (by the "Parish apothecary") of schools, lodging houses, and "houses in the most crowded courts and alleys." He also called for disinfection, control of smoke emissions, large-scale rebuilding in areas where the poor lived, with wider streets, plentiful water to clean the "kennels" daily, better scavenging (and not just on main streets), and privies that emptied into public sewers. He objected that the current "spirit of improvement" had its focus "in the best parts of the town." Surely it was "as much within the power, as it is unquestionably the duty of the legislature, aided by the minor authorities, to correct . . . the evils here complained of."[22] J. B. Davis agreed: "The frequent interposition of the legislature and the local authorities can alone carry on those systems of drainage, cleansing, making embankments."[23]

More strident was the Glasgow physician William Davidson, the principal fever authority Chadwick would quote in the *Sanitary Report*: typhus would "assail us so long as our cities contain so many narrow and filthy lanes, so long as the houses . . . are little better than dens or hovels, so long as dunghills and other nuisances are allowed to accumulate . . . so long as these hovels are crowded with inmates, and so long as there is so much poverty and destitution." We should demand, he thundered, legislation to "level these hovels to the ground . . . regulate the width of every street . . . the ventilation of every dwelling-house, that would prevent the lodging-houses of the poor from being crowded with human beings, and . . . provide for their destitution." To the cry that this would "interfere" with "liberty" he replied that "it might rather be designated an attempt to prevent the improper liberties of the subject; for what right . . . has any man to form streets, construct houses, and crowd them with human beings, so as to deteriorate health and shorten life because he finds it profitable to do so?" Even Charles Wing, writing on behalf of the ten hours' movement, urged that "sewers . . . be regularly made, and the streets formed into passable roads, instead of being left in an impassable state of mud and dirt."[24]

As Davidson's arguments indicate, to draw attention *to* "physical causes" was not necessarily to draw it *away* from destitution. Accordingly, the reports Kay, Arnott, and Smith offered in no way seemed schismatic, not, that is,

22  Henry Clutterbuck, *Observations on the Prevention and Treatment of the Epidemic Fever at Present Prevailing in the Metropolis and Most Parts of the United Kingdom* (London: Longman, Hurst, Rees, Orme, and Brown, 1819), 44–63.

23  J. B. Davis, *A Popular Manual of the Art of Preserving Health* (London: Whittaker, 1836), 29.

24  William Davidson, "Essay on the Sources and Mode of Propagation of the Continued Fevers of Great Britain and Ireland," in William Davidson and A. Hudson, *Essays on the Sources and Mode of Action of Fever* (Philadelphia: A. Waldie, 1841), 65–66; Charles Wing, *Evils of the Factory System Demonstrated by Parliamentary Evidence* (London: Saunders and Otley, 1837), cvi.

until spring 1840, when it began to become clear how Chadwick would use them.

The first critic of note was William Pulteney Alison, whom we met in chapter 2. Alison's *Observations on the Management of the Poor in Scotland, and Its Effects on the Health of Great Towns* appeared in January 1840, marking his entry into the Scottish poor law controversy. The thrust of Alison's critique was the effect of that policy on health; not surprisingly he took up the recent studies of the English Poor Law Commission. He was a gentle critic – Kay, after all, had been a prize pupil. But the London reports claimed too much for the pathogenicity of filth and neglected destitution as a cause of fever. Putrid matter might well be a predisposing cause of fever, but a correlation of fever with bad drainage (even that was questionable) did not mean putrid matter was "the immediate source" of fever: "Districts without sewers will, naturally, be not only the dirtiest, but the cheapest; they will be inhabited by the poorest and most destitute people, who will be huddled together in the greatest numbers in proportion to the space they occupy." Alison concluded: were "public authorities . . . [to] think it sufficient, in any situation where contagious fever is prevalent, to remove all *dead* animal and vegetable matter, without attempting to improve the condition of the *living* inhabitants, I am confident that their labour will be in vain." He clearly saw the ideological implication of the London conclusions: the view that filth was "adequate to the production of contagious fever" implied that fever could no longer be taken as a "test of previous destitution and suffering."

Alison maintained this civility in his Glasgow address to the British Association for the Advancement of Science in September 1840. There was plenty of evidence of the relative harmlessness to healthy and well-fed people of the gases of decomposition and of the association of fever with hunger. Asked "in very distinct terms" by the PLC whether "destitution without the filth, or . . . filth without the destitution . . . [was] more effectual in the production or extension of fever," he had replied cautiously. In Scotland, there was "no destitution without filth" but there was "filth without destitution . . . families living in close ill-aired rooms, of dirty habits, but regularly employed." During epidemics they seemed less prone to fever. He remembered the epidemic of 1818, attributed by many to dung hills on the outskirts of Edinburgh. Yet even with the dung hills gone, better scavenging, and new drains, fever remained. He accused Smith of the elementary error of confusing remittent fever, which almost everyone attributed to a malaria, with continued fever. By no means was he opposed to sanitary improvement – quite the contrary. He urged building regulations and a ban on dung hills near inhabited buildings. Yet in Edinburgh filth was neither "the most important, nor the most remediable, of . . . [fever's] auxiliary causes."[25]

25 W. P. Alison, *Observations on the Management of the Poor in Scotland, and Its Effects on the Health of*

By the end of 1840 the theme of "honest oversight" was giving way to one of "naive, sloppy, and indefensible oversimplification" in the medical press and cynical diversion in the general press.[26] Most important is an anonymous review of Alison's *Observations*, the London reports, and the great studies of Paris by Alphonse Parent-Duchâtelet, in the January 1841 number of John Forbes's *British and Foreign Medico-Chirurgical Review*.[27] The author was in fact William Tait, an Edinburgh surgeon and Alison associate.

Tait began by accusing Kay and Arnott of unsupported generalizations: "And this suffices to *prove* the influence of marsh-land!" he sneered, quoting one of Kay's extracts. That "such meager details . . . should have appeared to . . . justify the strong opinion which [Kay and Arnott] . . . express on the origin of contagious fever" was a matter of "extreme surprise": a "philosophical enquirer" would see these data as showing only that both fever and malaria were "common attendants on poverty"[28] Tait was even harder on Smith, whom he accused of confusing typhus with asphyxiation and intermittent with continued fevers, and of waffling on whether continued fever was contagious. Quoting a particularly florid passage, he wondered aloud, "It is astonishing to us who know Dr. Southwood Smith's great powers of mind and his acute and logical spirit, that he could have allowed such a passage . . . to drop from his pen." His explanation: "The enthusiasm of philanthropy and a vivid imagination . . . [had] secretly jumped to desired conclusions, while the cool and calculating eye of philosophy was closed in slumber." Speculations like Smith's took us "a century back in etiology."[29]

If Tait was harsher than Alison, he too would not represent the exclusion of destitution as anything other than bad science – he alluded simply to "a tendency" in the London reports "to regard too exclusively the local nuisances in the neighbourhood of the poor, to the neglect of their condition in respect to food, clothing, and employment." The corrective was Alison, who was only making the point, "neither new nor uncommon," that destitution was among the most important factors affecting the course of a fever outbreak.[30]

---

*Great Towns,* 2d ed. (Edinburgh: Blackwood, 1840), 10–11; idem, "Illustrations of the Practical Operation of the Scottish System of Management of the Poor," *Journal of the Statistical Society of London 3* (1840): 234–39.

26 By the end of 1841 Alison was less generous, insisting that the destitution–fever relation had "not been disputed by any medical authority" (whether Smith et al. were not conceived of as disputants or as authorities is not clear). He railed against naive statisticians who compiled great masses of figures and inferred much about "epidemic fever," an entity the best medical science was showing to be a melange of several diseases (Alison, "Further Illustrations of the Practical Operation of the Scotch System of Management of the Poor," *Journal of the Statistical Society of London 4* [1841]: 288, 305).

27 [William Tait], "Dr Alison, etc. on the Causes of Typhus Fever " *British and Foreign Medical Review* 11 (1841): 1–36.

28 Ibid., 5–9.

29 Ibid., 10–13.

30 "Allusions are occasionally made to these circumstances, but in a way, generally, which conveys the impression that they have attracted but little notice, and that a merely secondary importance,

A postscript to the review by the editor John Forbes makes clear how very sensitive the issue was. A blistering review like Tait's of a proposal to benefit the public might indeed be "culpable" if it were to "damp the zeal of those who are labouring to improve our towns, by giving the impression that by making sewers, removing filth, opening thoroughfares through densely-populated neighbourhoods, and inducing habits of cleanliness, they were not thereby removing the causes of diseases," Forbes wrote. But that was not the case: both the sanitarianism of Smith and Kay and the contagionism of Tait tended toward the same end of involving the medical profession in prevention. "The one says, that by cleanliness and ventilation you remove at once the cause of the disease: the other, that you remove the causes which propagate the disease when once it is in existence; for that whatever tends to concentrate the poison, or to weaken in any degree the vital powers, renders the victims more numerous." In balance, Forbes found the view of Tait (and Alison) "more persuasive to an extended benevolence." Those who linked fever to a malaria would "pursue but one object: the cleansing of the poisonous atmosphere of filthy, crowded rooms and streets: the contagionist would go farther and say that this is not enough, for unless you relieve that debilitated state of body and mind which arises from meager poverty, you leave unremedied one of the most powerful causes of the malady."[31]

Similar views appear in a spate of works on fever written in the years during which Chadwick's sanitary initiative was taking shape, many of them prompted by the Provincial Medical and Surgical Association's competition for the best essay on the nature and causes of continued fever. Several authors had substantial experience of fever among the poor. William Davidson was senior physician at the Glasgow Royal Infirmary; Alfred Hudson and Henry MacCormac were Irish dispensary doctors, in Navan and Belfast, respectively. Robert Cowan was Regius professor of medical police and forensic medicine at Glasgow. William Budd, later well known as a pioneer epidemiologist in recognizing the transmission of typhoid, was less experienced as an independent practitioner but had studied extensively in Paris and in Edinburgh with Alison.[32]

On the issues Tait raised, they spoke with remarkable unanimity. Several

---

is at the most, to be ascribed to them in contributing to the prevalence of fever" (ibid., 22–23). Tait included in this assessment the witnesses to R. A. Slaney's Health of Towns Select Committee, which had taken evidence in the spring of 1840.

31 Ibid., 36.

32 Cowan and Davidson are especially important here. In the *Sanitary Report*, Chadwick ingeniously enlists them as the major independent authorities for his case. On Cowan see Thomas Ferguson, *The Dawn of Scottish Social Welfare: A Survey from Medieval Times to 1863* (Edinburgh: Thomas Nelson, 1948), 97. The Thackeray Prize of the Provincial Medical and Surgical Association was to be given for the best essay on "the sources of the common Continued Fevers of Great Britain and Ireland" (Dale Smith, "Introduction," in William Budd, *On the Causes of Fevers*, ed. Dale Smith [Baltimore: Johns Hopkins University Press, 1984], 3–4).

cited Parent-Duchâtelet on the healthiness of Paris sewermen or gravediggers or the knackers of Montfacon.[33] Several cited Alison.[34] They avoided confusing the effects of asphyxiation with those of fever.[35] While accepting that the state of the air affected the generation and course of fever, several saw miasmatic explanations of the sort Smith offered as bordering on tautology. If filth caused fever, fever must exist in direct proportion to filth, for such was what one meant by cause and effect. Moreover, depending on what one assumed the filth poison was like, either there ought to be as many fevers as there were kinds of filth or only one kind of disease: single cause did not explain diverse effects.[36] Correlation did not imply cause; usually a correlation of fever with filth was also a correlation of fever with misery.[37] And each acknowledged destitution as a leading cause of fever:

"The influence of want of the necessaries of life . . . is perhaps more certainly assured by the fact, that most of the great epidemics of fever . . . have occurred in times of scarcity or other public calamity."

"Want, misery, and dirt, and undue exposure to atmospheric vicissitudes, are the powerful promoting causes of fever, and are much more influential in leading to it, than mere malaria or contagion; the latter indeed, under ordinary circumstances, is so insignificant a cause, as to be unworthy of much consideration."

"The connection of scarcity and privation with the occurrence of fever among the lower classes of the community, has been so often verified by the experience of epidemics, as now to be received as a general axiom."

"The most influential of all [causes of the 'diffusion' of epidemic disease] is poverty and destitution. In every one of the epidemic fevers which have ravaged Glasgow, its progress has been slow, unless extreme destitution has existed."[38]

Several recognized that the cyclicity of the industrial economy did cause unemployment, which led to want, and thus to fever.[39] Most saw the means to combat fever as a combination of sanitary improvement (especially ventilation) and provision of the necessaries in times of need. For Cowan, "food,

33  William Budd, "On the Causes and Mode of Propagation of the Common Continued Fevers of Great Britain and Ireland," in Budd, *On the Causes of Fever*, 70–80; Davidson, *Essay*, 85.
34  Alfred Hudson, "An Inquiry into the Sources and Mode of Action of the Poison of Fever," in William Davidson and Alfred Hudson, *Essays on the Sources and Mode of Action of Fever* (Philadelphia: A. Waldie, 1841), 109–10; Budd, *Causes*, 80, 101–3. Another common source was Alexander Tweedie, *Clinical Illustrations of Fever, Comprising a Report of Cases Treated at the London Fever Hospital, 1828–29* (London: Whitaker and Treacher, 1830). Tweedie, extremely skeptical of the malaria theory, was Southwood Smith's senior colleague at the London Fever Hospital.
35  Budd, *On the Causes of Fevers*, 80; Hudson, *Inquiry*, 142–43; Davidson, *Essay*, 44–47.
36  MacCormac, *Fever*, 50: "More room for speculation than reasoning"; Hudson, *Inquiry*, 139, 142–43; Davidson, *Essay*, 13, 17, 49–53.
37  Hudson, *Inquiry*, 143.
38  Selections are, respectively, from Budd, *Causes*, 103 (see also 117, 121); MacCormac, *Fever*, xvii; Tweedie, *Clinical Illustrations*, 78; Robert Cowan, "Vital Statistics of Glasgow, Illustrating the Sanatory Condition of the Population," *Journal of the Statistical Society of London* 3 (1840): 288–90.
39  Budd, *On the Causes of Fevers*, 117.

fuel, and clothing are the best preventives of fever"; for Hudson, "the true prophylactics" were "providing clothing and fuel, caus[ing] the light and air to be admitted into their crowded dwellings, and . . . relieving mind and body from the pressure of impending starvation, [which] will both render them less susceptible *of* disease *if* it approach them, and less capable of generating in themselves the poison."[40]

The view of sanitation as a cynical stratagem came not from within medicine, however, but from the *Times*, a dedicated opponent of the new poor law. In a November 1840 leader on a PLC circular inviting metropolitan guardians to use the new police act to cleanse insanitary premises, the *Times* accused the PLC of using sanitary activism to secure its survival. Certainly no one could object to an initiative "calculated to avert or diminish disease," but in this initiative, the PLC had laid open its "biases": it was "the completest demonstration of the iniquity of their system that we have recently chanced to meet with." Hunger was the great cause of disease, the paper claimed (on the authority of William Farr, "a far more disinterested" judge than the "medical hirelings" of the PLC). "Yet the commissioners, carefully concealing the fact that the increase of disease among the poor is mainly attributable to *starvation* (a damning test of their workhouse comforts, seeing that the emaciated pauper will rather pine in his own damp cellar than submit to their infliction) are bold enough to assert . . . that the prevalence of disease among the lower orders in close and crowded neighborhoods is to be ascribed entirely to the want of cleanliness and ventilation."

The PLC was "insulting the country by taking legal measures to *enforce cleanliness* for the protection of health, while they pertinaciously refuse to prevent the diseases and deaths *generated by their own miserable administration* in starving their workhouse victims, and in refusing outdoor relief." And of course it would bring up the problem in winter, when the well sealed shelter was the only antidote to cold for those who could not afford fuel or blankets. The last indignity was that occupiers were to pay for the cleansing: the law allowed "seizure of goods and chattels" in the event of nonpayment. The point was echoed in the *Provincial Medical and Surgical Journal*: Admitting "that want of cleanliness and of sufficient ventilation are active agents in the generation of disease," yet it was a "refinement in cruelty" to penalize "unfortunate sufferers" because of the "wretchedness in which they are reduced to live, by the operation of causes lying far deeper than it suits the commission to look into."[41]

40 Cowan, "Vital Statistics," 289; Hudson, *Inquiry*, 110; MacCormac, *Fever*, 192.
41 "[Poor Law Commission and Public Health]," *Times*, 25 November 1840, 4b–c; *Provincial Medical and Surgical Journal* 1 (1840): 199; cf. "Sanatory Measures," *Official Circulars of Public Documents and Information Directed by the Poor Law Commissioners to Be Printed, Chiefly for the Use of Boards of*

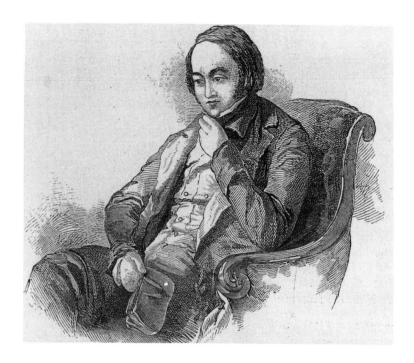

Edwin Chadwick at about age forty (with permission of the *Illustrated London News* Picture Library).

II

It would be wrong to think that Chadwick was the only one making fever theory do political work. Alison was too; fever theory was even more central in his campaign for a Scottish poor law. Alison and Chadwick had similar views of what a poor law should be, but opposite political problems. Faced with out-of-control costs in England, Chadwick was trying to justify a less generous relief policy; in Scotland, where there was effectively no right to relief, Alison was seeking to make the case for a more generous policy. In the Sanitary Inquiry each would exploit the other's authority. Alison would represent Chadwick and the PLC as independent poor law experts – who just happened to share his views. Chadwick had the rare experience of praise and support from an independent authority. Still, dealing with the Scots was complicated. The *Sanitary Report* would have little on Scotland: There was no lack

*Guardians and Their Officers* (1851; reprint, New York: Augustus M. Kelley, 1970), 10 November 1840.

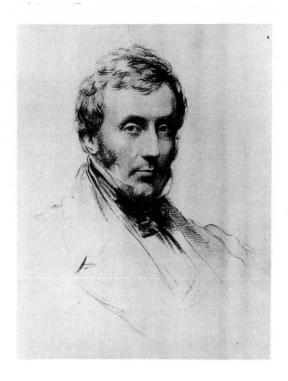

William Pulteney Alison (courtesy National Library of Medicine).

of Scottish evidence, but the Scots were so perversely insistent on making the Sanitary Inquiry serve their own agenda.

The queen's instruction of August 1839 had limited the Sanitary Inquiry to England and Wales. The possibility of expansion to Scotland arose initially in connection with the Edinburgh "fetid irrigation" scandal. In March 1839 Sir William Drysdale, a member of the Edinburgh Town Council, had called attention to the harmful consequences of diverting the streams that carried the town's street washings onto surrounding fields. While the practice was lucrative to suburban landowners, it was a nuisance for townsfolk, Drysdale argued, and surely a cause of fever. Drysdale had no trouble inflaming local passions, but Scots law held out no consummation. Individuals, not public bodies, suffered nuisances: a costly suit by an individual might fail (as one had three decades earlier). The only hope was for a general law giving towns power to control their surroundings in the name of the public good – just the sorts of powers the Sanitary Inquiry might lead to. Accordingly, in December 1839 Drysdale persuaded the Edinburgh town council to ask that the Sanitary Inquiry include Scotland: the Poor Law commissioners would come north, appreciate that the irrigated meadows were an intolerable nuisance, and go back to London and get a law passed banning them. Chadwick's wife, Rachel (Kennedy), was a friend of the Drysdales, and Chadwick did visit Edinburgh at the end of the month.[42]

About this time Alison became involved. Given his interest in fever, academic stature, vast knowledge of the health of Edinburgh's poor, and enormous popularity, both sides in the irrigation controversy had sought to enlist him. Alison would not be drawn. The irrigation was unpleasant but did not contribute significantly to fever: misery in the town was more serious than tainted air from distant fields.[43]

But Drysdale's campaign did coincide with Alison's decision to attack the Scottish poor law, in which relief mainly took the form of voluntary contributions administered by the local parish.[44] The approach might work well enough in stable, vibrant, and prosperous parishes, but not where there were many transients, or where parishes were weak and religious disciplines unrecognized – quite simply it was no adequate response to the industrial revolution. Like English towns, Scottish towns were awash with displaced people during the first half of the nineteenth century: crofters evicted by "rationalizing" landlords, kelpers and bleachers displaced by the new alkali industry, and lots of people from Ireland. Finding neither work nor relief in rural parishes they went to the towns.[45] Sooner or later many became dependent on medical charity. In substance, then, the Scottish system of poor relief was

42 C. Hamlin, "Environmental Sensibility in Edinburgh: The 'Fetid Irrigation' Controversy," *Journal of Urban History* 20 (1994): 311–39; Drysdale to Chadwick, 9 December 1839; PLC to Drysdale, 18 December 1839, *Scottish–PLC Correspondence,* PRO MH 19/196; Drysdale to Chadwick, 6 January 1840, UCL Chadwick Papers #655.

43 "Anxious as I am, for the credit, and even for the health in other respects of the inhabitants, to see such a nuisance removed, I must nevertheless express my conviction, that any money expended for that object will be found wholly ineffectual in diminishing the liability of the inhabitants to contagious fever." "Any one who has observed the vitiated state of the air of the closes, of the passages and stairs, and more especially of the rooms in those parts of the Old town . . . however strongly impressed he may be with the efficacy of foul air as a cause of the extension of fever, can hardly . . . think of resorting to the foul air of the marshes, more than a mile off, for an explanation of the extension of the disease by this means" (Alison, "Illustrations," 235–36).

44 R. A. Cage, *The Scottish Poor Law, 1745–1845* (Edinburgh: Scottish Academic Press, 1981), 84–85, 112–35; Audrey Peterson, "The Poor Law in Nineteenth Century Scotland," *The New Poor Law in the Nineteenth Century,* ed. Derek Fraser, 171–93 (London: Macmillan, 1976).

45 Prior to 1834 there had been much enthusiasm for the Scottish approach among the abolitionist school of English poor law reformers. See Stewart J. Brown, *Thomas Chalmers and the Godly Commonwealth in Scotland* (Oxford: Oxford University Press, 1982), 156; cf. David Monypenny, "Scottish Poor Laws," *Edinburgh Review* 59 (1834): 425–38; "Poor Laws of Scotland – Statement of Dr. Chalmers' Experience," *Edinburgh Review* 41 (1824): 228–58; "The Scottish System of Poor Laws," *Dublin University Quarterly* 3 (1834): 508–22, with [J. H. Burton], "Poor Laws and Pauperism in Scotland," *Westminster Review* 36 (1841): 178–90; "Poor Laws for Scotland," *Quarterly Review* 75 (1844): 125–48. On social conditions see Ian Leavitt and Christopher Smout, *The State of the Scottish Working-Class in 1843: A Statistical and Spatial Inquiry Based on the Data from the Poor Law Commission Report of 1844* (Edinburgh: Scottish Academic Press, 1979).

to dump debilitated bodies in the laps of medical men who often felt they could not say no. Its effect was to generate contagious fever among cold, starving people, who then transmitted it to the population in general.[46]

Alison proposed that parishes be required to raise a rate to fund relief to be provided in workhouses staffed by professionals. The proposal was deeply divisive: Alison would deprive the kirk of one of its chief communal functions; surely, unfeeling English Benthamites could have no sense of the spiritual dynamism of voluntary charity within a closely knit community. Rural land-owners balked at a new rate; urbanites delighted that towns would no longer be the sink for refugees. In the spring of 1840 rival organizations quickly crystallized. The issue of conflict was not Alison's still rough plans, but the prospect of an "official" investigation. Assuming the Scottish poor law did need some reform, should it be investigated by a local body steeped in Scottish values or, as the Alisonians would have it, by a panel of disinterested outside experts – say, the English Poor Law Commission?[47]

It was here that Chadwick's sanitary investigation became useful. On learn-ing that Edinburgh would request extension of the inquiry to Scotland, Alison asked that the petition not be limited to sewage irrigation. By early February he had coordinated a flood of petitions from other towns.[48] Chadwick was receptive but made it clear that his inquiry was limited to sanitary conditions. But perhaps, if it could be shown that pauperism was "intimately connected" to "the sanatory condition of the large towns," the Sanitary Inquiry might blossom into a general poor law inquiry, suggested P. D. Handyside, secretary of Alison's Association for Obtaining Official Inquiry into the Pauperism of Scotland, and Chadwick cautiously agreed. Ironically then, while Wakley and the *Times* were railing at the PLC's intrusion into medical matters, Alison, who shared their views on the social causes of fever, was welcoming the

---

46 Within a few years this would become a nucleus for the organization of Scottish practitioners. See "Association of Medical Practitioners in Scotland," *Home Office-Association of Medical Practitioners in Scotland Correspondence*, 1846, PRO HO 45/1663.

47 E.g., the resolution of the General Assembly of 31 May 1841: The church "would look with great apprehension and alarm to an Inquiry conducted by a Commission of a different character [than the church] and especially if composed chiefly or in great measure of parties not inhabitants of Scotland and unaccustomed to the habits and mode of living in this country." Quoted in "Me-morial of the Association in Second Report of the Committee of the Association for Obtaining an Official Inquiry into the Pauperism of Scotland," *Scottish Distress, 1840–41*, PRO HO 45/160. See the leader and "Poor Laws of Scotland," *Edinburgh Evening Courant*, 23 April 1840; "Man-agement of the Poor," *Scotsman*, 25 March 1840; "Pauperism," *Scotsman*, 2 May 1840; "Charity Workhouse," *Scotsman* 18 July 1840; "Town Council Proceedings," *Scotsman* 21 July, 5 August, 14 October 1840.

48 Drysdale to Chadwick, 13 January 1840, UCL Chadwick Papers #655. Edinburgh's petition (7 January 1840) referred explicitly to the irrigation; those from other towns simply argued that Scotland too "requires examination." Petitions, which also came from the Royal Colleges of Physicians and Surgeons in Edinburgh, were still arriving in late March, even though the extension had been granted on 24 January. *Home Office–PLC Correspondence*, May 1840, PRO HO 73/56; W. Fox-Maule to PLC, 28 January 1840, *PLC–Home Office Correspondence*, PRO MH 19/63; *Royal College of Physicians of Edinburgh, Minutes*, 4 February, 1840.

> 7.—Is the extension of the diseases described in question 1, ascribable in any or what proportion to want of any of the necessaries of life; or to other causes than those specified in questions 4, 5, and 6 if so, distinguish those other causes so far as you are able, and the extent of diseases resulting from them?
>
> *[handwritten annotation: although poverty predisposes yet the Irish wakes are the greatest source of extension as the wants of the poor are well attended to in this parish in all known cases.]*

The revised question 7 in a completed copy of Chadwick's Scottish survey. In June 1840 Alison's poor law reformers succeeded in having the forms revised to refer specifically to "necessaries of life," but it was the original innocuous version referring only to "other causes" that appeared in the front matter of the *Sanitary Report* (reprinted with permission of University College London, Chadwick Papers #45).

Sanitary Inquiry *precisely because* it was in the hands of these English experts possessed of great experience and "absolute neutrality."[49]

It was May before Chadwick could launch a Scottish inquiry. As there were no poor law unions, the first problem was simply to locate informants, ideally medical practitioners familiar with the condition of the poor. To these went a packet of the Smith, Kay, and Arnott reports. Unlike the English informants, they also received a questionnaire. The questionnaire indicates the evolving concept of sanitation: for the first time, the hydraulic idea was prominent. It was not enough that there be sewers; it was important that they be "well supplied with water to dilute, and sufficiently sloping to carry off all such refuse . . . [and] sufficiently *closed* to confine noxious exhalations." Local government reform was important, and Chadwick was coming to see how much the impediments to improvement were legal and financial, not conceptual. But most important is question 7:

Of the diseases described in question 1 ["various forms of continued fever, and other contagious febrile diseases"] are any or what proportion ascribable to other causes than those specified in questions 4, 5, and 6 [i.e., external conditions, including drains, internal structure, and cleanliness, and internal economy, crowdedness, pigs, and so forth]? If so, distinguish those other causes so far as you are able, and the extent of diseases resulting from them.

49 P. G. Handyside to Chadwick, *Scottish–PLC Correspondence*, 18 May 1840, PRO MH 19/196; "[First] Report of the Committee of the Association for Obtaining an Official Inquiry into the Pauperism of Scotland," 26 April 1841, in *Scottish Distress, 1840–41*, PRO HO 45/160, 2, 6, 9. Cf. "[Poor Law Commission and Public Health]," *Times*, 25 November 1840, 4b–c. *The Times* speaks of the PLC as "opening a Poor Law intrigue with various parties in Scotland, with the view of eventually bringing that country under their domination."

Earlier questions had addressed most of the factors Kay had drawn from the metropolitan medical officers' responses; the "other causes" were economic causes of fever. The inclusion of such a question makes clear that Chadwick was willing to go some way to accommodate Alison. Already he had admitted to Handyside that while the inquiry was "chiefly directed to those physical and removable agencies by which disease is caused," it might be "necessary to distinguish the extent of the disease so caused from disease . . . *arising from the state of poverty and of the destitution of the proper means of subsistence.*"[50] That distinction was appropriately a medical decision.

But "other causes" was still too vague for the Scots. Soon after the questionnaire went off, Chadwick had a polite query from Handyside asking that question 7 be revised to raise the destitution–fever issue directly. Chadwick obliged: "Other causes" became "want of any of the necessaries of life." New questionnaires were posted to informants with instructions to disregard the previous ones.[51] But Chadwick went further: in early July he wrote an anonymous leader praising Alison's "masterly pamphlet." This had shown that epidemics "arise from the frequent destitution of the population for whose relief there is no adequate provision." He chastised those like Lord Haddington, a practitioner of fetid irrigation (and opponent of the inquiry), for sacrificing "the health and welfare of a community" in order to maintain his rental income. The Scots, he noted, simply wanted what England had: "some efficiently administered, compulsory provision for the relief of destitution."[52]

Scottish medical men responded enthusiastically to Chadwick's invitation, though most were contributing more to Alison's campaign than to Chadwick's. While acknowledging the need for sanitary improvement, they tended to reiterate the centrality of destitution as a cause of disease.[53] Throughout

---

50 Draft response, Chadwick to Handyside, 18 May 1840, *Scottish–PLC Correspondence*, MH 19/196. Chadwick had received Alison's pamphlet in January (Drysdale to Chadwick, 13 January 1840, UCL Chadwick Papers #655).

51 "Sanitary Inquiry. Request for Information from Medical Men in Scotland," *PLC Appendices to Minutes*, 19 June 1840, PRO MH 3/2; Handyside to Chadwick, 18 May, 6 June, 15 June 1840; draft Chadwick to Handyside, undated May 1840, 13 June 1840, *Scottish–PLC Correspondence*, MH 19/196. Chadwick did edit Handyside's suggested text: "If you have reason to think that the extension of contagious fever among the Poor is to be ascribed to their state of poverty, or frequent or occasional destitution of the proper means of subsistence, of clothing, fuel, etc., – as much as, or more than, to the existence of a malaria, arising from defect in drainage, or bad construction of their dwellings, you will have the goodness to state that opinion and the grounds for it, distinguishing as far as you can, the extent to which both descriptions of causes appear to contribute to that unfortunate result." Chadwick also made it plain that the terms of analysis were geographic and structural, not epidemiological or ethnic (he generally eschewed the blame-the-Irish invitation), economic, occupational, and so on. "Circular Letter," *Report to Her Majesty's Principal Secretary of State*, xvii.

52 The leader, from an unnamed newspaper for 6 July 1840, is signed by Chadwick and titled in his hand "Sanatory Inquiry Being Extended to Scotland." It includes early evidence collected for the Sanitary Inquiry and quotes at length from the Smith–Kay–Arnott studies.

53 A great many respondents are listed in the Poor Law Commission, *Official Circulars*, 1 September

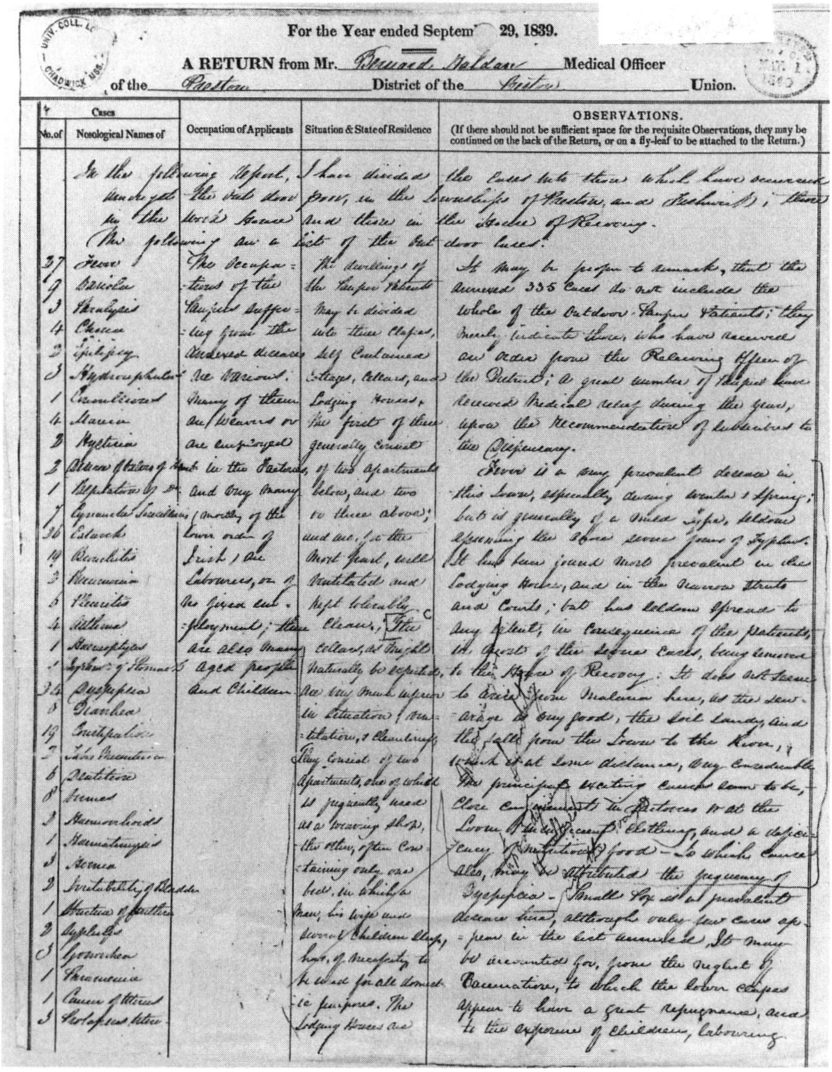
For the Year ended Septem[ber] 29, 1839.

A RETURN from Mr. Bernard Haldane Medical Officer of the Preston District of the Preston Union.

| No. of Cases | Nosological Names of | Occupation of Applicants | Situation & State of Residence | OBSERVATIONS. (If there should not be sufficient space for the requisite Observations, they may be continued on the back of the Return, or on a fly-leaf to be attached to the Return.) |
|---|---|---|---|---|

A completed return on local causes of disease by Bernard Haldane, one of the poor law medical officers of Preston Union, made as part of the Sanitary Inquiry. Haldane has written that "the fever does not seem to derive from the malaria here. . . . The principal exciting causes seem to be, – close confinement, in factories or at the Loom, an insufficiency of clothing, and a deficiency of nutritious food." Chadwick has marked the passage and made a note to query – "Qy" – the claim (reprinted with permission of University College London, Chadwick Papers #45).

1840 Chadwick and Alison were working closely. In September, Chadwick attended the British Association's Glasgow meeting, site of the great debate between Alison and Thomas Chalmers on whether food or moral discipline was the road to Scotland's salvation. With Alison and Robert Cowan (and Arnott and the Liverpool sanitarian W. H. Duncan), Chadwick toured grimmest Glasgow.[54] As the local reports came in, he supplied copies to Alison, who drew on them in his attacks on Chalmers.[55] Beyond this, he kept quiet: given the Scottish contempt for all things English, his endorsement of a new poor law would have backfired utterly. In the *Sanitary Report* itself Scotland was treated no differently from England and Wales. All the same, though Chadwick was willing enough to help Alison get a proper poor law – even to the extent of recognizing the possibility that destitution *might* cause fever – he had little stomach for Alison's do-gooderism: it violated anyone's first principles of political economy. Chadwick's view of the world was in fact much closer to that of Alison's opponents: the problem with the Highlanders who had descended on Edinburgh and Glasgow was really laziness – they were less willing to work even than the Irish.[56]

Indeed, at least some in the beleaguered church were beginning to sense the political potential Chadwick saw in sanitation: it was a route to social betterment compatible with the religious–economic discipline of the Chalmersian community. Here the main thinker was the Reverend George Lewis of Dundee, whose ideas would figure centrally in the General Assembly's May 1841 response to Alison.[57] On the one hand, Lewis clung to Chalmers's principle that comfort was a function of character, which he took as the opposite of Alison's philosophy. In Dundee, rising wages had depressed "the character of the population." If money harmed the morals of the industrious poor, how much worse must be the effects of public stipends on the indigent? Without "character," "comfort" led only to drink. Sanitation and "innocent amusements," such as music lessons and literary and scientific societies, were ways

---

1840. Most of their reports did not make it into the volume of Scottish *Local Reports*, but survive in *Scottish–PLC Correspondence*, MH 19/196.

54 Neil Arnott, "On the Fevers Which Have Prevailed in Edinburgh and Glasgow," *Sanitary Condition of the Labouring Population. Local Reports for Scotland, P.P., House of Lords*, 1842, 28, 8; Chadwick to William Shuttleworth, 8 January 1847 in "Appointment of Local Surveyor and MOH, Liverpool," *Home Office Files Miscellaneous*, PRO HO 45/1824. On the great debate see *Glasgow Saturday Post, and Paisley and Renfrewshire Reformer*, 26 September 1840.

55 "Reply by Dr. Alison to a Member of the Committee Opposed to the Official Inquiry," Appendix in *Second Report of the Committee of the Association for Obtaining an Official Inquiry into the Pauperism of Scotland*, in *Scottish Distress, 1840–41*, PRO HO 45/160, 26–45. Alison cited the local reports of de Vitre on Lancaster, Howard on Manchester, Duncan on Liverpool, and Tufnell on Kent and Sussex.

56 Chadwick to Macvey Napier, 2 March 1845, UCL Chadwick Papers #2181/8; Chadwick to the Reverend Whitwell Elwin, 22 October, 8 November 1841, UCL Chadwick Papers #694.

57 "Reply by Dr. Alison to a Member of the Committee Opposed to the Official Inquiry," 22–26.

to combat drink (indeed, sanitation was an especially valuable way, inasmuch as it acted independently of talent or intelligence).[58] But sanitation was more than diversion – it could be the high road to morality. Lewis offered a thoroughgoing environmental determinism: Chalmers's solution – more churches – was no longer viable; the only hope was in sanitary infrastructure. Place a middle-class housewife in the "vennels" of Glasgow, "her notions of cleanliness and decencies will rapidly degenerate." Relocate her to "her own self-contained house . . . with her own lobby and her own front door, in the eye of every passer-by, her ideas of cleanliness and decency will undergo a rapid improvement." Some fever might be God's will, but all could not be, for the effect of the malaria was also "to undermine the vigour of manhood itself, sow the seeds of premature decay, and render the wretched resource of strong drink little less than a necessity to repair the languid frame and wasted spirits." Lewis believed that all religions and factions could unite on sanitary reform. He saw it as no less critical than the defeat of Napoleon had been (and likely to be just as costly).[59]

Both Lewis and Chadwick had sensed that a sanitarian analysis upheld the status quo. In England or in Scotland, the misery of the poor was not to be attributed to the existing poor law, much less to the class relations of industrial capitalism. The answer was structures. Build what ye will whatever it cost, but tamper ye not with class relations! Surely, sewers and water were the bread and circuses of the Victorian age.

Whatever compromises one might make secretly, at all costs Chadwick had to prevent Alisonianism from infecting the English debate on the harshness of the new poor law. In the *Sanitary Report* itself he would dismiss the destitution–fever idea as a quaint belief dispelled by modern science. Lewis is the most frequently cited Scottish author. The front matter of the *Sanitary Report* included the original question 7, with its "other causes" rather than "want of any of the necessaries of life."[60]

58 George Lewis, *The State of St. David's Parish, with Remarks on the Moral and Physical Statistics of Dundee* (Dundee 1841), title page, 29–31, 35–36. The General Assembly called for "sanatory regulations and the providing for large towns of open spaces or parks whereby the health of the inhabitants may be promoted, the craving for artificial stimulants, arising from a state of the body not healthful, or deprived of the natural stimulation of exercise or recreation in the open air, may be lessened, and the tendency to diseases and early mortality diminished" (quoted in "Memorial of the Association in Second Report of the Committee of the Association for Obtaining an Official Inquiry into the Pauperism of Scotland," *Scottish Distress, 1840–41*, PRO HO 45/160).

59 George Lewis, "Prevailing Evils Examined in Detail. Physical Destitution," *Lectures on the Social and Physical Condition of the People Especially in Large Towns, by Various Ministers of Glasgow* (Glasgow: Collins, [1842]), 54–56, 64–66, 74–75.

60 *Report to Her Majesty's Principal Secretary of State*, xix. The revised version is published in Poor Law Commission, *Official Circulars*, 10 September 1840. Chadwick was also sending Lewis's pamphlets to his protégé the Reverend Whitwell Elwin (Chadwick to Elwin, 22 October 1841; Elwin to Chadwick, 8 November 1841, UCL Chadwick Papers #694) and distributing copies of the anti-Alison report of the General Assembly of the Church of Scotland (Chadwick to Home Office, 6 April, 17 June 1840, *PLC–Home Office Correspondence*, PRO HO 73/56).

Still, Alisonianism pervaded the volume of Scottish *Local Reports.* Most reporters did not present Alisonian approaches as an alternative to Chadwickian sanitarianism. But Alison's own report, "Observations on the Generation of Fever," did. In the volume, it was sandwiched between two reports from Neil Arnott. The first, "On the Fevers Which Have Prevailed in Edinburgh and Glasgow," was breathtakingly arrogant. Arnott devoted only two of his twelve pages to the two greatest towns in Scotland and ignored the wealth of fever data compiled by Scottish medical men over the years. He reiterated the conclusions of 1838, expressed his wonder that the Scots who had debated the causes of misery and disease in the Glasgow British Association for the Advancement of Science (BAAS) meeting ignored the "malaria of filth," and found in his brief local tour that "all appeared confirmatory of the view of the subject of fevers submitted to the Poor Law Commission by those who prepared the report in London."[61]

Condescension is the hallmark of Arnott's second report. A "careless reader" might think there was disagreement between London and Alison. But surely not. Swept up in a good cause, Alison had been hasty and oversensitive. He had written "perhaps before he had fully examined the reports to which he referred." Surely everyone knew destitution harmed health (though, by the way, bad air was much more important)! That England had a poor law and hence no destitution, while Scotland, with no proper poor law, had a destitution problem, accounted for Alison's crotchets. He could not imagine disagreeing with anything Alison had "fully considered" and "deliberately expressed" and urged adoption of a proper poor law in Scotland.[62]

While parts of the report are in the form of a letter to Alison, Arnott is really addressing readers of the volume of local reports. Chadwick's key points come through clearly: Scotland should emulate England in poor law, one must read destitution–fever claims in light of current political needs, and (therefore) destitution can be dismissed as a significant cause of disease. Readers who went on to the other Scottish reports would know they should be skeptical. All this talk of starvation? Just Scots politicking.

Alison's views were not, as Arnott had claimed, hastily and imprecisely stated, but carefully qualified, widely shared, and supported by many examples. But Alison and his friends were not in much of a position to protest Chadwick's use of their reports. In March 1842, a few months before the issuing of the *Sanitary Report,* the Poor Law Commission suddenly discovered that those with Irish or Scottish credentials were not "duly qualified," in the view

---

61 Arnott, "On the Fevers Which Have Prevailed in Edinburgh and Glasgow," 1–12.
62 Neil Arnott, "Remarks on Dr. W. P. Alison's 'Observations on the Generation of Fever,' " in *Scottish Local Reports,* 34–39. The London reporters were offered a response on the grounds that Alison had criticized them; on the grounds that Arnott had conceded the harmfulness of destitution, Alison chose not to reply (Chadwick to Alison, 18 August 1840; Alison to Chadwick, 14 September 1840, PRO MH 19/196).

of learned counsel, to serve as medical officers in English unions. No one at the PLC would defend this ruling on the merits of the issue; it was to imply no judgement of the quality of Scottish universities or licensing bodies. The tone of response to the torrent of petitions and letters was friendly dismissal: "So sorry. Can do nothing, hands tied. Law, you know." Within a year Sir James Graham, the home secretary, overruled the opinion, but at the time of the *Sanitary Report,* it appeared that Chadwick, by a move of raw power, had neutralized what might otherwise be a powerful opposition.[63]

It is true that the destitution–fever claims of Scottish medical men had political significance, but it would be wrong to think of them as *merely* political. Such views antedated the poor law crisis. They derived from principles of constitutional medicine, confirmed repeatedly in investigations of epidemics. Indeed, for Alison, political action followed from medical knowledge and was a form of medical practice. Alison did get his inquiry, the Royal Commission on the Poor Laws of Scotland of 1843–45. A balanced commission, it led to an unsatisfactory compromise.[64] But Arnott's haughtiness had a longer-lasting effect. Scottish medical men would continue to see public health as social policy; Alison would block Chadwick's attempts to take the 1848 Public Health Act north.[65]

63 "Minute of the Commissioners, Respecting the Admissibility of Scottish and Irish Medical Practitioners to Union Medical Officers in England," *Ninth Annual Report of the Poor Law Commission, with Appendices, P.P.,* 1843, 21, [468.], Appendix B4, 224–26; petitions, April–May 1842; Graham to PLC, 23 August 1843, *PLC–Scotland Correspondence,* PRO MH 19/196. See also Ruth Hodgkinson, *The Origins of the National Health Service: The Medical Services of the New Poor Law, 1834–1871* (London: Wellcome Historical Medical Library, 1967), 67–71; Irvine Loudon, *Medical Care and the General Practitioner* (Oxford: Clarendon Press, 1986), 113, 183; Henry Rumsey, "The Medical Care of the Poor in England, Part I," *Essays on State Medicine* (London: Churchill, 1856), 177–78; Anand Chitnis, *The Scottish Enlightenment and Early Victorian English Society* (London: Croom Helm, 1986), 136–40.

64 Cf. Cage, *The Scottish Poor Law,* 135–36; Brown, *Thomas Chalmers,* 288–96, 350; William Hanna, *Memoirs of the Life and Writings of Thomas Chalmers D.D.,* 4 vols. (Edinburgh: Constable and Co., 1852), IV, 196–216; Ferguson, *The Dawn of Scottish Social Welfare,* 245; Leavitt and Smout, *The State of the Scottish Working-Class in 1843,* 153.

65 An 1848 committee of the Royal College of Physicians in Edinburgh on the Health of Towns or Improvement Bills opposed bringing Scotland under the General Board of Health: "Although they have a high respect for the individual members of the General Board of Health in London, yet the confident expression of opinion which those gentlemen have officially made on several important questions touching the diffusion of epidemic diseases, which the Committee regard as very difficult and doubtful – and on which they know that some of the most experienced practitioners in Scotland hold a very definite opinion – have by no means tended to increase their expectation of the efficacy of measures, applicable to Scotland, for restraining the diffusion of epidemics, which may proceed from that source." Quoted in Ferguson, *The Dawn of Scottish Social Welfare,* 147. See also ibid., 79; Brenda White, "Scottish Doctors and the English Public Health," *The Influence of Scottish Medicine,* ed. Derek Dow, 82–83, 85 (Park Ridge, N.J.: Parthenon, 1988).

III

Arnott's implied corollary, that since Scottish science was political, English science must be pure, was of course quite wrong. In the summer of 1840, all the while Chadwick was placating and manipulating the Scots, he was trying to suppress starvation scandals.

In late August 1840 a letter appeared in the *Times* complaining of cruel treatment that led to the death of a workhouse pauper. In June, Samuel Daniels, a fifty-six-year-old consumptive whitesmith, had left Stratford workhouse to escape the combination of heavy work and lack of "sufficient food to support nature." On returning to Chelsea he had found no work, and he died in early July. A dispensary doctor had registered the death as due to "low living and want of sufficient nourishment." As his widow stated at the inquest, "Doctor said deceased was consumptive; deceased had not got proper necessaries."

The author wrote because such cases were "much more numerous than is generally imagined." Noting Daniels was a consumptive, he observed that "in this disease the higher class of patients are directed to take a mild, nutritious diet, to avoid cold, and to live in a pure, open air. The physician points them to the south of England, or Italy." Daniels, however, had been "shut up in a workhouse, sent to pick stones with a bag suspended round his neck, and fed upon a diet which had a tendency to produce the distressing diarrhoea to which the consumptive are liable." Was this "necessary"? he then asked.

May not these poor people, and there are hundreds of them in different stages of consumption, be allowed to live in rooms and cottages of their own choice, with a few shillings a week, without any artificial aggravation of their sufferings, or violation of their natural feelings? Their days on earth are numbered; and can any man or class of men in England desire that they should be put to torture while they live, to uphold a system, and to expiate the crime of having saved no surplus after a life of toil, or the misfortune of having lived in England until the workhouse system was established?[66]

The Daniels case was only one of many starvation scandals in 1840–41. How much hunger affected death rates in the "hungry forties" would be hard to say, but it was politics, not demographics, that brought the issue so often to public attention. Already "starvation" had been a catchword of the anti–poor law movement and the Chartist press; it was becoming increasingly central in the public relations of the anti–corn law movement.[67]

66  "Alleged Death from Starvation: Singular Inquiry," *Times*, 26 August 1840, 7; William Farr to *Times*, 31 August 1840, 5e. For further assertions and denials see C. Fowell to *Times*, 25 August 1840, 3 c; R. H. Hobbs to *Times*, 1 September 1840, 3f.
67  See, for example, W. Cooke Taylor, *Notes of a Tour in the Manufacturing Districts of Lancashire*, 3d ed., with a new introduction by W. H. Chaloner (1842; reprint, New York: Augustus M. Kelley, 1968), 38: "The fact is, that the mass of the population is on the very brink of sheer destitution, and that thousands are absolutely starving." In 1841 *The Anti Corn Law Circular* changed its name

What makes the Daniels letter significant is its author: William Farr, statistician to the registrar general, one of the best known figures of mid-Victorian public health. The letter linked Farr with Thomas Wakley, West Middlesex coroner as well as Finsbury M.P. and *Lancet* editor, who had conducted the inquest. Though isolated in Parliament, Wakley was powerful in the metropolitan vestries and a virtuoso of sarcasm. The new poor law was one of his many great hates, an animating animus. Together the two were well placed to mount a medical critique of the new poor law. Farr's stock was rising, his first two reports on causes of death having been well received. To the extent that credibility in public health rested on some statistical bedrock, it was Farr who had the best claim to that credibility.

Though Farr had been no great friend of the new poor law, his venom was unexpected, and Chadwick himself bore some responsibility for provoking it, having attempted to humiliate Farr.[68] In Farr's first report to the registrar general (for the second half of 1837), 63 of over 148,000 deaths were attributed to starvation. Commenting on the returns, Farr had observed that "hunger destroys a much higher proportion than is indicated by the registers . . . but its effects, like the effects of excess, are generally manifested indirectly, in the production of diseases of various kinds." He noted also that parliamentary inquiries had shown the inadequacy of the diet of agricultural laborers.[69]

This statement implicated the poor law, whose first purpose was to prevent starvation. If people starved, something wasn't working: either workhouse diets were too lean or deterrence was too effective. One might have been pleased that there were so few starvations, and Farr's claim about the pervasiveness of hunger was but a passing comment in a long report, unsupported and probably unconfirmable. But Chadwick chose to make an issue of the matter. He was right in sensing a potential public relations problem. To the

to *The Anti Bread Tax Circular* and shifted its focus from abstractions of political economy and tariff retaliation to the more immediate matter of hunger. It printed a steady stream of reports on starvation and political poems, some of them critical of the poor law. The emergence of this criticism is important because Chadwick had long-standing connections with the Mancunian manufacturing community, whence came the leadership of the movement. Finer, *Chadwick,* 187; John Morley, *The Life of Richard Cobden,* 2 vols. (London: Macmillan, 1908), I, 169–70, 202, 249, 264; J. L. Hammond and Barbara Hammond, *Lord Shaftesbury,* 3d ed. (London: Constable and Co., 1925), 54.

68  Under the heading "Relief of Destitution" the entire correspondence was printed by Chadwick in Poor Law Commission, *Official Circulars,* 9 March, 18 May 1840. The correspondence is reprinted in D. V. Glass, *Numbering the People: The Eighteenth Century Population Controversy and the Development of Census and Vital Statistics in Britain* (Farnborough, Hants.: Saxon House, 1973), 42–67. Ostensibly Chadwick writes on behalf of the Poor Law Commission to Registrar General T. H. Lister, yet the controversy is clearly between Chadwick and Farr. See also John M. Eyler, *Victorian Social Medicine: The Ideas and Methods of William Farr* (Baltimore: Johns Hopkins University Press, 1979), 25–26; C. Hamlin, "Could You Starve to Death in England in 1839? The Chadwick–Farr Controversy and the Loss of the 'Social' in Public Health," *American Journal of Public Health* 85 (1995): 856–66.

69  Farr, "[First] Letter to the Registrar General," in *First Annual Report of the Registrar-General, P.P.,1839, 16,* (187.), Appendix P, 75.

medically ignorant or to those with a grudge against the establishment, starvation was an easy enough diagnosis to make whenever some impoverished person died. The lay registrars might naively accept such claims (the Registration Act did not require medical certification of cause of death). And of course there were medical men who would insist on seeing predisposing causes like hunger as the most important causes of disease and death. Richard Baron Howard of Manchester had already defended that claim (though Chadwick probably did not yet know of Howard's book), and Farr's comment certainly suggested a similar perspective.[70] Farr needed to be straightened out sooner rather than later. So at the end of September 1839, as the Sanitary Inquiry was getting under way, Chadwick wrote to T. H. Lister, Farr's supervisor, for details of the sixty-three cases.

Chadwick had reason to suppose Farr would be receptive to fatherly admonition. He had lobbied for the registration bill and for Farr's appointment as statistician. Farr did supply details. Over half of deaths were of infants. In many cases their mothers had died or been too weak or ill to nurse them effectively. Among the adults, some had succumbed to cold, often when drunk. In only one case had a request for relief been refused; in several, victims had refused relief. To call all this starvation was very misleading, Chadwick complained to Farr in February 1840: these deaths did not implicate the poor law authorities as neglectful.

But Farr was not contrite. He argued that starvation was a broad economic category: "Want of food implies a want of everything else . . . as firing, clothing, every convenience, every necessary of life, is abandoned at the imperious bidding of hunger." Thus those who died from cold died from deprivation, quite as much as those who died from lack of food. The infant deaths might be understood similarly; infants "starved in the cold nights of winter, and on the coarse, innutritious, inadequate subsistence of impoverished parents." A death was appropriately attributed to "starvation," argued Farr, if the person would presumably have lived had the substance in question been provided.[71]

Chadwick felt that he had absolved the PLC of blame for the starvation deaths and that Farr was guilty of stretching "starvation" beyond customary use. He published the correspondence in the Commission's Circulars, a series he had invented at the end of 1839 as a way to manage the commission's image.[72] Henceforth Farr would notify the PLC of deaths registered as starvations. On receiving such notifications, PLC staff would review the evidence, and reinterview witnesses to discover whether there had been a failure in poor law administration. Had the person really died of starvation? Had someone

---

70  Gibson, "The Public Health Agitation," 66, 71.
71  For other examples of this image see Taylor, *Notes of a Tour in the Manufacturing Districts of Lancashire*, 48, 79.
72  On the circulars see Chadwick to Lord John Russell, 9 January 1840, UCL Chadwick Papers #1733.

failed to give aid? Starvation, the commissioners decided, was an acute condition. Possession of any assets ruled out starvation, since the person would have been able to buy food. Invariably these inquiries found the poor law guiltless.[73] They were rarely publicized; in the hands of Wakley or a *Times* leader writer, their tendentiousness would have been embarrassing.

As Chadwick recognized, "starvation" was no mere diagnosis. In a land which recognized a right to relief, it was also an accusation of wrongful death. "Starvation" was irretrievably political; hitherto loosely defined, it had been used against the PLC; in defining it precisely and narrowly, he was seeking to make it work for him. Necessarily in doing so he was transforming ideas of rights and responsibilities, and necessarily he collided head on with the medical radical Wakley, dedicated to an antithetical redefinition of rights and responsibilities.

The chief forum of Wakley's medical populism was neither the *Lancet* nor the House of Commons but the West Middlesex coronership, to which he had been elected in spring 1839. As Wakley saw it, the coroner's job was to help society decide whether a death was acceptable to community standards. The coroner was neither advocate nor judge but inquisitor, free to raise the most far-reaching questions of responsibility, and an inquest was not so much an antecedent to a criminal trial as an opportunity for the people to say whether culpability in its broadest sense was present. It made no difference that a death had occurred in circumstances that were legal and customary: if these violated public sensibility, the inquest should register that outrage. Among the targets of Wakley's show trials were flogging in the military and the game laws, as well as the new poor law. On taking office he had circulated a list of the sorts of cases in which inquests were appropriate, as for example, "when persons die who appear to have been neglected during sickness or extreme poverty" or "when lunatics or paupers die in confinement" (e.g., workhouses). The radical metropolitan electorate shared his sensibilities; the Daniels inquest followed a petition from thirty Chelsea residents.[74] Accordingly, Wakley found the resolution of the Chadwick–Farr controversy especially galling. Rather than being sent to the PLC to be covered up, apparent starvations should go before the coroner and receive the people's justice.

Thus in England as in Scotland Chadwick was challenged by those who

---

73  "An Abstract of the Circumstances of Alleged Deaths from Want Occurring in the Year 1840 and of the Results of Inquiries Relating Thereto. In Mr. Chadwick's of 22 September 1841," *Home Office–PLC Correspondence*, PRO HO 73/56. See, for example, the cases of Bridget Berry, James Jolson, Elizabeth Stewart, Mary Kitching, and Mary Stephenson, and the Yeadon starvations, June 1840–February 1841, *Leeds–PLC Correspondence*, PRO MH 12/15225; also Power to Chadwick, 1 January 1840, *Power–PLC Correspondence*, PRO MH 32/64; Sir J. Graham to PLC, 7 September 1841, *PLC–Bolton Union Correspondence*, PRO MH 12/5594. Also see "Daniels Inquest," 8 June 1841, *PLC Miscellaneous Correspondence*, PRO MH 19/224.

74  S. Q. Sprigge, *The Life and Times of Thomas Wakley* (London: Longmans, Green, 1897), 318–19, 381–82, 399.

would make disease and death among the poor the basis of a thoroughgoing critique of liberal society. The response in both cases was to sever disease from the domain of the social by attributing it to mysterious poisons that acted randomly, at least with respect to the most politically sensitive social conditions. The strategy is especially plain in one of the few starvation reviews to be publicized, the case of Elizabeth Friry from autumn 1840. Friry was reported to have died of "want . . . of sufficient nourishment." The PLC's review was conducted by Kay and Sir Edmund Head, another assistant commissioner. Kay tried to convince Friry's medical attendants that she had died from a disease, an "idiopathic" fever, not from starvation. The case hinged on what one meant by "typhus." Wakley used the term in its traditional generic sense – an *"irritative fever –* fever *symptomatic* of impoverished blood, the want of food, warmth, all the necessaries, and all the comforts of life." Drawing on the new French view of typhus and typhoid as discrete clinical entities (with, one might presume, distinct causes), Kay steered attention away from whether Friry had had food to the obscure pathognomic signs of typhoid. For Wakley the question was "Had she had good food, would she have lived?" For Kay it was "Did she have characteristic intestinal lesions?" Wakley respected Kay but saw here "a predetermination to torture the facts."[75]

## IV

A further complication was R. A. Slaney's select committee on "the Health of Towns," which took evidence in the spring of 1840. Slaney has often been seen by historians as stealing Chadwick's initiative and then ruining it by promoting premature and poorly drafted legislation.[76] But he was not a rival: he had neither talent nor desire to control a new province of public administration. Nor was his inquiry derivative of Chadwick's; indeed he is better understood as enlarging and enriching Chadwick's inchoate notion of sanitary condition, and of making much more overt its place in the condition-of-England question. He opened new areas of inquiry, like the safety of urban burial grounds and the competence of the Greater London sewers commissions, which would become standard concerns of Chadwickian sanitarians. The tone of sanitarianism changed, too, as Slaney's old-fashioned philanthropy washed off some of the new poor law harshness. Chadwick took much from Slaney; arguably the *Sanitary Report* reflects the agenda of Slaney's committee more than that of the 1838 reports or the queries of November 1839.

Robert Aglionby Slaney, M.P., was a Shropshire Whig squire. He had not

---

75 "Examination in the Case of Elizabeth Friry," *Lancet,* 1840, ii, 348–49.
76 In 1841 Lord Normanby introduced bills founded on the committee's report. These met with opposition and were withdrawn; see chapter 8.

set out to investigate "sanatory" matters: in early February he had asked for a select committee on "the causes of discontent." It was a long-standing concern: Slaney had been watching urbanization and industrialization destroy the social fabric of England and feared that process must end in chaos. Finding Slaney's request too sweeping, Lord John Russell had urged him to stick to "sanatory" causes of unrest.[77]

Besides medical men like Arnott and Smith, Slaney's witnesses included union relieving officers, the surveyors and clerks of sewers commissions, field investigators for the Royal Commission on Hand-Loom Weavers, a few progressive northern industrialists, and two critics of the Edinburgh sewage irrigation (and, unavoidably, one of the irrigators). While almost every witness was asked about drains, Slaney invited witnesses to consider a great range of causes and solutions to the condition-of-England problem, including school ventilation, playgrounds, and public walks. One witness was much concerned about the lack of cricket grounds.[78] Yet the incoherence was only apparent: Slaney was in control. Trained, like Chadwick, as a lawyer, he knew well how to lead witnesses to the right points and to get the right answers. He, too, had clear ideas of the bounds of legitimate social reform, and they did not include allowing poverty to be a disease. The issue of hunger was to be treated as Southwood Smith had treated it, not as a problem in its own right but as a circumstance that might exacerbate the effects of bad air.[79]

The "health" in Slaney's inquiry was no longer tied to fever prevention, but was a placeholder for morality. Drawing on traditions of constitutional medicine, witnesses explained how filth affected health by instilling habits that damaged "the moral tone," which was, after all, part of the "tone" of the nervous system. Thus, according to Joseph Fletcher, investigator for the Royal Commission on Hand-Loom Weavers, the lack of sporting grounds led young men to "sweethearting," which in turn injured the "constitution." Slaney held such constitutional changes to be hereditary, and some medical witnesses, like Arnott, agreed.[80]

77 On Slaney see Paul Richards, "R. A. Slaney, the Industrial Town, and Early Victorian Social Policy," *Social History* 4 (1979): 85–101; Brundage, *Making of the Poor Law*, 55; Cowherd, *Political Economists*, 130, 168, 170; and chapter 8. On the inquiry see Gibson, "The Public Health Agitation," 43, 47; Peter Mandler, *Aristocratic Government in the Age of Reform* (Oxford: Oxford University Press, 1990), 178.

78 Joseph Ellison in "Select Committee on the Health of Towns, Minutes of Evidence," *P.P.*, 1840, 11 (384.), qq 1635–37; on playgrounds and places for walking see Samuel Byles, Neil Arnott, Joseph Fletchter, James Williamson, Edmund Ashworth, J. R. Wood, ibid., qq 221, 595, 1237–38, 1315–17, 1736, 1849–51, 2191–92.

79 See especially Slaney's questioning of John Clarke, medical officer of St. Olave's Southwark (ibid., qq 460–62): "They are not able, by the wages they earn, to get the kind of food that would fortify them against the attacks of disease?" "No." "Where people get only an insufficient supply of food, is it not necessary that they should be guarded from disease, by a better mode of ventilation, and sewerage, and draining?" "Yes." See also James Williamson, ibid., q 1682.

80 Ibid., qq 565–67, 935–40, 1243–44, 2224–25.

As well as drawing forth a long list of dreadful conditions and imperative reforms, Slaney used the committee to investigate the several Greater London sewers commissions. He had already decided that bad drains and sewers were the greatest sanitary problem, a view Chadwick would arrive at only by the end of the decade. It was necessary, therefore, to find out how good sewers came to be and why in some places and not others. The seven sewers commissions were artifacts of the sixteenth century. They were not strangers to politics or criticism, but their doings had not heretofore been implicated in this "condition-of-England" question, and they had no reason to think that within two years they would be vilified, blamed for nearly every disease and for the pervasive "demoralization" of the laboring classes.[81]

Slaney interviewed clerks and surveyors from the Kent, City of London, and Tower Hamlets commissions, who made up about a third of all witnesses. Some of his questions concerned impediments to sewer building, factors Parliament might change to help the commissions do their work. How were sewer projects planned and financed? Could they be built more quickly? But Slaney was also the sanitary accuser. What were the commissions doing to remove disease-generating filth, he wanted to know, a question that presumed that the sewers commissions bore the awesome responsibility of protecting the nation against disease.[82] Such questions perplexed witnesses. Mission statements were a thing of the future, but the commissioners and officers did not see themselves as guarantors of health. As one of the more articulate put it, sewers were a matter of property, not of health. Water would run downhill and accumulate, inconveniently, in low places; conflicts among landowners resulted; the commissions resolved them by technical and financial means.[83]

This preoccupation with sewers and the identification of sewer builders as archvillains were new. Henceforth, holding the sewers commissions to a new standard of accountability would become one of the sanitarians' main stratagems. Chadwick would echo the condemnation in the *Sanitary Report*, and the same troop of clerks and surveyors would be marched in for a dressing down before the Royal Commission on the Health of Towns in 1843–44 and the Royal Commission on the Sanitation of the Metropolis in 1847–48.

The picture that emerges from the Slaney testimony differs little from other social investigations. What is remarkable is the invocation of medical authority implicit in "health of towns." A medical problem seemed to imply a medical solution, perhaps a "board of health" like those established during epidemics to get nuisances off the streets and keep victims out of circulation. But here the threat was not disease, but a vast revolutionary anger that other authorities seemed unable to deal with: not the church, which hardly commanded the

81 "Select Committee on Metropolis Sewers," *P.P.*, 1823, *5*, (542.); "Select Committee on Metropolis Sewers," *P.P.*, 1834, *15*, (584.).
82 Beriah Drew, "Select Committee on the Health of Towns," qq 1539–41.
83 James Peeke, Beriah Drew, ibid., qq 1481, 1512, 1517–24, 2064–65.

loyalty of the rebellious elements; nor education, itself a hostage to religious controversy. Perhaps then the newly scientific medicine? In attacking those "nuisances" that were supposed to cause disease, might one equally attack the moral degradation that nurtured revolution? In retrospect it must seem outlandish – to begin an inquiry into the causes of revolution and end up in "public health"? It was one thing to look for political solutions to medical problems – that was what Alison was doing – quite another to think that political problems might have medical solutions.

By 1842 Chadwick would have adopted most of Slaney's "broad-church" public health. As late as August 1840, however, he was still focusing on the narrower issue of "labouring classes." He hoped William Farr would give him crucial information on deaths from "epidemic, endemic or contagious diseases" in key occupational groups: hand loom weavers, factory workers in the northern cotton and woolen industries, colliers, metal workers in Birmingham and Sheffield. He proposed to compare the mortality rates of workers and others in the same localities.[84] The *Sanitary Report* would thus continue the demonstration begun in the 1833 factory report. It would at once disarm arguments about the unhealthfulness of work and focus disease prevention efforts on the employed work force rather than the querulous poor. In light of Chadwick's recent humiliation of Farr, it is an imperious request, but perhaps he felt he had made the public health pecking order clear. Suffice to say there is no record of a reply and no such analysis in the *Sanitary Report*.

V

The final shaping influence on the *Sanitary Report* was the Graham–Peel agenda. For much of 1841 work on the report had lapsed as Lord Normanby vainly sought support for drainage and building regulation bills based on the Slaney report. In midyear the weak Whig administration, damaged by its links to the new poor law, gave way and the Tories returned to government for the first time since the parliamentary reform crisis over a decade earlier. The new prime minister, Sir Robert Peel, and the home secretary, Sir James Graham, shared the centrist policies of their predecessors, if perhaps with more emphasis on order than on reform. Graham expected violence within the year (the Plug Plot riots of August 1842 would prove him right). Accordingly, when Chadwick returned to the *Report* in the fall, the effect of bad sanitary administration in encouraging "dangerous classes" and of sanitary reform in

---

84  Chadwick to William Farr, *Registrar General–PLC Correspondence*, 18 August. 1840, PRO MH 19/191. On continued interest in the correlation of deaths with occupations see PLC to Assistant Commissioners, *PLC Appendices to Minutes*, 23 November 1840, PRO MH 3/2; Chadwick to Dr. Forbes, 26 August 1840, *PLC Miscellaneous Correspondence,* PRO MH 25/1; Robert Baker to Chadwick, 17 November 1841, *PLC–Leeds Correspondence*, PRO MH 12/15225. Farr's data were in fact very little used in the *Sanitary Report*.

neutralizing them became a key theme.[85] From the fall–winter of 1841–42 come his anathemas against bone pickers and scavengers, seen as idle thieves rather than diligent recyclers.[86]

This new tone is clearest in correspondence with the new chaplain of the Bath workhouse, the Reverend Whitwell Elwin, and the Manchester police commissioner, Sir Charles Shaw. Elwin would be the most cited informant in the *Sanitary Report* (six citations). His predecessor had been a cause célèbre, fired for protesting the brutal treatment of workhouse inmates. Elwin, by contrast, preached a penal rigor that made even Chadwick flinch. "A poor law must be worked rather roughly," he wrote. True, yet some deterrents – like putting women to stone breaking – simply would not fly politically, Chadwick replied. Elwin understood the *Sanitary Report* as dealing with the causes of pauperism in general, not simply the role of disease. Like the Chalmersites, he saw these mainly as moral: a filthy environment was simply a sign of preexisting moral degradation.[87] Chadwick had contacted Shaw in connection with the Constabulary Commission, but increasingly his vast intelligence of political and moral activity in the unruly Northwest seemed pertinent to the *Sanitary Report*. Shaw had complete data on the quasi-criminal scavengers, and knew that do-gooder relief usually just bought gin.[88] In Chadwick's view these men seemed best to appreciate the argument and importance of the *Sanitary Report*. He hoped both would review it for the quarterlies, though he was unable to arrange that.[89]

The publication of the *Sanitary Report* in the summer of 1842 (signed 9 July, it was available in early August) is also the stuff of legend. One of these is that the *Report* appeared under Chadwick's name alone. It was, we are told, too true, therefore too radical; the equivocating commissioners feared causing

---

85 Finer, *Chadwick*, 212; Lewis, *Chadwick*, 39. The usual view, drawn from Chadwick's later report, is that Graham allowed Chadwick to continue simply to keep him busy. Whether or not this is true, Chadwick certainly went to great lengths to bend the report to the government's concerns. With a field staff of trustworthy assistant commissioners, the PLC was already used as a source of intelligence on working-class political activity; see PLC to Home Secretary, 27 January 1840, in *PLC–Manchester Correspondence*, MH 12/6039.

86 Reports from Superintendents of Metropolitan Police on Ending the Trade in Bones, *PLC Miscellaneous Correspondence*, April 1842, PRO MH 19/224. On joint Chadwick–Graham concerns see Stanley H. Palmer, *Police and Protest in England and Ireland* (Cambridge: Cambridge University Press, 1988), 421–22, 455–62.

87 Elwin to Chadwick, 17 December 1841; Elwin to Chadwick, 19 October 1841; Chadwick to Elwin, 22 October 1841, UCL Chadwick Papers #694. Elwin felt his experience "amply sufficient to show how large a portion of the sickness of the lower orders is produced by their own reckless and dirty habits, how much misery and indigence is of their own choosing" (Elwin to Chadwick, 16 November, 23 December 1841). Despite the usual characterization of Chadwick as an environmental determinist, this view is fully compatible with much in the *Sanitary Report* (and with Kay's classification of crowded housing as a voluntary cause of disease).

88 Shaw to Chadwick, 21 April 1842, UCL Chadwick Papers #1794.

89 Shaw to Chadwick, 1 April 1842, UCL Chadwick Papers #1794; Macvey Napier to Chadwick, 22 August 1842, UCL Chadwick Papers #1465. See also Shaw to Chadwick, 28 September, 14 October 1841, UCL Chadwick Papers #1794.

offense. That it appeared at all is said to have been due to a compromise between Chadwick's supporter Nicholls and G. C. Lewis and Sir Edmund Head, his enemies on the commission. The source of the story is Chadwick's unpublished but widely circulated "vindicating" letter of 1847, composed when he and the commissioners were in the midst of a nasty divorce over the Andover workhouse scandal. Parts of the legend are true. The commissioners did discuss how, and even whether, to issue the report. But parts of the legend are wrong and others are misleading.

Most importantly, the PLC *did* take responsibility for the *Sanitary Report*. Chadwick's text was embedded in the *Report to Her Majesty's Principal Secretary of State for the Home Department, from the Poor Law Commissioners on an Inquiry into the Sanitary Condition of the Labouring Population of Great Britain; with Appendices*. That document consists of twenty-one pages of front matter; then Chadwick's report itself, with its appendices; and the two volumes of *Local Reports*, one for England and one for Scotland, which include chapters by the assistant commissioners and the reports of the "eminent" practitioners. In the front matter the commissioners list these local reports individually and announce that *they, not Chadwick,* are presenting *these* to Parliament and that *these reports alone* satisfy the charge given in 1839. But because it would be hard to use such data in "undigested" form, they had asked Chadwick "to peruse the information which we had received . . . and, by comparing the different statements with such authentic facts bearing upon the question as he might collect from other sources, to frame a report which should exhibit the principal results of the inquiry which we were instructed to conduct."[90] Then, following the questionnaires Chadwick sent out in 1839 and 1840, is the title page of the *Report on the Sanitary Condition of the Labouring Population of Great Britain* by Edwin Chadwick. It was the commission's custom to publish major investigative reports under the names of the staff members who wrote them – thus Kay got proper credit for his 1839 report on the education of pauper children. To have withheld such acknowledgment and presented the report as the work of the commission would have been much odder. Nor is it clear that the commissioners objected to Chadwick's report: Lewis called it Chadwick's best work; Nicholls was also impressed.[91]

90  *Report to Her Majesty's Principal Secretary of State*, ix. This front material is not included in Flinn's modern edition. Strictly speaking, Flinn's statement that "Edwin Chadwick . . . presented to the House of Lords his *Report on the Sanitary Condition of the Labouring Population of Great Britain*" is wrong. Cf. Edwin Chadwick, *Report on the Sanitary Condition of the Labouring Population of Great Britain* ed. M. W. Flinn (Edinburgh: Edinburgh University Press, 1965), 1. See "Poor Law Commission Minutes," 9 July 1842, PRO MH 1/34.
91  Richardson, *Health of Nations*, liv; Finer, *Chadwick*, 212; Lewis, *Chadwick*, 40; G. C. Lewis to G. Grote, 13 March 1842, *Letters of the Rt. Hon. Sir George Cornwall Lewis, Bt. to Various Friends, Edited by His Brother the Rev. Sir Gilbert Frankland Lewis* (London: Longmans, Green, 1870), 119–20. For the substance of this see Nicholls to Lewis, 26 February 1842, National Library of Wales, Harpton Court Mss; Nicholls, Chadwick's ally among the commissioners, found the report

But nor should we think that all was well in sanitary reporting. The commissioners' introduction may be read as an effort to embarrass Chadwick. To recognize the *Local Reports* as the real thing and Chadwick's text merely as a "digest" was to present his work as secondary; it was also to call attention to how closely the "digest" reflected the material digested (as well as to the "authenticity" of the "facts" he had derived from "other sources"). In fact, Chadwick's text is not mainly a digest, and certainly not of the local reports. On the destitution–fever question, several local reporters contradicted Chadwick's claims, a fact he ignored in the *Sanitary Report*. It is not at all clear that Chadwick expected the local reports to be published, much less to be presented as the *Sanitary Report*.[92]

Why would the commissioners embarrass Chadwick? Certainly relations were not good in 1842. Chadwick had just been passed over for a commissionership for the second time. He felt left out of policymaking, betrayed by the commissioners' flexible and pragmatic administration of the law, which, he felt, emasculated it utterly. He criticized them publicly; indeed, he was circulating a brief denouncing their administration as illegal and accusing them of suppressing reports that did not confirm their policies.[93] The *Local Reports* showed Chadwick doing that very thing – misrepresenting evidence from the field.

Lending credibility to this view is the fact that precisely this criticism – of a discrepancy between digest and digested – is the theme of the most detailed review of the *Sanitary Report*, published in the radical weekly, *The Spectator,* in mid-September. Of Chadwick's *General Report,* the reviewer complained that it was "crotchety" and "put forward with a sort of Papal infallibility – the Poor Law people against the world." The Slaney report was more useful. A week later the reviewer focused on the local reports. These were better "in freshness of observation" and several other respects than Chadwick's text. Then came the accusation:

It was no doubt far from Mr. Chadwick's intention to garble the documents submitted to him, or even to select their information in order to advance any views of his own as to the theory of disease, or to mislead Parliament into legislating for sanitary purposes. But the person who attentively examines these Reports will draw conclusions different from those which he would gain from Mr. Chadwick's volume; for a fair proportion of the

"clever" and full of "good matter" (as did Lewis) but wholly derivative of medical writers. He agreed that the commissioners could not sign it, though it is not clear why.
92 Although he quotes from local reports, he does not cite them or even speak generally of them, while he does send readers to his own appendices. In describing the conduct of the inquiry, he does not mention the local reports at all, though at least some of them had already been printed and circulated.
93 Anthony Brundage, *The Making of the New Poor Law: The Politics of Inquiry, Enactment, and Implementation, 1832–1839* (New Brunswick, N.J.: Rutgers University Press, 1978), 100. On Chadwick's earlier misrepresentations see Finer, *Chadwick,* 64, 201. On Chadwick's status and concern about poor law compromises see Finer, *Chadwick,* 188–90, 243.

medical authorities as regards number, and we think a convincing proportion as regards weight, consider that *poverty* and its concomitants are the real cause of the infectious diseases which affect the poor; and that the action of dirt, bad drainage, and bad ventilation (though highly proper things to be remedied by legislation), is slight to the operation upon the human system, compared to the depressing effects of hunger, scanty clothing, and the mental anxiety of destitution.

The reviewer echoed Alison, noting that some Scottish reporters had "interpreted the *sanitary* objects of the Commissioners into a full inquiry into the condition of the poor." He or she took issue with Chadwick's contention that wages were adequate to good housing and health, especially during periods of depression. But the crux of the matter was dishonesty: here was "a person clothed with an official character, collecting information in virtue of that character drawing up a Report which receives the sanction of his own and his superiors' public position, and is intended to lay the foundation of a legislative measure, suppressing opinions opposed to his peculiar views." The reviewer endorsed sanitary reform, but it had been "morally wrong" of Chadwick to suppress opposing views, and unwise as well: he had "armed" the opponents of sanitary reform "with a charge of dishonesty, which cannot be confuted."[94]

The review has the marks of an inside job. It strains credulity to think that within three weeks of publication a reviewer would have waded through well over a thousand pages of sanitary reports to make this criticism of incompatibility with regard to destitution and fever: someone has pointed to this particular inconsistency. Lewis seems the likeliest candidate, even though the arguments have a strong Wakleyan flavor.

Usually Chadwick resisted provocation. Not this time.[95] The claims were "untrue and libellous, and publicly as well as privately injurious," he began. His vindications were several. First, that few still believed destitution caused fever, and none went so far as Alison (who did not, in fact, claim that). He did not deny failing to include this opinion in his text but asserted that it was already in the local reports, "printed uniformly with the General Report, as easily accessible." He noted (rightly) that it would have been impossible to address destitution–fever arguments from Scottish reporters without meddling in Scottish poor law politics. Had he presented such views without comment, he would have been taken as approving them. Nor could he challenge each such claim, but had to follow the guide of "preponderant experience." He then denied claiming the harmlessness of destitution: "That absolute destitution . . . must aggravate diseases, is, so far as I am aware, questioned by no one." But a proper sanitary inquiry must be "confined to the means of im-

94 "Report on the Sanitary Condition of the Labouring Poor," *The Spectator* 15 (1842): 760–61; "Local Reports on the Sanitary Condition of the Poor of Great Britain," ibid., 928–30.
95 Edwin Chadwick, "Mr. Chadwick's *Sanitary Report*," ibid., 1001–4.

proving, not what may be termed the pecuniary condition, but the sanitary condition of the population." And because the destitution argument was or might be used to weaken the case for sanitary improvement, it had been necessary to refute it. He then reasserted the report's conclusion, that prosperity would not prevent or even diminish "epidemic disease" (a much broader term than fever, conveniently including smallpox, a disease not usually linked to destitution), and concluded by protesting the "wanton detraction by which I have been assailed to a greater extent than other officers in the same service."

In response *The Spectator* reiterated its charge. Whether destitution–fever was right or wrong was not for a digest writer to say: that person was to distill large quantities of data for easy use by others. It objected also to the artificial narrowing of "sanitary." Such an inquiry should be guided by the real phenomena of illness, not by arbitrary distinctions among presumed causes.

Like the metropolitan reports of 1838 the *Sanitary Report* caused less of a stir than is usually believed. Polite notices with extracts appeared in a few major newspapers. With the exception of the *Quarterly,* the major reviews did not cover it (Napier commissioned a review for the *Edinburgh,* but found it subpar and did not publish it). Part of the lack of interest was due to bad timing. Chadwick's report appeared at the outset of the Plug Plot riots. While civil order itself hung in the balance, the need for sewers could hardly compete.[96] One should also be skeptical of claims of massive sales. While the report may have sold well for a blue book, most copies were for presentation: as with the metropolitan reports three copies went to every union.[97]

But let us turn now from context to text.

96  See *Times,* 27, 30, 31 August, 2 September 1842; *Morning Chronicle,* 12, 30, 31 August, 1, 7, 8, 9 September 1842; *Athenaeum,* 13 August 1842, 725–26; *Manchester Guardian,* 31 August 1842; *Blackburn Gazette,* 27 August 1842. Among provincial and Scottish papers, *The Lancaster Gazette, The Lancaster Guardian and General Advertiser, The Leeds Intelligencer, The Leeds Mercury, The Caledonian Mercury,* and *The Edinburgh Evening Courant* do not appear to have reviewed the report.

97  *PLC Appendices to Minutes,* 22 August 1842, PRO MH 3/3; Chadwick to S. M. Phillipps, 15 March, 12 July 1842; Phillips to Chadwick, 19 March 1842, in *PLC–Home Office Correspondence,* PRO MH 19/64; Stationery Office to PLC, 25 July 1842, *PLC–Stationery Office Correspondence,* PRO MH 19/198. Depending on how one interprets this last, the press run negotiated on 25 July was either 9050 or 10,500. About 500 were to be sold; something on the order of 5000 were reserved for distribution to Parliament and to poor law officialdom. The main evidence of massive circulation is Flinn's statement that Chadwick claimed (in a letter to Brougham of 24 July) that 20,000 copies had already been sold (M. W. Flinn, "Introduction," *Sanitary Report,* 55). My own reading of the letter suggests that the reference is to a different report on which the two had collaborated, the "Extracts" from the reports of the investigative Poor Law Commission of 1832 (Chadwick to Brougham, 24 July 1842, UCL Chadwick Papers #378); cf. Finer, *Chadwick,* 48, 98, 209–10; Lewis, *Chadwick,* 60.

# 5

## The *Sanitary Report*

Edwin Chadwick's *Sanitary Report* of July 1842 is often seen as the great book of public health, but what kind of book is it? Usually it is seen as an exposé of conditions. In the standard view Chadwick is a simple, good man who sees clearly and speaks honestly. With his "indomitable courage, keen insight and a thirst for knowledge . . . [Chadwick] was forced by his inquiring nature into the middle of the morass. Knee deep he made his notes and put his questions. A master of detail, he displayed his facts with clearness and backed them with unanswerable statistics." He looked where no one had wanted to, found obvious problems with obvious solutions – the absence of good water and air, the presence of "filth" and therefore of disease. Chadwick was but a public servant providing information for policymakers. The *Sanitary Report* was to be neither tract, nor essay, nor treatise. Its only ideology was truth; it would "dispel by the hard light of its revelations the darkness of ignorance which hid from bourgeois eyes the domestic condition of the workers." He was good because he spake that truth about disease and dirt, water and sewers – again and again, however little people wanted to hear it. To have kept silent would have "meant more cholera deaths, more suffering." All should share sanitary appliances, "necessaries" hitherto available only to the rich, he insisted. Hence he was forcing the birth of a new kind of government based in truth and action: "His energy meant devastating and unanswerable reports upon which immediate action had to be taken."[1]

The medical historian who works through the *Sanitary Report* will be struck by how little it deals with disease. There are allusions to disease outbreaks, but little effort at epidemiology or etiological inference, a bit more on comparative mortality. Knowing Chadwick's reputation one might expect a treatment of sewers and water, and there is some of that. But there is a great deal

1 Maurice Marston, *Sir Edwin Chadwick (1800–1890)* (London: Leonard Parsons, 1925), 93, 150–52; R. A. Lewis, *Edwin Chadwick and the Public Health Movement, 1832–1854* (London: Longmans, Green, 1952), 12, 46; David Roberts, *Victorian Origins of the British Welfare State* (Hamden, Conn.: Archon Books, 1969), 99. The hyperbole has gone, but recent scholars have not substantially challenged this picture.

more about morality and "character": about illegitimacy, crime, labor unions, sedition, family values, domestic economy, dress, vagrancy. Why all this extraneous stuff? Doesn't Chadwick realize he is writing in an age of increasing urban mortality? "Cut to the cholera, Chadwick," we are likely to say.

Are we perhaps being anachronistic in expecting "public health" or even "sanitary condition" to be overtly medical? Or is Chadwick, like a good modern liberal, thoroughly and thoughtfully exploring the social environment in which disease occurs? Neither, I think. Instead, the themes of disease prevention and public medicine function rhetorically in providing the authority for reorganizing society: given the incontrovertibility of disease prevention as a social good, and the authority of science to recognize the influence on disease incidence of all manner of undesirable aspects of social and personal life, one obtains, in the name of public health, a license to reorder society.

We must learn, then, to see the *Sanitary Report* as a political document. The problems it addressed were only incidentally problems of health or even of decent living conditions, and the stakes were much larger than piped-in water and good sewers. At risk were the survival of the state in the face of revolution, and the grand question of whether the class relations of liberal industrial society could work. It was a systematic attempt to dehumanize the poor, particularly those attracted to the politics of class. The Sanitary Inquiry advanced Chadwick's career (by inventing a field in which he could be the authority) and helped the hated Poor Law Commission to survive. The initial claim of fever preventable by "sanitary reform" diverted attention from the charges of Thomas Wakley and others that the new poor law itself bore responsibility for fever. In sanitary reform the commission found a new and positive field of endeavor, and a way to emasculate the threatening medical profession as well as other rival authorities in engineering and public administration. Finally, Chadwick offered Peel and Sir James Graham an innocuous yet viable way for moderate governments to respond to the polarized condition-of-England question.[2]

Ostensibly, the *Report* is a summary of evidence, a common format in parliamentary reports. Chadwick's general points are exemplified in quotations (248 of them, some several pages in length) from informants or published accounts. But while Chadwick ends with a set of conclusions purportedly distilled from the great vat of data, by no means should the report be read as a long inductive argument. It is better seen as the masterpiece a journeyman

---

2 "He [Carlyle] does not, indeed, very clearly shadow out what he means by that question, or indicate of what other elements than the education question and the emigration question it consists. If, however, there be one question which may be called A CONDITION OF ENGLAND QUESTION, it is surely the question as to the sanatory condition of the people of England in respect to the situation and construction of their dwellings, and we are glad to be able to state that that question, which he and other political writers have overlooked, has not been neglected" [Chadwick], "Sanatory Inquiry Being Extended to Scotland," leader in an unnamed newspaper for 6 July 1840, University College London [UCL] Chadwick Papers, #112.

policy analyst crafts for his new patron, Peel. In it he displays several skills of political persuasion: he offers suggestive general inductions from preselected facts, demonizations of the "other," veiled ad hominems against key opponents, thorough and ingenious explorations of precedent, magnificent systems to solve social problems, the erudition of the obscure source (and the ignoring of familiar, yet unacceptable sources), and finally masterful management of the scope of the inquiry.

The rubric of empiricism was the means to these political ends. Because he was simply a compiler of information on the utterly new topic of sanitary condition, Chadwick need not engage with any predecessors except at his pleasure and on his terms. He could attack major figures in contemporary social policy (i.e., Malthus, Thomas Chalmers, W. P. Alison) without naming them – their views dissolved, as if by the natural force of empirical inquiry, without having ever been put on the table for criticism. Indeed, what is most remarkable about the *Report* is the absence of intellectual and political context. Though Chadwick quoted innocuous bits from Villermé and Parent-Duchâtelet, he left out their substantive work on central topics of his inquiry and virtually ignored the rest of French hygiene. He ignored also the English and Scottish literature on fever, cholera, population, and working class and occupational health – the works, for example, of Gaskell, Thackrah, and even his associate Kay. Not all of this was ideologically unacceptable, and many of these works, Gaskell's for instance, included careful, quantitative studies of the health of groups of laborers.[3]

That image of empiricism, with his control of the domain of the sanitary, allowed him to treat only those causes of social problems that he wished to deal with – for example, road pavements but not food prices – without needing to show them as prior to or more significant than other causes. When those other causes became too persistent, he could simply exclude them as outside the inquiry as if to do so somehow made them impotent or nonexistent.

This chapter is a review of the themes and arguments of the *Sanitary Report*. The *Report* consists of eight chapters, plus an Introduction and a Recapitulation of Conclusions (see illustration of contents of the *Sanitary Report*). I shall follow a tripartite division that, broadly speaking, reflects Chadwick's order of presentation. Chadwick's first two chapters are the familiar tours of insanitary Britain. The long middle section (and a late chapter on "lodging houses") deals mainly with the relations between environment and "character." The final section examines institutions for the application of expertise:

3  On Thackrah and Kay see chapters 1 and 2 of this book. See also Philip Gaskell, *The Manufacturing Population of England* (London: Baldwin and Craddock, 1833). On the French hygienists see Ann LaBerge, *Mission and Method: The Early Nineteenth-Century French Public Health Movement* (Cambridge: Cambridge University Press, 1992).

Organization of contents of Edwin Chadwick's *Sanitary Report* of 1842.

Chadwick's legal training, administrative experience, and Benthamite predilections made him most at home here. It is not a tightly organized work. On occasion his syntax is ambiguous. His statistics are inconclusive, his arguments do not always mesh, and his generalizations are sometimes undermined in the very passages he is summarizing. The section on "Bad Ventilation and Overcrowding of Private Houses," a prominent theme in the fever literature, is a mere two pages and deals substantively with neither subject; there are similar discussions of the effect of building materials in the third and sixth chapters, and separate subsections on "overcrowding of private houses" and "overcrowding of private dwellings." The arrangement of topics often seems arbitrary: "land drainage" includes a tirade against the water sellers and scavengers of Paris, while the main discussion on fever is in "Domestic Mismanagement."[4] There is no focused discussion of causes of fever, the ostensible occasion of the report.

I

The case that Britain is hideously and dangerously insanitary, and that a Benthamite program of systematic sewering could remedy that state appears mainly in the first two chapters of the *Sanitary Report*. To the extent that a case is made that insanitary conditions cause disease, that also occurs at the outset.

Chadwick began with a table, drawn from William Farr's data, of the death rate from preventable diseases, by county. He noted the costs of disease in lost labor and debilitating injury and pointed to improvements in naval hygiene to show the feasibility of prevention. And he insisted that the evidence pointed to one cause: "atmospheric impurity, occasioned by means within the control of legislation, as the main cause of the ravages of epidemic, endemic, and contagious diseases among the community, and as aggravating most other diseases."[5] The term was broad and vague – it could refer to overcrowded houses or humid marsh air. That "atmospheric impurity" harmed health few would have doubted; that it was the key cause of disease would have required much more proof, and this Chadwick did not offer. He said nothing of the reports of Arnott, Kay, and Smith. With the documents that shaped it thus hidden, the *Report* could appear theory-free. But while the claim of atmospheric cause is put forth as a generalization from the evidence,

---

4 Even friendly critics found the going tough: "We cannot say that he [Chadwick] shows much skill in the grouping and arranging of his facts and views" ([F. B. Head], "Report on the Sanitary Condition of the Labouring Classes," *Quarterly Review* 71 [1842–43]: 423).
5 Edwin Chadwick, *Report on the Sanitary Condition of the Labouring Population of Great Britain*, ed. M. W. Flinn (Edinburgh: Edinburgh University Press, 1965), 79. To be cited as Chadwick, *Sanitary Report*.

Chadwick made only rudimentary gestures at deriving it. In practice it was an axiom.

If disease is a product of atmosphere it is also a product of place and may be influenced by structures. Chadwick's first chapter is on the "General Condition of the *Residences* of the Labouring Classes Where Disease Is Found to Be the Most Prevalent" (italics mine). For Chadwick structures, not persons with unique histories (or even populations), are the significant loci, for they either promote or inhibit the all-powerful "malaria," the only significant cause of disease. Thus, one may speak of healthy or diseased places or structures without reference to the persons who occupy them: humans are but a litmus test of environmental condition. But usually one need not look for that confirmation; health can be discerned from the outside, from streets, drains, and dung heaps.

This chapter is a tour of insanitary Britain. Chadwick begins in Cornwall; twenty-six quotations later, he reaches Glasgow, conveniently the apotheosis of filth. Chadwick is ostentatiously empirical, marshaling quotations purporting to represent conditions in all corners of the land. Letting the evidence "speak for itself," he offers few comments, needing only to state what is to be the obvious induction. The argument is hidden, presupposed in the statement to be confirmed. For example, what one learns from the "tour" of filthy residences is that there are plenty of examples of them; that they are associated with disease, Chadwick suggests; that they are preferentially associated with disease he does not bother to argue.

The theme is ubiquity: the dung heaps, marshes, reeking privies that are to inspire our vicarious revulsion are everywhere. The tiny parish of Breadsall represents rural England, while Truro represents the "condition of the town population" and Windsor demonstrates "that the highest neighbourhoods in power and wealth do not at present possess securities for the prevention of nuisances dangerous to the public health." Yet already there is much unclear about what "sanitary condition" encompasses. Despite its title, the chapter's focus is not housing; many passages are more concerned with external filth (dung heaps), or with pervasive dampness from poor drainage. Some do not deal with disease at all; many deal with diseases other than fever and attribute them to deplorable conditions in general, even to destitution. John Fox describes agricultural laborers in Dorset as "badly fed, badly clothed, and many of them habitually dirty, and consequently typhus, synochus, or diarrhoea, constantly prevailed." He adds that these people were "very poor, very dirty, and usually in rags, living almost wholly on bread and potatoes, scarcely ever tasting animal food, and consequently highly susceptible of disease and very unable to contend with it."[6]

Many of the instances of malign atmosphere are in the section entitled "The

6 Ibid., 81–84, 87.

Sanitary Effect of Land Drainage." There Chadwick cited reports from medical officers on undrained places with disease and on well drained places without disease. Generally, correspondents were vague as to what diseases were caused by wetness or "incipient moisture."[7] He related a visit from a medical officer who suddenly rushed off, convinced from a change in weather and the draining of a canal that fever would be awaiting him when he got home (Chadwick does not say whether it was).[8] Finally there were Dr. Edward Harrison's tales (from 1804) of sheep getting "rot" (which he equated to typhus) from walking a miry road. A beast removed from the flock had not been stricken; those "left to graze in the ditches and lane" had. Certain conditions of temperature and moisture could make a pleasant meadow deadly. Sheep could " 'be tainted in a quarter of an hour, while the land retains its moisture and the weather is hot and sultry.' " A shepherd must know that " 'if after providing drained pasture and avoiding 'rotting places' in the fields, all his care may be frustrated if he do not avoid, with equal care, leading the sheep over wet and miry roads with stagnant ditches.' " The same precautions would be "equally applicable to the labouring population who traverse such roads," Chadwick added.[9]

Far from a careful summation of contemporary knowledge either on epizootics or on human diseases associated with moist land, this was an epidemiology of superstition, of fears of a malign, perhaps a willfully malign, nature. A person or animal has sickened and we seek some plausible, environmental malignance to bear responsibility. While Chadwick expressed surprise at the importance of land drainage ("of a magnitude of which no conception had been formed"),[10] medical writers had long been concerned with the problem. Intermittent and remittent fever were invariably associated with wet soils and had been since Hippocrates. The seventeenth-century fen drainage had been promoted in part for reasons of health. Indeed, the environmental sensibilities and disease theories to which Chadwick appealed would have been as familiar to his readers as worries about carcinogenic chemicals are to us. Centuries of hygienic lore advocated good air, dry soil, and removal of decomposing dung – but also sufficient food, clothing, and shelter.

In this second chapter, "Public Arrangements External to the Residences by Which the Sanitary Condition of the Labouring Population Is Affected," Chadwick was moving even further from diseases in persons. He tried to show the effects of good sewers with two dubious epidemiological demonstrations. William Baker of Derby had traced fever in adjoining houses along an unfilled

---

7 I.e., "Although malaria does not produce diseases of any *decided character*, yet, during a wet spring or autumn, there are always cases of inflammation of the lungs or bowels, and rheumatism, both in acute and chronic forms." Ibid., 152; see also 157.
8 Ibid., 155.
9 Ibid., 158.
10 Ibid., 150.

ditch. Though Baker stated the relationships among the stricken, he did not consider the possibility of contagion: their disease arose from air contaminated by a "succession of foul and stinking pools."[11] A Mr. Crowfoot, "one of the most eminent of the medical practitioners in Suffolk," noted the lower mortality rate of Beccles, in a bad site but with good sewers, than in nearby Bungay, with a good site and no sewers. Selecting suggestive cases was a characteristic approach. There was the barest pretense of a general induction, much less of a testing alternative hypotheses.[12]

The section "Street and Road Cleansing: Road Pavements" was mandated on the grounds that "the external condition of the dwelling powerfully and immediately affects . . . internal cleanliness and general economy."[13] Street cleaning was a well-recognized public responsibility. Hundreds of local acts from 1750 onward had given towns power to keep streets clean and free of obstructions.[14] Why, then, were they so full of holes and why did efforts to clean them so often lead only to piles of malarial muck? The answer was a lack of "science." Parliament was to blame for bad streets, as it had "presume[d] that no science, no skill is requisite for the attainment of the objects, or presume[d] both to be universal."[15]

"Science" was Chadwick's all-purpose authority. More than empirical inquiry or a testing of what had been taken for granted, it meant rational systematic action. Chadwick conceived of "scientific administration" in much the same way that Frederick Winslow Taylor would later conceive of "scientific management." In the case of roads, science indicated drains. In towns, drains must carry more or less of the wastes that befouled the streets. If one asked why that refuse were not more regularly removed, the answer was that it was too costly to cart (in part because the streets were so befouled by it). How could removal be made cheaper? By suspending it in water and letting it drain away through sewers. Why was this not done? Because the sewage would pollute streams. Here Chadwick paused. A problem existed, but one surely "inappreciable . . . in comparison with the ill health occasioned by the constant retention of several hundred thousand accumulations of pollution in the most densely-peopled districts."[16] Luckily, not only was it a minor evil, but also an avoidable one, for sewage could be used to fertilize pasture or arable land, as in Edinburgh, where the "Foul Burn," carrying the street drainage of the old town, fertilized the sands of Portobello.

11 Ibid., 99–102.
12 Ibid., 102–3. The rates, 1:69 versus 1:67, are nearly the same. Chadwick does not consider alternative explanations of death rates.
13 Ibid., 111.
14 Frederick H. Spencer, *Municipal Origins: An Account of English Private Bill Legislation Relating to Local Government, 1740–1835; with a Chapter on Private Bill Procedure* (London: Constable and Co., 1911).
15 Ibid., 109–10.
16 Ibid., 120–21.

If it were so profitable, why was sewage irrigation not widely used, and why did many Edinburghians (like Chadwick's friend Sir William Drysdale) so object to it? Because, answered Chadwick, it was not being done scientifically and the proceeds were not going to the public. A regional, holistic, scientific perspective would make clear that irrigation could be done safely and profitably by using steam power to pump sewage farther and allow its use on more land. Thus sewage farms would solve the street cleaning problem, which solved the dirty house problem, which in turn solved the disease problem.

This is typical of what might be called Chadwick's Benthamite mode: he retreats from the problem of the diseased person — who barely enters the discussion — to increasingly more general levels that presumably determine that problem — house, street, town, region. At each level, the impediment to the obvious solution appears on the next level. Once one arrives at the ideal level of analysis — here the drainage basin — solutions are comprehensive: they satisfy all legitimate criteria, require no significant trade-offs, and, if one does proper accounting, have no ultimate costs (initial capital may be needed), since the solution to one problem is the solution to all associated problems. A simple improvement may trigger a cascade of benefits: a harder, smoother road surface would allow use of lighter vehicles pulled by fewer horses, which would cause less wear of pavement, less need for cleaning of streets, less health and property damage from dust, cheaper commodities, and so on.[17]

## II

In the long middle section of the *Report* Chadwick did deal with people. One had to: their behavior dictated what would be the effects of a technology. Knowledge of that behavior guided rational technological change.

That concern is first evident with regard to water. Chadwick confessed himself shocked; earlier investigations had not disclosed a widespread water scarcity. He wrote of people waiting through the night for water, getting water from puddles or even from "the prints made by horses' feet."[18] But what must such a life be like? Thus far, Chadwick had been more interested in drains and dung heaps than in the people affected by them. The issue of people's interaction with water arose with regard to whether water need be laid on to every dwelling or merely made available at a nearby common tap. Chadwick held that each residence needed its own water because the alternative was exhausting and inhumane: "The whole family of the labouring man in the manufacturing towns rise early . . . they return to their homes late

17 Ibid., 131–32.
18 Ibid., 135, 140.

at night. It is a serious inconvenience, as well as discomfort to them to have to fetch water at a distance out of doors from the pump or the river on every occasion that it may be wanted, whether it may be in cold, in rain, or in snow."[19] But such a subject's eye view is rare – and disingenuous, for the beneficiaries of convenience and comfort are not solely (or mainly) the water drawers themselves, but capital accumulation and political stability. Productive, employable time was spent waiting to fill water containers.[20] And crowds at pumps, especially of girls, threatened order and morality: bad language was learned, squabbles arose, and assignations were made.

The case of squabbling girls in water queues is an instance of what is arguably the main concern of Chadwick and of all condition-of-England writers: the relation of physical to "moral" condition. In the *Report*, the humans who populate such discussions are almost always objectified entities. Chadwick's determinism excludes subjectivity; what counts is behavior: political passivity, frugality, sobriety, responsibility. Perhaps this is more style than substance, but it does distinguish Chadwick from many others, including Southwood Smith, who approached reform with evangelical concerns. For them the (subjective) state of the soul was primary, and behavior relevant only as a measure of it.

In one of his "overcrowding" sections, Chadwick explained how he came to give so much attention to morality in a report ostensibly about the physical causes of disease. It came from informants: as well as being seen as a direct cause of disease, "overcrowding is also frequently noticed as a cause of extreme demoralization and recklessness, and recklessness, again, as a cause of disease."[21] In fact, Chadwick was no longer much interested in the disease, but in the recklessness itself. Finding a third of the men in a marshy rural district rheumatic, he deemed it "evident that the prevalence of damp and marsh miasma from the want of drainage, if it did not necessitate, formed a strong temptation to, the use of ardent spirits."[22]

One effect of this recognition was to circumvent the destitution–disease claim. One might admit destitution as an immediate cause of disease, but attribute destitution to "recklessness," and "recklessness," in turn, to some hypothetical exposure to physical causes. But it was a general political argument: any behavior Chadwick wished to discredit could be explained away as a pathological effect of a bad environment. In a section on ventilation, for example, he explained that breathing vitiated air led to "nervous exhaustion" among London tailors, which in turn led to a need for stimulants (gin during work), which only augmented the exhaustion. Here, not only intemperance,

19 Ibid., 141.
20 Ibid., 142.
21 Ibid., 190.
22 Ibid., 196.

but also the very mental competence (and political program) of radical metropolitan artisans might be attributed to poor ventilation.[23]

Such was the thrust of a late chapter, "Lodging Houses." Lodging houses were not originally part of the topic of the inquiry. From a miasmatic standpoint, there was no reason to think the urban miasma more deadly to transients than to families in crowded tenements. Yet many informants associated lodging houses with disease and felt that they ought to be regulated or even eliminated. Chadwick accepted their contagionist explanation: though a town may be "highly advanced in . . . general drainage, and its arrangements for house and street-cleansing may be perfect," unless its lodging houses were properly policed, "it will be liable to the continued importation, if not the generation, of epidemic disease." Yet the focus, both for Chadwick and for many of his correspondents, was "moral depravation": crime, political agitation, and illicit sex – dangerous people. Several did not mention disease at all: Thus, Birmingham, where the lodging houses were the "resort of the most abandoned characters . . . sources of extreme misery and vice." Or Brighton, where the filth was transferred from physical environment to human inhabitants: "The streets in this neighbourhood have for many years been an intolerable nuisance. . . . They are the resort of tramps, begging impostors, thieves, and prostitutes of the lowest description, who daily and nightly take their rounds through the town." Or in the Tees valley, where even well built lodging houses were "a source of physical and moral disease."[24]

More than most others, these passages exhibit the revulsion–fascination that characterized sanitary inquiry. One can taste the spit and feel the shudder with which these writers utter their "disgusting"'s or "deplorable"'s. For Chadwick and some of his correspondents lodging houses were "receptacles," a word otherwise used for a container for refuse or dung.[25] Yet however much the writers blanch, they are mesmerized with the awful and exotic (the sanitarian sublime). They describe some things, push readers to imagine the rest.

The most dramatic proof of "how strongly circumstances that are governable govern the habits of the population, and in some instances appear almost to breed the species of the population," is the case of cesspool emptiers, water carriers, and those unofficial scavengers who gleaned a living sifting through street muck. Most of the evidence came from Paris, where these "turbulent

23 Chadwick implies that any artisans working in close quarters were ill and politically irresponsible. Tailors, cobblers, and other artisans made up the core of London radical politics. Contemporaries would have associated tailor shops in particular with the Westminster tailor Francis Place, who had risen from a sweatshop worker to a sweatshop proprietor. Place, Benthamite, Malthusian, political power broker, was Chadwick's rival for a poor law commissionership. Chadwick is thus able to get in a subtle dig at Place's own sanity and to suggest that this hero of the common man might be harming his own employees. Westminster radicalism is thus made a product of nervous exhaustion and gin.
24 Ibid., 411–15.
25 Ibid., 412.

bodies of men" were "degraded and savage . . . ready to throw away their wretched lives on every occasion . . . conspicuous actors in the revolution of 1830." He quoted a prefect of police, petrified at walking among these "men with naked arms and haggard figures, and sinister looks . . . hideous aspect . . . [and] hoarse and ferocious cries." No longer are these beings human: "They had neither human tastes nor sympathies, nor even human sensations, for they reveled in the filth which is grateful to dogs, and other lower animals." There were refuse parasites in Britain too: 598 in London, 302 in Manchester, 100 in Bath. They were criminals and haunters of workhouses, not the fevered laboring poor who were to have been the subject of the report.[26]

This theme of filth-bred life was stock in trade of the armchair explorer of social exotica.[27] But how did people get this way? Chadwick does not say. Indeed, while the passage is to illustrate the effect of environment on innocent victims, he is at the same time pointing a finger. These people are evil: they are presented as freely choosing their way of life. Take their diet, for example, according to a witness: " 'I have seen them take a bone from a dung-heap, and gnaw it while reeking hot with the fermentation of decay.' " Indeed, in a backhanded way Chadwick admitted that these people were behaving exactly as the political economists would have them do. In a rational economy refuse would find its highest use; these canny laborers had found an unexploited niche. Yet he could not accept it – even if these able-bodied workers had to be shut up in workhouses, it was imperative to "force a change to other occupations of a less degrading character." And, having noted that such people were an "idle, dissolute class," always "prowling about the stables, yards, backs of premises and lanes," one informant mentioned as an afterthought that replacing such labor with an automatic mode of filth removal might also benefit "health."[28]

The problem Chadwick was reckoning with was general. Mainly, he was making a case for environmental determinism. Whatever the problem – immoral sexual activity or political agitation – it was to be seen as a product of physical conditions. The power of this deterministic argument lay in its universality. Even gentlefolk would act like sinners unless they had their necessary sewers. Civilization itself was no stronger than the thin wall of the pipe sewer. Yet fully to convey the enormity of determinism one had show that conditions could obliterate all traces of original humanity, leaving depraved and completely alien souls.[29] Thus, at some point the poor were no longer in-

26 Ibid., 162–65.
27 Chadwick would later cite a metaphor used by Walker, a Thames Police magistrate, in testimony to the Poor Law Commission, to describe the effects of the environment on human beings: "If you will have marshes and stagnant waters you will there have suitable animals, and the only way of getting rid of them is by draining the marshes" (ibid., 202).
28 Ibid., 164–65.
29 Chadwick would cite the observations of the Reverend Whitwell Elwin of Bath. Elwin noted how quickly the effects of structure were felt: "A person accustomed to fresh air, and all the

nocent victims, but truly depraved beasts. As Chadwick said little of *how* physical conditions produced moral effects (he left that to imagination), readers were simply given a correlation – revolting conditions and despicable people.[30] By no means was the determinism conundrum unique to Chadwick, but other reformers found more coherent responses. Believing in the essential goodness of humans, Southwood Smith, for example, usually managed to avoid depravity-mongering. To the evangelical Lord Ashley depravity was something we all struggled with. Bad conditions exacerbated it; he saw a duty to help others overcome it.

These opposing images – innocent victims of environment, yet also repulsive evil agents – appear in many sections of the *Report*. Bad structures, for example, generated a population "prone to passionate excitement . . . apt instruments for political discontents; their moral perceptions . . . obliterated . . . characterised by a 'ferocious indocility which . . . destroys their social nature, and transforms them into something little better than wild beasts.' " Examples included an Edinburgh man murdering his wife in "a fit of passion," people who admitted that they'd last washed when last in prison, in Glasgow "a thousand children who have no names, whatever, or only nicknames, like dogs."[31]

Particularly threatening to social stability were women and youths, the former through sex, the latter through political agitation. Chadwick's focus was men. Sanitation was to end the need for support of widows and orphans by preventing men's premature deaths. Since they *are* the problems, women and youths do not also have full status as victims of problems; indeed, in some places he hints that women, children, and infants are welcome to shuffle off this coil when they choose: if fatal disease were only to strike them as frequently as it struck men, there would be no problem. The men, however, have responsibilities.

One of the chief subjects in a rambling section, "The Want of Separate Apartments, and Overcrowding of Private Dwellings," was precocious or im-

---

comforts of civilized life, goes into a miserable room, dirty, bare, and, above all, sickening from the smell. Judging from his own sensations, he conceives that nothing but the most abject poverty could have produced this state of things, and he can imagine nothing necessary to a cure but a way for escape. A very simple experiment will correct these erroneous impressions. Let him remain a short time in the room, and the perception of closeness will so entirely vanish that he will almost fancy that the atmosphere has been purified since his entrance. There are few who are not familiar with this fact; and if such are the effects of an hour in blunting our refined sensations, and rendering them insensible to noxious exhalations, what must be the influence of years on the coarser perceptions of the working-man?" (ibid., 203).

30  At base, the problem arises in trying to give moral phenomena physical causes. When Arnott and Kay had distinguished causes of fever "independent of habits" from causes "originating in habits," they had been making a distinction of moral responsibility based on a long-standing distinction between those things which people freely chose and those which happened to them. "Moral" and "physical" were accordingly mutually exclusive categories; "moral" could not be made to derive from physical without ceasing to be truly moral.

31  *Sanitary Report*, 198–99.

proper sexual activity or simply sexual knowledge, mainly among women. Overcrowding had been a standard issue for fever writers, who worried about concentrated effluvia, but in the *Sanitary Report* it referred to shared beds and was usually a euphemism for incest.[32] The Ampthill union clerk told of a family of eleven in two rooms, seven sleeping in one bed. "How could it be otherwise . . . than that they should be sunk into a most deplorable state of degradation and depravity?" Surely "their degraded moral state is mainly attributable to the wretched way in which they have lived and herded together."[33] A Romsey medical officer reported twenty-one people in a two room cottage, fourteen sleeping in one room. "Here are the young woman and young man of 18 or 20 years of age lying alongside of the father and mother, and the latter actually in labour. It will be asked what is the condition of the inmates? – Just such as might be expected." Robert Baker, the Leeds factory inspector, told of "brothers and sisters, and lodgers of both sexes . . . occupying the same sleeping room with the parents, and consequences occur which humanity shudders to contemplate." From his experience of more than 100 visits, Riddal Wood of the Manchester Statistical Society had many stories of "persons of different sexes sleeping promiscuously": mothers and grown sons, man and wife's sister, a girl remaining in her chemise during his visit, seeing nothing wrong in that. In such cases "the sense of decency was obliterated"; such sleeping arrangements led to prostitution, Wood believed.[34]

The most detailed illustration of environmental determinism concerned not overcrowding, but the effects of bad cottages. It was the story of a visit (by whom is not clear) to an ex-servant, married and living in a wretched cottage. "For her station," this woman

had received a very excellent religious and moral education. Before her marriage she had been distinguished by the refinement with which she sung national airs, and for her knowl-

---

32 Of nine passages on overcrowding, only one raises the issue of disease from this source. The effects of different kinds of cottages on "moral condition" was explicitly one of the issues of the inquiry; one respondent translated this into the "comparative character of the female inmates and children"; cf. J. Woodman, in Robert Weale, "On Cottage Accommodation in Bedford, Northampton, and Stafford," *Sanitary Condition of the Labouring Population. Local Reports for England and Wales, P.P.,* House of Lords 27, 1842, 131–32; *Report to Her Majesty's Principal Secretary of State for the Home Office on the Sanitary Condition of the Labouring Population of Great Britain* (London: Clowes, 1842), xii, xv.

33 *Sanitary Report*, 190–91. Like many of the stories Chadwick included, this one was less than compatible with his doctrines. There had been no problem with this family, and the father had been a good worker, until the cottage had been pulled down and the family forced into a workhouse. At that point the husband deserted the family, the eldest daughter gave birth to an illegitimate child, and another daughter was sentenced to transportation. Yet the clerk nevertheless maintained that workhouse had improved the "grossly filthy habits and . . . disgusting behaviour" of this family. Ampthill was notorious as a site of resistance to the new poor law (Charles May, "Report to the Poor Law Commission on Outrages," *Poor Law Commission [PLC]–Ampthill Correspondence*, 1835, Public Record Office [PRO] MH 12/1). The phrase "herding together" was common and portrays the poor as making the rational choice to become animals.

34 *Sanitary Report*, 191–93.

edge of the Bible and of the doctrines of her church. Her personal condition had become of "a piece" with the wretched stone undrained hovel, with a pigsty before it, in which she had been taken. We found her with rings of dirt about her neck, and turning over with dirty hands Brown's Dictionary, to see whether the newly-elected minister was "sound" in his doctrine.

The passage asserts not only the influence of conditions, but also their primacy over education and religion. This was a central issue in Scottish poor law reform. It is the gratuitous detail – "Brown's Dictionary" and "sound" doctrine – that transforms a general argument into a joke at the expense of Thomas Chalmers.[35] Here the marks of mature Christianity – for Chalmers the key to betterment – are hallmarks (even causes?) of degradation.

The general effect of such an approach is to invalidate the subjectivity of those who lived in overcrowded dwellings or poorly built cottages.[36] Its particular effect was to exclude women from the category of sufferers of sanitary conditions. Chadwick neither blames women for such problems nor sees them as victims; that issue is moot, for they are objects. In the felicific calculus of Bentham, the problems that they somehow embody – illegitimacy, prostitution, and immorality – belong to the society (and the economy) generally. If there must be a particular *one* who suffers problems, that one is the working-class man as the presumptive economic and political unit. In effect, then, women become "sanitary conditions": in conjunction with certain aspects of structure, they are the generators of certain forms of social instability. One stabilized the workhouse or prison by eliminating or segregating women. Clearly that was impracticable in the laborer's dwelling, but the crowdedness

35 Ibid., 196. This passage follows a similar story from "a lady who is my informant." It is possible, though I think unlikely, that the "I" who narrates the story is not Chadwick, but someone else who had been informed by the lady. If it is Chadwick telling the story, it is unique in being the only case of his using his own experience as evidence in the report. *The Dictionary of the Bible*, by the eighteenth-century Haddington minister John Brown (1722–87), went through twelve Scottish editions by 1862. Brown anticipated Chalmers as an evangelical critic of the Scottish church. Elsewhere (199), Chadwick took direct issue with Chalmers's claims: "I consider that the use of the whiskey and the prostration of the education and moral habits for which the Scottish labourers have been distinguished is, to a considerable extent, attributable to the surrounding physical circumstances, including the effects of bad ventilation." See also 200: "No education as yet commonly given appears to have availed against such demoralizing circumstances . . . but the cases of moral improvement of a population, by cleansing, draining, and the improvement of the internal and external conditions of the dwellings . . . are more numerous and decided. . . . The most experienced public officers acquainted with the condition of the inferior population of the towns would agree in giving the first place in efficiency and importance to improvement, and that as against such barriers moral agencies have but a remote chance of success."

36 In only one of nine passages was there any effort at reflecting a subjective perspective. Wondering how an agricultural laborer's family packed twelve into a twenty-four by sixteen foot cottage, preserved "common decency . . . [and avoided] unutterable horrors," a Durham canon asked the man: " 'Pray,' said I, 'do you not think that this is a very improper way of disposing of your family?' 'Yes, certainly,' was the answer, 'it is very improper in a Christian point of view; but what can we do until they build us better houses' " *(Sanitary Report*, 191–92).

problem for Chadwick does translate into the need for woman-neutralizing structures.

The problem of rambunctious youth arose in regard to the question of how much society would save by adopting preventive measures. The main savings would be in lowered costs for the support of widows and orphans left by prematurely dying male workers. A study of the average age of men who left widows and orphans showed that had they lived an expected life span they would have been able to support their children to responsible adulthood.[37] Yet widows posed still further social costs. If they remarried, they would usually choose men in the same work as the previous husband(s). These would then die, having fathered even more children, who would then compete for the few jobs and without fatherly influence turn to crime or political agitation.[38] It is an odd argument, this parade of dying husbands, and serves mainly as the warrant for Chadwick's claim that the "vice and crime" of callow youths must be reckoned among the costs of sanitary neglect.[39]

By "vice and crime" he meant mainly political and labor agitation. He cited his own Constabulary Commission work:

Older men, we were assured by their employers . . . perceived that . . . large capital, was not the means of their depression, but of their steady and abundant support. They were generally . . . above the influence of the anarchical fallacies which appeared to sway those wild and really dangerous assemblages. . . . On expostulating . . . with middle-aged and experienced workmen on the folly as well as the injustice of their trade unions, by which the public peace was compromised by the violences of strike after strike, . . . the workmen . . . invariably disclaimed connexion with the proceedings. . . . The common expression was, they would not attend to be borne down by "mere boys," who were furious, and knew not what they were about. The predominance of a young and violent majority was general.

These juvenile delinquents were victims of a degeneration that affected moral and intellectual ability as well as physical size. They could not be taught, were "torpid . . . irritable and bad tempered." These facts showed how "the noxious physical agencies . . . [also acted] as obstacles to education and to moral culture; that in abridging the duration of the adult life of the working classes

---

37 Chadwick does not consider situations, increasingly frequent in factories, in which labor of women and children supported men. It may also be noted that the suggestion that the widowing of the wives of working men was sufficiently common to be a problem does not fit well with his claim that place and structure, not work, caused disease, but he does not seem aware of that problem – he says little about a sex differential in mortality rate.

38 *Sanitary Report*, 269–70. The result will be "three widows instead of one, and three sets of stunted and unhealthy children dependent for . . . various periods . . . and competing for employment at the same place, instead of one set of healthy children arrived at the age of working ability for self-support." Here Chadwick does use Malthusian modes of analysis and raise Malthusian concerns. The number of marriages is the crucial variable, and Chadwick implies that it is better for these young people not to get jobs, so they will not marry so early.

39 *Sanitary Report*, 254.

. . . they substitute, for a population that accumulates and preserves instruction and is steadily progressive, a population that is young, inexperienced, ignorant, credulous, irritable, passionate, and dangerous, having a perpetual tendency to moral as well as physical deterioration."[40]

This assault on the legitimacy of the emerging labor movement is the context of much of Chadwick's discussion of occupational health. In large measure, his views in the *Sanitary Report* extend the perspective of the 1833 Factory Commission. They may also reflect his increasingly close ties with the manufacturers' outlook: In 1838 he had married Rachel, daughter of John Kennedy, a major cotton manufacturer and one of the founders of the Manchester Statistical Society. Chadwick did see a warrant for state interference in dusty trades, if only to protect ratepayers, who would otherwise have to support widows and orphans. He urged also that employers be made responsible for accidents as they were in the best position to prevent them.[41] Yet in most cases he went to great lengths to refute claims of work-induced disease. Given the poor law philosophy of pushing people into work, it would not do to find that work was killing workers, just as it would not do to find that lack of food was killing them. He hoped the *Report* would "disabuse the popular mind of much prejudice against particular branches of industry arising from the belief that causes of ill health really *accidental* and removable . . . are *essentials* to the employment itself."[42] He blamed workers: in lead manufacture, damage to health was due to workers' "recklessness." In any programs to aid them, "such workmen . . . [were] to be regarded and treated as children, for they are children in intellect." In the case of noxious trades, sobriety was the "best means of withstanding the effects of the noxious agencies which they have to encounter. Amongst the painters, for example, the men who are temperate and cleanly suffer little . . . but if any one of them become intemperate, the noxious causes take effect with a certainty and rapidity proportioned to the relaxed domestic habit." Where an occupation–mortality link was undeniable, one might nevertheless posit factors outside the workplace. Disease among Durham coal miners was attributable to the crowding of too many people into unventilated sleeping rooms or to their walk home.[43]

---

40  Ibid., 266–68.
41  Ibid., 261–62, 271.
42  Ibid., 181, 183.
43  Ibid., 320, 203, 176–77, 258–61. Chadwick quoted (183) the instruction given to the medical inspectors in the 1833 factory commission. Upon finding cases of "excessive . . . effects of labour" they were to "investigate minutely the concurrent causes of ill health . . . to examine and report the state of the drains in and about the factory: the state of the neighbourhood of the factory as to dryness or dampness, cleanliness or filthiness: the state of the houses and neighbourhood in which the children and adult workpeople take their meals and exercise (if they leave the factory), and where they sleep: the state of the air within the factory, and which the workpeople usually respire, whether it be fresh or whether it be not fresh, owing to deficient ventilation, – whether it be pure, or whether it be rendered impure by effluvia floating in it, and if so, what the effluvia are: what organs of the body are likely to be injured, and what, from careful examination, you find to be

The main discussion of fever occurred not in connection with work but with wages, or rather, since Chadwick believed that laborers' wages were adequate and even too high, with "Domestic Mismanagement." Proof of "depraved domestic habits" came from a comparison, by Charles Mott, assistant poor law commissioner for Lancashire, of prudent and imprudent families living on the same streets, doing the same work, getting the same wages. Mott listed ten respectable and ten dissolute families in similar circumstances. Chadwick quoted the conclusion of Wood of Dundee on such findings: "We have on the one hand, filth, destitution, and disease, associated with good wages; and on the other, cleanliness, comfort, and comparative good health in connexion with wages which are much lower. . . . Filth, fever, and destitution in many families is occasioned, not by their small incomes, but by a misapplication or a prodigal waste of . . . their otherwise sufficient wages."[44] Mott saw himself demonstrating the independence of character; to Chadwick it showed only that low income was no excuse.

This section includes Chadwick's attack on William Pulteney Alison's view of poverty as a cause of disease. Chadwick claimed that his investigation found little support for the view that epidemic disease was "occasioned by extreme indigence, or that it can be made generally to disappear simply by grants of money. In the great mass of cases . . . the attacks of disease are upon those in full employment, the attack of fever precedes the destitution, not the destitution the disease."[45] While insisting that he represented "the majority of the medical officers" Chadwick quoted only one authority to support the claim, Dr. William Davidson, physician to the Glasgow Fever Hospital. Studying the "physical habit" or "constitution" of admittees to the hospital, Davidson had found only a tiny minority to be "emaciated or unhealthy in appearance."[46] Chadwick failed to mention that Davidson himself did not see this "influence of delicacy of constitution" as relating to the destitution–fever claim, which he took to be well established.

The evidence on this point was indeed too great to ignore. Chadwick reinterpreted it, blaming the weather: "Wet or bad seasons, which suspend agricultural industry and much labour in the towns, is [sic] usually of a character of itself to predispose to disease, if not to produce it." The closest Chadwick would come to admitting deprivation as a cause was that it might prevent the poor from buying soap to remove the filth that caused the miasma. He admitted that the oft observed winter mortality peak (an observation more compatible with a deprivation than a decomposition explanation) showed the

---

actually injured; the temperature of the air, the highest, the lowest, and the average temperature, and the condition of the air as to dryness and moisture" (see chapter 3).

44 Ibid., 206–9.

45 Ibid., 210. This was a straw man. The view that poverty was the sole cause of fever was held by few if any.

46 Ibid., 210–11, 216.

effects of "cold, wet, and crowding," but took the observation to indicate the need for drainage (of these three "wet" was the most "remediable"; heat was off limits as a marketable commodity).[47] And, Chadwick finally noted, the matter was moot: deprivation (or rather, since wages were adequate, "mismanagement of expenditure in respect to supplies of food . . . [and] also in respect to clothing and fuel") as a cause of fever did "not come within the immediate scope of the present inquiry," which he understood to be "the evils affecting their sanitary condition, that come within the recognized provinces of legislation or local administration."[48] However much Chadwick might wish it otherwise, food prices and wage rates had been and were "recognized provinces of legislation."

In fact, the main disease from which Durham miners or journeyman tailors or other artisans died was not fever but consumption. Indeed, among the groups Chadwick considered, the ratio of respiratory deaths (including consumption) to fever deaths ranged from two to one to ten to one.[49] Yet despite its prominence consumption remained on the periphery of public health for most of the century. Chadwick excluded it from the *Report* (except in connection with ventilation and temperature change) on the grounds that "investigation of the whole of the contributory causes to the production of the immense mass of mortality occasioned by that disease, would be beyond the time or means allowed for the present inquiry."[50] In short, consumption was left out because it was too important.

In a mortality-driven public health the exclusion of consumption would have been indefensible. In many places and among many groups it was a much greater cause of mortality than fever. It struck people in their working years and as a chronic condition represented a greater burden on society than did brief bursts of fever. But consumption could not be fully recognized as a public health problem; the conditions of its emergence seemed none other than the totality of conditions of life for many people. Throughout the *Report*, Chadwick appealed to a threshold concept. Once it was reached, the poor but healthy artisan suddenly became acutely ill. In consumption there seemed no clear border between health and illness. Even more than fever, it was a classic debility disease, a concomitant of hard work, poor food, wet and cold, crowdedness, dirt and dust. Fever might be incidental to the industrial world; the same could not be said of consumption.

Oddly, what is often seen as Chadwick's most vivid demonstration of the priority of physical over economic causes of disease, the comparison by the Manchester Statistical Society of mortality in the industrial Northwest and in

47  Ibid., 213.
48  Ibid., 218.
49  Ibid., 167–71, 256.
50  Ibid., 174.

rural Rutlandshire, did not for him have that significance.[51] Instead, the lower mortality in Rutlandshire than Manchester showed that "moral causes, inducing habits of sobriety," were more important than wages, which were much higher in Manchester.[52] It is important to consider why, given this opportunity to document the urban demographic penalty, Chadwick turns away from structural factors.

There are several reasons. First, Chadwick had already claimed in principle that morality was determined by structures. Second, the survey itself and the society that commissioned it tended to be concerned with presumably independent moral variables: Riddal Wood, the investigator, was interested in whether dwellings were "well furnished" and "comfortable." Third, the data were by no means wholly compatible with a physical conditions explanation; one could not equate rural with sanitary and urban with insanitary. Yet the main reason for the prominence of moral (and rational) competence is that such arguments were essential in refuting Malthus.

Chadwick does not mention Malthus, as he had not mentioned Alison, but he did devote much space to arguing that Malthus's "positive checks" – epidemics, famine, and "vice" – did little to stem the rate of population growth. On the contrary, where mortality was high, births were also high, "more than sufficient to replace the deaths, however numerous they may be."[53] The records of Geneva, where two-and-a-half centuries of registration data were available, showed that "the increased duration of life had been attended by a progression in happiness: as prosperity advanced marriages became fewer and later; the proportion of births were reduced, but greater numbers of the infants . . . were preserved." This perspective reflected the optimism he shared with Nassau Senior, his coauthor of the poor law report: if people had something to look forward to, then the prospect of happiness, not the fear of disaster, might motivate them to reproductive prudence.[54]

---

51 Ibid., 220–24. Again, he skirted the possibility that work might kill: were these data analyzed by "particular trades . . . the case of classes with still lower chances [of survival] would have been presented," but as the inquiry was concerned with general solutions, he had not done so. He did, however, defend factory over domestic manufacture, maintaining that factories were drier and warmer than homes. The argument was drawn from a comparison of Manchester and Bethnal Green. This is one of the few places where Chadwick takes an interest in infant mortality, which is appealed to here to distinguish the effects of place from the effects of labor. We would now probably say that Chadwick was finding a "healthy worker effect," which showed less what the health conditions of factory labor were than that a certain level of health was needed to carry on such labor. He told of "weakly children . . . put into the better managed factories as healthier places for them than their own homes."

52 Ibid., 221–22. Rents in Rutlandshire, however, were less than half what they were in the Northwest; hence even Chadwick's claim about the relative unimportance of wages is compromised.

53 Ibid., 243.

54 Ibid., 241–42. Chadwick spoke of "an impression of undefined optimism . . . frequently entertained by persons who are aware of the wretched condition of a large portion of the labouring population; and this impression is more frequently entertained than expressed, as the ground of inaction for the relief of the prevalent misery from disease, that its ravages form the natural or

Chadwick's concern with the destitution–fever issue was itself part of his critique of Malthusianism. Were Malthus right, disease would increase as a society approached its maximum population (one might equally see rising fever rates as proof of his principle). Malthus had distrusted industrial growth, believing it unsustainable. To find then that disease hit not the weak but the healthy, and for reasons easily avoidable; to show that upon its eradication people would reproduce *more* responsibly, raising their own wages and prospects of happiness, was to vindicate the factory system.[55]

The pull of rising expectations rather than the push of misery was to drive progress, then. But how to induce those expectations? On the one hand, environmental determinism suggested that higher expectations would accompany better housing, which, Chadwick was convinced, most people could afford. But it explained also, how, from long living in squalor, they had become accustomed to low expectations and standards. This was the old "comfort or character" problem that was at the heart of the Scottish poor law debate. It would not do simply to give more or larger or cheaper housing: the problem was to develop a disciplinary architecture that would more rapidly suppress the old habits and foster the new expectations. That, and not more money, was what the people needed. Wages were already too high, but investment in sanitary improvement would give their workers "a higher standard of health and comfort . . . at a less expense than that in which they now live in disease and misery."[56] The proof of that claim were the new model prisons inspired by John Howard. They showed how much healthier a population might be, living in the "same atmosphere, on a less expensive diet than that of the general labouring population, but provided with clean and

positive check, or . . . a 'terrible corrective' to the pressure of population on the means of subsistence."

55 A final point in the section is of interest as the only part of the *Sanitary Report* that those pushing for the ten hours' bill found useful to their case: this was the observation of the literal degeneration, in strength and stature, of people who lived in towns. Children did not grow as large as their parents had. The Spitalfields weavers, according to Dr. Mitchell, were "decayed in their bodies; rapidly descending to the size of Lilliputians. You could not raise a grenadier company amongst them all." That the observation was made on hand loom weavers, rather than factory hands, is significant (though Chadwick did refer to the difficulty of the army in finding healthy recruits in Manchester). The hand loom weavers were seen by the PLC as an obsolete group, whose welfare did not reflect the ordinary operation of the factory system. That they might be weak and puny was not wholly surprising. For the workers pushing for a ten hours' bill, however, this degeneration reflected wages and working conditions prevalent throughout the factory system; for Chadwick it reflected only "noxious influences" and the "depressing effect of adverse sanitary circumstances." He did worry that the weakening of the labor force threatened the nation's economic strength. Especially when we note the spur to public health activity that would take place when this fact, and these arguments, reappeared in connection with the raising of an army to fight the Boer War, it is worth considering why in 1842 this degeneration, though documented by others than Chadwick, evoked little reaction (ibid., 251–53).

56 Ibid., 276.

tolerably well-ventilated places of work and sleeping-rooms, and where they are required to be cleanly in their persons."[57]

But could one go to structures that acted automatically? Chadwick explored these issues most fully in the section "Employers' or Owners' Influence in the Improvement of Habitations and Sanitary Arrangements for the Protection of the Labouring Classes in the Rural Districts." Detached dwellings were desirable. "Much social disorder" arose from the "close contiguity of residences." Where many families were under one roof a "discipline almost as strong as that of a man-of-war" was needed. Technologies of sociability – public wash houses, pumps, ovens – were dangerous: best "to avoid any arrangement which brings *families* into close contact with each other." Lacking "a degree of education," the people (women) would brawl over priority.

Chadwick offered brief moral tales of families fallen or redeemed by architecture. In one case, for example, from Peter Lowe of Stafford Union, failure to fix a damaged roof "expose[d] the family to every vicissitude of the weather; the liability of the children so situated to contagious maladies frequently plunges the family into the greatest misery." Then, "the husband, enjoying but little comfort under his own roof, resorts to the beer-shop, neglects the cultivation of his garden, and impoverishes his family. The children are brought up without any regard to decency of behaviour, to habits of foresight, or self-restraint; they make indifferent servants; the girls become the mothers of bastards, and return home a burden to their parents." By contrast, the chairman of the Bedfordshire Union wrote of the results of moving families into better cottages: "The improvement has arisen . . . from the parties feeling that they are somewhat raised in the scale of society. The man sees his wife and family more comfortable than formerly . . . he is stimulated to industry, and . . . *becomes aware* that he has a character to lose. . . . He strives more to preserve his independence, and becomes a member of benefit, medical, and clothing societies; and frequently, besides this, lays up a certain sum . . . in the savings' bank." There follow an investment in education, improved church attendance, and so on.[58]

Employers doubling as landlords were to be the principal executors of these changes, and Chadwick devoted a great deal of space to counseling and reassuring them. "There appears to be no position from which so extensive and certain a beneficial influence may be exercised as that of the capitalist who stands in the double relation of landlord and employer," wrote Chadwick. Model housing projects seemed uneconomical only because gains in workers' health and morality were left out of the accounts. But rent could be deducted from wages, and the character of tenants overseen. Tenants would gain in

---

57 Chadwick's other main example was another controlled institution, the navy (ibid., 279, 284–85).
58 Ibid., 33–35, 323–25.

"neatness and cleanliness by their being known and being under observation."[59]

All manner of other public structures and arrangements (beyond sewers, and water, and smooth streets) could foster the same ends. Chadwick told of a plowing contest diverting a debauched crowd of fair-going agricultural laborers, and of a Chartist demonstration undermined by the opening of the zoo and botanical garden to the working classes. Front gardens and public green space were valuable not so much because fresh air and exercise were healthful: parks were the alternative to "drunkenness and gross excitement, whether mental or sensual"; in the cottage gardens children might play "under the eye of their mothers" and avoid bad language and bullies.[60] Much could be done by redesigning the workplace. At the innovative one-story textile factory of James Smith of Deanston in Catrine, Ayrshire, Chadwick delighted in the Panopticon-like supervision such a design afforded: "The bad manners and immoralities complained of as attendant on assemblages of workpeople of both sexes in manufactories, generally occur . . . in small rooms . . . secluded from superior inspection and from common observation." But in Smith's works, "the young are under the inspection of the old; the children are in many instances under the inspection of parents, and all under the observation of the whole body of workers, and under the inspection of the employer. It was observed that the moral condition of females . . . stood comparatively high . . . there were fewer cases of illegitimacy and less vice observable." Whatever the initial cost, there were "countervailing economical advantages to the capitalist . . . [in] this same facility of constant general supervision." (Chadwick treated the better known New Lanark experiment of Robert Owen fleetingly, noting that it was "by no means essential to such improvements that the labourers should become proprietors of their occupations.")[61]

Employers were also to abandon the practice of paying wages in pubs on Saturday nights (as well as encouraging intemperance, this led to imprudent food buying, and in turn to irregular diet and ultimately to disease); to fire workmen who got drunk (distinguishable by uncleanliness and "pallid" complexion); to make employees wash (dirtiness was "not necessary to any occupation . . . not the necessary consequence of poverty," and they could wash in the warm condensate of steam engines); and to inspect their dress, since "the personal appearance . . . through the self-respect, [affected] the morality." William Fairbairn, of Manchester, inspected his employees' Sunday dress – it was easier than inspecting their houses.[62]

59 Ibid., 300, 306–8, 326.
60 Ibid., 337–38.
61 Ibid., 302, 306–8. Smith, also an expert on agricultural drainage, would later become one of the first group of engineering inspectors under the Public Health Act of 1848.
62 Ibid., 309, 316, 320, 322.

III

The second great shift in the report was from dangerous classes to archaic institutions. How could English (here Chadwick ignores Scotland) laws and institutions be adapted to solve the great sanitary problem? Who would pay? Who would be in charge? All questions any self-respecting disciple of Bentham was primed to answer. Such is the focus of parts of chapter 5, and the long chapter 7: "Recognised Principles of Legislation and State of the Existing Law for the Protection of the Public Health."

If done in accord with "science," the necessary works (water, a water closet, house drains, and main sewers) would cost a bit more than a penny a week, he claimed, much less than the cost of privy cleaning alone (ten shillings/year/tenement).[63] But the improvements were to be paid for not from savings on privy cleaning, but from the surplus working people now spent on the spirits they would cease to desire once the improvements were in place: "The cost of one dram per week would nearly defray the expense of the structural arrangements of drainage, etc., by which some of the strongest provocatives [sic] to the habit of drunkenness would be removed."[64]

It was a principle of Chadwick's Benthamism that a rational administration was an economically optimal administration and an article of faith that preventing disease was ultimately cheaper than supporting those it left destitute. But how to show that? Calculations of the costs of neglect and the extraordinary benefits of improvement would become regular features in calls for sanitary reform, but Chadwick himself did not make them in a consistent way.[65] How large the costs of sanitary neglect were depended on what indirect effects one included, and on this matter there were no well accepted rules. Within the vast determinate edifice Chadwick had sketched out, one could make a plausible case that the benefits of complete sanitary reform would be extraordinarily far reaching and would be felt for generations to come. Few seem to have been bothered that the utilitarians seemed able to cook up any "bottom line" they wished. Some who flaunted such calculations admitted that they found them slightly obscene. Christian duty itself was sufficient authority for disease prevention; the audits were always for others, less charitable.[66]

---

63  Ibid., 288–91.
64  Ibid., 292.
65  In the *Sanitary Report* the main factors are cost in poor relief to widows and orphans, cost of lost wages, medical costs (including fever hospital investment) for provision of the sick poor, and then the large and indeterminate cost in crime and social instability.
66  *Sanitary Report*, 272–74. Chadwick quotes the Reverend George Lewis of Dundee: "Apart altogether from the waste of human life, and the indescribable suffering and sorrow which annually fall upon the working classes of Dundee from this periodical scourge, and viewed only as a mere matter of profit and loss to the mercantile and monied interest of Dundee, it were easy to dem-

In chapter 7 Chadwick first set out to show that sanitary improvement was legitimately within the province of legislative interference, and also that only through legislative interference could its uniform application, and accordingly its success, be assured. Parliament already oversaw urban improvement through innumerable local acts for paving, lighting, and cleaning as well as for harbor, bridge, and market building. In allowing towns to make building bylaws, it had acted to prevent fires. It regulated the workplace. What the law did not supply was uniformity: much legislation was local, and to escape its demands builders fled to suburbs. Workers suffered the results: "increased fatigue and exposure to weather in traversing greater distances to sleep in a badly-built, thin, and damp house." Yet at the same time any impediments to building would lead to overcrowdedness. Even uniformity was insufficient without comprehensive planning. Water supply had to be adequate to drainage, streets laid out to ensure a "free current of air," and new housing provided for those displaced by improvement projects who would otherwise simply worsen the crowding of remaining dwellings. All this might be coordinated by "an impartial authority" that would "obtain and, on consultation with the parties locally interested . . . settle plans for regulating the future growth of towns . . . with due protection of the landowners' interest."[67]

Chadwick found precedents for public action to protect health and remove nuisances. His proposals were not radical; constitutional objections to them had long since been overcome. There were statutes establishing sewers commissions, regulating noxious trades, requiring light and ventilation, banning river and air pollution and overcrowding.[68] In some boroughs, a leet jury of local tradesmen still circumambulated the town once or twice yearly to present to the magistrates the nuisances it found. The English common law of nuisance – "anything by which the health or the personal safety, or the convenience of the subject might be endangered or affected injuriously" – could be powerful. Anyone could make use of this law: Blackstone held that a sufferer of a nuisance could remove it without waiting for a slow court. There were precedents for a concept of nuisance that would even include "things . . . offensive to the sense, from which no injury to the health or other injury can

onstrate that the expenditure of several thousand pounds per annum in providing the means of cleanliness to this town, in the better cleansing of its streets, but above all, of its back closes, courts, and lanes . . . would have been rewarded by a saving to the community of a vast sum, which the ravages of disease and death have been, for the last few years, compelling Dundee to pay in a way its inhabitants think not of." "But how shall we estimate the pecuniary loss of 1,312 deaths? It seems a strange thing to go about estimating the money value of that which money did not give, and cannot restore when taken away; yet as there are those who understand better a profit and loss account than the arguments of religion and humanity, we shall attempt to estimate the money loss."

67 Ibid., 340–42, 346–47.
68 Ibid., 350–54.

be proved than the often overlooked but serious injury of discomfort, of daily annoyance, as by matters offensive to the sight . . . by filth, by offensive smells, and by noises."[69]

Could it be that the idea of a "medical police" came from Tudor Parliaments, not absolutist German princes? In fact, as Chadwick realized, the statutes were mostly unenforceable, the leet courts had negligible enforcement powers, and the quagmire of common law was little help, since classes of activities or things were not nuisances per se: each "nuisance" had to be independently proved.

The problem lay less in laws than in institutions of execution and enforcement. Particularly serious was the failure of local administration: boroughs, improvement commissions, parishes, road or turnpike authorities, sewers commissions. Here Chadwick had three concerns: first, that they were irrationally conceived, both spatially and in terms of powers and responsibilities; second, that their executive officers were incompetent; and third, that even had those officers been competent they were powerless: "impartial authority" was badly needed.

In the administration of poor relief the ancient parish had given way to the modern union. The municipal corporations had been reformed in 1835, but other local institutions still represented a patchwork of tradition and makeshift legislation that not only harmed health but impeded economic development. Land drainage, for example, was known to increase agricultural production, reduce fever, and facilitate commerce. Yet perverse landowners who would not see their own interests and political (or ecclesiastical or civil) boundaries that violated natural drainage basins often made what was technically straightforward practically impossible.

Among these indefensible traditions were those governing the duties and perquisites of officers. Chadwick attacked the surveyors to the Greater London sewers commissions at length. High fees and labyrinthine procedures effectively meant that the public sewers were not serving the needy public. Not only were such officers oblivious of a responsibility for health, their gas-emitting sewers – "latent sources of pestilence and death" – made conditions worse. Under such circumstances, the public was right to oppose sanitary improvement. A new science of public administration would replace "the

---

69 Ibid., 349, 354. Nuisances, Chadwick explains, are classified as public and general – a nuisance to the realm; common – a nuisance to all passersby; or private – a nuisance to one's property. A common nuisance can entail commission or omission. A private nuisance requires civil action; against a public nuisance one seeks an indictment. Using such definitions, Chadwick implied that common law ought to be equated with common good. In regard to mill proprietors whose dams flooded farmland, for example, he wrote, "In many . . . such cases, the use of property, with such attendant consequences, would be found to be in contravention of the existing public rights." It was only "the expense and delay and uncertainty of the legal procedure [that] . . . sustained such invasions on the surrounding property and on the public health" (ibid., 365).

influence of petty and sinister interest" with "officers of superior scientific attainments," who would be responsible for everything relating to "under-drainage and surface-drainage, road structure and repair."[70]

Chadwick is usually seen as a centralizer of administration, yet "science" was more important: "In proportion as science is securely allied to local administration is its respectability enhanced and the attainment of its objects ensured."[71] Hence it was essential that districts be large enough to hire skilled engineers. Far from being subject to central dictate, engineers needed great discretion to adapt public works to local situations. A local engineer might be permitted to act as a sort of technological magistrate to resolve the inevitable planning disputes.[72]

What sort of unit of local government should protect the public health? The institution Chadwick had in mind was a cross between a sewers commission and a poor law union. It should embody some popular representation, yet not too much: the "shopocracy" of small property holders was less likely to appreciate the need for improvement than were owners of large property. There should be ex officio seats for relevant experts. These would not be boards of health like those authorized during the 1832 cholera and long used by Continental towns in fighting plague. Boards of health were temporary, and the needs of towns constant. Usually they were advisory rather than executive; theoretical rather than experienced. Worst, they were the classic forum of the futile deliberation of medical men.

Doctors were not to be excluded from public health, but their role was secondary. The twenty-three hundred union medical officers best knew the living conditions of the poor; they were to have power to require removal of the nuisances they found. There was also to be an independent district medical officer, who, free from the need to kowtow to powerful clients, could back up the local man.[73] That person might also inspect factories, schools, lodging houses, and so forth, and monitor epidemics. (In situations where

70  Ibid., 367–76. Such an administration would also levy a combined rate: much of the antipathy of ratepayers Chadwick attributed to the annoyance of multiple, and therefore frequent, demands.

71  Ibid., 384.

72  "The appointment of persons having the scientific qualifications and position of civil engineers might serve to supply a want which is generally found to be the chief impediment to the drainage of land subdivided amongst numerous small holders, namely, the means of reference or appeal to some authority deriving confidence from skill and impartiality to determine on the need of works, and the mode of executing them, or to arbitrate; and on the compensation due from damage arising from them. Given such an authority, and in those small, but, from their great number, most important cases, where the expense of an application to Parliament is out of the question, it might be safe to say, by a general provision, that the inhabitants of a town may procure springs of water, and make, deepen, and scour drains through the circumjacent district; that regulations may be made for arching over or covering the sewers to the proper distances from the towns; for the purchase of ground, and for the erection of works for rendering the refuse of the towns available for agricultural purposes: that power might also be given to lay pipes in the highways, to put plugs for the supplies of water against fires, and for watering the roads" (ibid., 393).

73  Ibid., 402–4.

these epidemics resulted from occupation, Chadwick reiterated, the particular causes would be "found to be removable, and not essential to the occupation itself.") Mainly, however, fever prevention required institutions in which engineers could act: "The great preventives – drainage, street and house cleansing by means of supplies of water and improved sewerage, and especially the introduction of cheaper and more efficient modes of removing all noxious refuse from the towns – are operations for which aid must be sought from the science of the civil engineer, not from the physician, who has done his work when he has pointed out the disease that results from the neglect of proper administrative measures, and has alleviated the sufferings of the victims."[74]

The discussion included Chadwick's fiercest attack on doctors, though he had made most of the points earlier. Doctors were easily duped. However great their clinical or pathological knowledge medical men were "frequently found to be destitute of any knowledge of the pervading cause in which they are themselves enveloped." Without opportunity to compare disease in different situations, they made unsound inferences on the basis of insufficient evidence. That had happened in the factory agitation. Medical men who did not work exclusively with an occupation in the full range of places and environments where that work was carried on were unwarranted in attributing disease to that work:

A working person . . . presenting himself with the symptoms of a consumption, the medical man has no means of detecting *the* one of many causes by which it may have been occasioned, and the individual patient himself is more likely to mislead than to inform him. Unless his attention were accidentally directed to it, or unless the medical investigator had himself the means of observing the different personal condition of the different sets of persons following the same occupation in town and in country, it is highly probable that the evidence that the disease is not essential to the occupation would escape him.

Similarly, on the deprivation issue, medical men were "extremely liable to deceive themselves . . . by what they call the evidence of their own eyes": they saw squalor, but did not ask about wages. Even their "various contradictory opinions on diet, and the older views on the innocuousness of miasma," could be referred "to the circumstances under which the medical observers were placed."[75]

Notwithstanding significant restatements and judicious silences, Chadwick's conclusions did recapitulate his key points. He had shown, he claimed, the pervasiveness of "various forms of epidemic, endemic, and other disease caused, or aggravated, or propagated chiefly . . . by atmospheric impurities produced by decomposing animal and vegetable substances, by damp and filth, and close and overcrowded dwellings." (In fact, he had done little to show

74 Ibid., 396.
75 Ibid., 181, 215, 409.

that these were the main causes of such diseases.) On the key issue of disease and destitution, he stated that "high prosperity in respect to employment and wages, and various and abundant food, have afforded . . . no exemptions from attacks of epidemic disease, which have been as frequent and as fatal in periods of commercial and manufacturing prosperity as in any others." Few would have disputed the first clause, but it was not what Chadwick had been arguing.[76] To recognize that employment and good food could not *prevent* disease was not to exonerate destitution as a significant cause of disease. The second clause was controversial, but also unwarranted – the *Report* included no analysis of the relations of fever to cycles of prosperity and distress.

Nothing in the conclusions hinted that Britain was in the midst of economic distress. On occupational disease Chadwick was silent. He did not repeat his charges that medical men and surveyors were incompetent, nor call for a building program to ease overcrowded housing. He did, in several statements, reiterate the profound implications of physical conditions on political stability: water was important not because it was used for drinking or cooking but because "formation of all habits of cleanliness is obstructed by defective supplies of water." He reiterated that "adverse circumstances" (bad physical conditions) produced "an adult population short-lived, improvident, reckless, and intemperate, and with habitual avidity for sensual gratifications," and that "these habits lead to the abandonment of all the conveniences and decencies of life, and especially lead to the overcrowding of their homes, which is destructive to the morality as well as the health of large classes of both sexes." His remedies were drainage, the water carriage and recycling of wastes, establishment of local authorities whose boundaries coincided with drainage basins, the application of science to public works, lengthy periods for repaying public works loans, and uniform legislation in Scotland and England.[77]

## IV

It will be clear that the report of July 1842 was both broader and quite different in focus than that commissioned in August 1839, which was intended simply to discover whether the conditions that purportedly led to fever in the metropolis existed elsewhere. They did. To them Chadwick had ascribed not only disease but social problems generally. He had outlined a redemptive vision, based on a novel technological system that required novel public institutions. But he had taken up questions far beyond epidemiology and poor law policy: matters of the sphere of equality, the legitimacy of democracy, and the best way of circumventing revolution.

---

76 Ibid., 422. The statement might also be given an interpretation contrary to Chadwick's intention, as implying that work caused disease.
77 Ibid., 422–23.

Why the transformation? Partly because new ideas emerged from the inquiry, like the potential of sewage recycling, and of an hydraulic system of urban sanitation; partly because, as in fever etiology, medical men (particularly Scottish medical men) had been unenthusiastic about his claim that sanitation was the most important fever preventive; partly because poor relations with William Farr prevented any serious epidemiology. But mainly because the matters Chadwick dealt with were the critical matters of the day. Matters were worse in the summer of 1842 than in the spring of 1838. Five years of economic distress made for a desperate people. One in five in industrial Lancashire was receiving relief. Many were organized in Chartist groups, some of these armed. Class war seemed imminent. His old patrons, the Whigs, were out of power and unlikely to return soon. The new bunch, Peel and Sir James Graham, owed him nothing. Their concern was order. Chadwick shared it. Finding that Whig justices of the peace would not enforce introduction of the new poor law, he had lobbied successfully for a Royal Constabulary Commission, established in 1837 with himself as the main member. All through the sanitary inquiry he still saw himself as a constabulary commissioner and was looking to the authoritarian regimes of the Continent for models of effective policing.[78]

Chadwick saw "sanitation" as a politically more viable route to stability than any of the alternatives being pushed on Peel's government. The widely held faith in the civilizing effects of education was accompanied by passionate disagreement over who would run the schools and what would be taught. The ten hours' and anti–corn law movements promised social renewal, yet the partisans of each were opposed to the other. Restricting the working hours of children (and by connection adults) appealed to landed interests but threatened industry. Lowering food prices by removing protection, simple justice to Cobden and the northern manufacturers, seemed to threaten the very existence of home agriculture. Neither approach commanded a majority; corn law repeal would ultimately split the Tory party.

Sanitary improvement, on the other hand, was both innocuous and powerful; in principle it offended no parliamentary constituency. By insisting that the morality of the people was a function of their drains, Chadwick had made the case that his reforms were the key to preventing revolution. He had distanced sanitarianism from the factory and corn law movements by showing on the one hand that work was harmless and wages were fine, on the other that hunger was not a significant health problem. He damned Chartists, damned all manifestations of democracy, in favor of a sanitary technocracy. Matters would be much better " 'by avoiding the metaphysical, and by pursuing a quiet but strong course of physical improvement (in which I would

---

78 Stanley H. Palmer, *Police and Protest in England and Ireland* (Cambridge: Cambridge University Press, 1988), 421–26.

submit that it is most important that the Government, and the natural leaders should take and keep the lead),' " Chadwick would write to John Russell a few years later.[79] To a degree it worked. In debates on public health bills in 1847 and 1848, the point arose repeatedly. "By such measures they would be able to change . . . the condition of large bodies of the population of great towns, and to make them contented and cheerful," noted Robert Slaney.[80]

But how was the *Sanitary Report* to have this mollifying effect? Even if a law were passed, years would go by before new sanitary systems could be built and work their physical and moral miracles. Yet even before that time (and even if sewers and waterworks were never built), the very existence of a government report finding the need for them might ease conflict. Privately, Graham worried that the agitation that led to the August riots was distracting the laboring classes from those programs the government was preparing for their improvement.[81] Thus the sanitary idea itself had public relations value.

Yet if Chadwick had meant to project the image of the government as friend to the noble poor, why then all the depravity-mongering in the middle of the *Report*? One may say that Chadwick's discourse simply reflects the polarization of the times and the view of a middle-class poor law bureaucrat. But this gives Chadwick too little credit. What we must keep in mind is that we are not accompanying Chadwick's doctors on a reconnaissance of darkest England, but are readers in the hands of a skillful author. Chadwick is a broadcaster, not simply a recorder of images. His intended readership was not, after all, those sufferers of insanitation, but those who managed the poor: union officials, members of Parliament, even middle-class ratepayers. Sanitation, it is true, would protect them from disease, but more importantly it would neutralize the unruly masses. Hence the soap opera quality of the report: Chadwick's alternation between chaos and control, horror and security. With his informants, we observe, retch vicariously, spout medicomoral truths. We share their revulsion, indignation, or pity – all in the safety of the printed page. The narrative is not open-ended. It has a plot, heros and villains, and a happy ending: a system of house drains spiriting all wastes into public sewers will exterminate these human vermin.

But why, we may ask, would Chadwick see utility in heightening class tension? Principally, I think, because that was necessary to discredit Chartism: to identify a group of subhuman filth victims who happen to be revolutionaries was to invite his readers to announce that they were none of those things.

79  Chadwick to Lord John Russell, December 1848, quoted in R. A. Lewis, *Edwin Chadwick and the Public Health Movement, 1832–1854* (London: Longmans, Green, 1952). See also Oliver MacDonagh, *Early Victorian Government, 1830–1870* (London: Weidenfeld and Nicolson, 1977), 141.

80  Slaney in *Hansard's Parliamentary Debates 3rd series, 98,* 1848, 769; also see Lord Campbell in ibid., *99,* 1848, 1405.

81  *The Life and Letters of Sir James Graham,* ed. Charles Stuart Parker, 2 vols. (London: John Murray, 1907), I, 333–36.

Hence the centrality of environmental determinism. It was both the main point on which Chadwick enforced a distinction between "us" and "them" and equally the source of order. They, products of filth, had absurd ideas instilled by filth; those ideas must be absurd because they oppose the ideas that we, the true, independent, rational, humans, have. But, because they were determined and not independent beings, it was easy enough to wash those ideas right out of their heads. Thus, sanitation was simultaneously a mechanism for fostering fear and for neutralizing it. The *Sanitary Report* is then an ideological manifesto, not an empirical survey of conditions affecting health. Far from representing any kind of radicalism it was thoroughly conservative in seeking to solve a problem through minimal changes maximally acceptable to established interests.

Chadwick's philosophy – that true humanness derives from water closets – may seem ludicrous and his proposal to make sanitation the antidote to Chartism, simplistic and even transparent. Yet within two years, sanitation would become a popular social movement – it seemed simple, promising, unequivocally good. Almost every reformer could find a reason for being a sanitary reformer too.

How did that happen? What we must explore next is how much of this "public health" was common to an incipient public health community – those medical men and poor law officials concerned with disease and with what for lack of a better term we can call social welfare. We have seen that on the narrow question of fever theory, many medical men refused to focus solely on sanitary reform. Some rejected the political economy in which Chadwick grounded his distinctions of legitimate and illegitimate public intervention. But what of their views of class, or gender, or morality, or politics?

# 6

## Chadwick's Evidence: The *Local Reports*

What did others, particularly medical men, think about the interrelations of disease, environment, social stability, morality, and public policy? The two volumes of *Local Reports,* understood by the Poor Law commissioners as the true *Sanitary Report,* are an opportunity to see how a few who shared Chadwick's interests viewed the issues he considered in the *Sanitary Report.* How far did a common sensibility prevail?

There are 27 local reports on England and Wales, 18 on Scotland, ranging from 2 to more than 60 pages. These represent only a portion of the data gathered in the Sanitary Inquiry. They are the source of 68 (27 percent) of 248 block quotations in the *Sanitary Report.* It will be recalled that in the case of England and Wales, Chadwick had solicited information from three classes of informants. First were the 2300 or so union medical officers, who were to describe the diseases they commonly encountered and state their causes. Second were the Poor Law Commission's (PLC) field agents, the assistant commissioners, who were to review conditions in their districts, paying special attention to the effects of housing on morality. In practice, they were the main users of the medical officers' returns; some of their reports were essentially digests of those returns. Third were the eminent practitioners in the various towns. In Scotland the inquiry was conducted almost entirely through appeals to local medical men. Assistant poor law commissioners contributed 15 reports, while most others are by medical men or medical committees, as in Aberdeen and Birmingham. Although a few (like one on Scottish nuisance law) are topical, most are on towns or regions.

This is not a complete or coherent class of documents. Coverage is uneven – there are no reports for major towns like Bristol, York, Newcastle, or Dundee; the longest is on the Scottish mining town of Tranent (population four thousand). Wales is virtually ignored. Those who wrote were pursuing a variety of ends. For the assistant poor law commissioners, these reports were an official duty. Still, only a few made an effort to cover their districts comprehensively, and some used the occasion to air irrelevant crotchets. Recruiting town practitioners (ten English reports, thirteen Scottish) proved difficult.

Uninvited practitioners felt snubbed as non-"eminent." A good deal of work was expected for which there was no pay.[1] Many more offered to report than did (though some reports were omitted, including many from Scottish practitioners, as, perhaps, too brief or informal).[2]

Some who did report had things to say that Chadwick would rather have not heard. William Pulteney Alison of Edinburgh, R. B. Howard of Manchester, and Edward de Vitre of Lancaster wrote at least in part to highlight their disagreement with Chadwick's fever theory. Some other Scots, Charles Baird of Glasgow, James Sym of Ayr, Somerville Scott Alison (no relation) of Tranent, and William Stevenson of Musselburgh, echo Alison and appear to be writing as part of his crusade to reform the Scottish poor law. As a group the writers are not particularly "eminent," though W. H. Duncan (Liverpool) later became that city's first medical officer of health. Robert Baker of Leeds was a longtime friend of poor law administration. Howard and Scott Alison achieved some fame as hospital staff, but the renown of most others will have been mainly local.[3]

Clearly the local reports were influenced by Chadwick. He set the agenda and sent the Smith, Kay, Arnott reports as models of local sanitary inquiry. Nonetheless, except for a few Scottish reporters who kept to Chadwick's questionnaire, the authors do not share common format or content. Some were puzzled as to what Chadwick wanted, opening their responses with phrases like "If I rightly understand." It seemed information was wanted on the so-called condition-of-England question, especially as embodied in the built environment, but in what detail, or how well supported? Some had trouble finding a testable hypothesis: the "filth–disease" link seemed too vague to test or too obvious to need confirmation. The metropolitan reports were little help: four quite different approaches, each hasty, inconclusive, and in-

---

1 *Report to Her Majesty's Principal Secretary of State for the Home Office on the Sanitary Condition of the Labouring Population of Great Britain* (London: Clowes, 1842), xi; *Poor Law Commission [PLC] Index to Correspondence*, 1840, Public Record Office [PRO] MH 15/5; E. C. Tufnell to PLC, 29 November 1839; PLC to Tufnell, 7 December 1839; PLC to Assistant Commissioners, 18 December 1839, *PLC Appendices to Minutes*, PRO MH 3/2; Chadwick to Tufnell, 7 December 1839, *PLC–Tufnell Correspondence*, PRO MH 32/70; Mott to PLC, 7 December, 30 December 1839; R. B. Howard to Chadwick, 14 January 1840; Chadwick to Howard, 24 January 1840, *PLC–Manchester Correspondence*, MH 12/6039; James Williamson to Chadwick, 29 December 1840, *PLC–Leeds Correspondence*, PRO MH 12/15225; Power to Chadwick, 13 December 1839, 12 May, 9 December 1840; Chadwick to Power, 20 December 1839; *PLC–Power Correspondence*, PRO MH 32/64; W. Gilbert to PLC, 8 December, 18 December 1839, *PLC–Gilbert Correspondence*, PRO MH 32/27; E Twistleton to PLC, late November 1839, *PLC–Twistleton Correspondence*, PRO MH 32/72.

2 The Scottish reports are in PRO MH 19/196. A report of Arnott's was left out (Arnott to Chadwick, 31 July 1842, University College London [UCL] Chadwick Papers #193). There are 71 responses from parties offering to furnish reports in the *PLC Index to Correspondence*, PRO MH 15/5.

3 On Howard see *Gentleman's Magazine*, n.s. *30* (1848): 323–25; on Scott Alison see *The Roll of the Royal College of Physicians of London*, ed. William Munk, 8 vols. (London: Royal College of Physicians, 1878–1988), IV, 97–98.

complete. And, in the multicausal traditions of constitutional medicine, it was quite plausible to think that the causes (and preventives) of disease were unique to each locality.

For them, as for Chadwick, health was not merely medical: morality and social harmony affected it, as well as environment. Some ranged more widely, including economic and political factors on which Chadwick had been prudently silent. The reports vary enormously: variously they bear marks of great labor, or deep compassion, or careful inference, or shrewd equivocation. However much they impressed *The Spectator's* reviewer, they were no sound basis for sanitary legislation – the inquiry was too broad, and lacking in any test of the hypothesis of filth as the cause of fever. On the contrary, it was effectively an invitation to wallow in tautology: filth was filthy, squalor squalid, wretchedness wretched, corruption corrupting.

I shall examine the local reports in terms of five questions: First, what was the scope of public health and why? Second, what were the causes of disease, particularly fever? Third, what concept of human did reporters assume, and how did they characterize the "labouring classes"? Were these humans, or some classes of them, products of environment? How much were *they* like *me*? Fourth, how did they understand society: the roles of men, women, and children; of churches, factories, the market, the state? Last, what are their environmental sensibilities? I shall focus mainly on the medical reports, those of both poor law medical officers and "eminent" practitioners.

Underlying these questions is one of problem definition, of how a society distills unsatisfactory and conflictual situations – here the complex of situations labeled poverty and disease – into well-defined problems. Determinations must be made of whose problem, whose fault, what causes, and finally, where to tinker to solve or prevent such problems from recurring. Chadwick, Peel, and the local reporters all recognized complications of urbanization and industrialization. They did not agree which aspects deserved the label "problem" (are high wages a problem or a solution?), or to whom they should be assigned (were they personal, public, or matters of relations between private parties?), or in what category of problem (medical, religious, educational, economic?) they belonged. And some of what was truly problematic must be left to the market, or the course of nature, or divine will. Even when they agreed that a public problem existed, they might disagree on where in the network of cause and effect to seek a solution. At the 1840 Glasgow meeting of the British Association Arnott heard disease blamed on drink, lack of poor rates, and lack of education. These were not exclusive causal hypotheses, but only different views of where intervention would be feasible, proper, and effective.[4]

4 Neil Arnott, "On the Fevers Which Have Prevailed in Edinburgh and Glasgow," *Sanitary Condition of the Labouring Population. Local Reports for Scotland, Parliamentary Papers [P.P.]*, House of Lords, 28, 1842 [to be cited as *LRS*], 6–7.

One might expect close correspondence between diagnoses and prescriptions, but this is often not the case. One had to consider the propriety, practicality, and implications of a solution. To acknowledge hunger or overpopulation as key problems (and key causes of other problems) was not necessarily to believe that governments (or churches or philanthropists) should provide food or institute programs of population control. An example of the gap between problems and solutions is a survey of sixteen Glasgow elders on the causes and remedies of destitution, appended to Charles Baird's local report.[5] As causes of destitution, twelve mentioned intemperance; nine, insufficient employment; six, low wages; five, lack of education; four, fever or other disease; three, early marriage; three, Irish immigrants; three, high cost of food; two, lack of domestic economy. As remedies, eight recommended greater parish relief; eight suggested better education; seven, temperance; three, more benevolent oversight from the upper classes; two, corn law repeal; one, establishment of a workhouse; one, emigration; one, savings banks; and one, a "medical police for the suppression of contagious diseases, and the regulation of houses occupied by the poor, and the removal of nuisances."

Wages, work, prices, decisions to marry, the influx of the Irish poor – all these seemed either impracticable or inappropriate to adjust. Increasingly medical and environmental intervention seemed the route of least resistance. To those of us for whom disease prevention is a quintessentially medical matter – the tracking down and rooting out of some microbe – it may seem odd to find disease thrown in with customs, economic policies, institutional inadequacies, ethnic antagonisms, and personal habits as a cause of social problems. It may also seem odd to find disease acquiring its legitimacy as a public problem only through links with broader matters of destitution and "demoralization."

## I

Most informants, particularly the medical men, understood that they were being asked for their views on "public health." They recognized, too, that medical matters were inextricably mixed up in the great social questions. They did not share a common view of what public health was or how it fit with other social policies. As the inquiry was not tied to a particular epidemic, they emphasized prevention and description, rather than matters of organizing the treatment and isolation of victims. Here they drew upon two traditions of medical thought: the Hippocratic legacy of medical topography and the Enlightenment concept of a medical police.

---

5 Charles Baird, "On the General and Sanitary Condition of the Working Classes and the Poor in the City of Glasgow. Appendix A. Analysis of Reports (or Answers to Queries) made by City Missionaries, Elders, and Others, to C. R. Baird," *LRS*, 195–200.

Among those who understood Chadwick's requests in terms of a neo-Hippocratic medical topography was John Adamson, the St. Andrews reporter. Adamson delineated the "general causes which may be supposed to affect the health of the community" – its soil, topography, temperature, winds, and rains; then its layout and buildings, housing and working conditions, and finally the habits of the peculiar breed of human that occupied the place. This last included "stock" or predominant constitution, as well as culture, occupation, economic situation.[6] Together, these accounted for health.

Medical topography traditionally had been mainly descriptive. It alerted practitioners to problems they would meet and guided "delicate" persons in selecting a residence. It provided no framework for ranking causes of illness or determining which depended on which others. Nor did it do much to inspire prevention. So long as there was no presumption that these were remediable conditions, medical topographers might identify such factors as nutrition or occupation as causes of illness without accusatory overtones.

The Continental medical-police tradition offered a more activist legacy. Those who appealed to it (mainly Scots, the first British chair in medical police having been established after great strife at Edinburgh in 1806) endorsed many of the interventions Chadwick would call for and more besides.[7] Baird of Glasgow suggested a broad list of responsibilities:

> to inquire into the causes of disease and mortality, and to adopt all salutary and necessary measures for promoting the health, cleanliness, and comfort of the inhabitants; [to have] . . . power to remove all slaughterhouses, shambles, etc., producing noxious and offensive effluvia; to prevent interment in crowded burying-grounds in the immediate vicinity of inhabited houses; to open up ill-ventilated lanes, closes, or courts; to make sewers or drains where none exist, but are required, and to enlarge or improve those which are defective; to pull down houses unfit for the habitations of human beings; to regulate the construction of houses for the poorer classes . . . to see that these houses are kept clean; to erect public conveniences; to regulate lodging-houses . . . to provide an ample supply of water, and generally to attend to and promote the public health.

Jenks of Brighton included food adulteration and exposure to sunlight, which, he felt, prevented a tubercular diathesis. W. H. Forrest of Stirling thought a

---

6 John Adamson,"Report on the Sanitary Condition and General Economy of the Labouring Classes in the City of St. Andrews," *LRS*, 267. See also G. S. Jenks, "On the Sanitary State of the Town of Brighton," *Sanitary Condition of the Labouring Population. Local Reports for England and Wales, P.P.*, House of Lords, 27, 1842 [to be cited as LREW], 57. On this tradition see James C. Riley, *The Eighteenth Century Campaign to Avoid Disease* (London: Macmillan, 1987).

7 Brenda White, "Scottish Doctors and the English Public Health," *The Influence of Scottish Medicine*, ed. Derek Dow (Park Ridge, N.J.: Parthenon, 1988), 81. On the tradition of medical police see also George Rosen, "Cameralism and the Concept of Medical Police," and "The Fate of the Concept of Medical Police, 1780–1890," in his *From Medical Police to Social Medicine: Essays on the History of Health Care*, 120–41, 142–58 (New York: Science History, 1974); *A System of Complete Medical Police: Selections from Johann Peter Frank*, edited with an introduction by Erna Lesky (Baltimore: Johns Hopkins University Press, 1976).

medical police ought to undertake "the building of new houses for the poor." Scott Alison of Tranent listed care for the aged and insane, an isolation hospital, ventilation and the prevention of dust in collieries, public whitewashing and drains, investigation of accidents, and enforcement of restrictions on children's and women's labor. William Chambers, the prominent Edinburgh publisher and local worthy, thought medical police, "in the strict sense of the term," included the relief of dire poverty.[8]

"Medical police" was a creation of benevolent despots (needing cannon fodder). Could such an institution really be adapted to constitution and common law, to liberalism, political economy, evangelical activism, and perceptions of Malthusian overpopulation? No. Invocations of medical police were in terms of the rights of "free-born Englishman" (which Scots were demanding too). Exactly what these rights were was the question. Take the grand issue of state interference with property. Chadwick, despite pushing for a broad construction of the common law of nuisance, was uncomfortable interfering with property. Enlightened landowners would appreciate sanitary improvement as essential to the maintenance of great and well capitalized estates; state action would be needed only to deal with pesky petit bourgeois obtuseness. Many of the reporters were more aggressive. They appealed to analogy (e.g., if municipal governments had the right to prohibit sale of putrid meat, why not to "forbid the renting of rooms in which putrid, damp, and noisome vapours are working as sure destruction as the worst food"?).[9] A few, like Scott Alison of Tranent, vastly expanded the concept, invoking Cobbett's doctrine that health was the landless laborer's only property and as much deserving state protection as any other property right.[10]

In this age of political economy, appeals to rights and property were grounded even more in economics than in moral philosophy or common law. The assistant poor law commissioner Alfred Power agreed that health warranted a prohibition on excessive occupancy of rooms, even though this was "not a proper subject for legislative interference." But he worried that "by too rigid a course [of regulation], capital may be driven from the building of

---

8 Baird, "Glasgow," *LRS*, 194; Jenks, "Brighton," *LREW*, 86; W. H. Forrest, "Report on the Sanitary Condition of the Labouring Classes of the Town of Stirling," *LRS*, 266; S. Scott Alison, "On the Sanitary Condition and General Economy of the Town of Tranent, and the Neighbouring District in Haddingtonshire," *LRS*, 122–26; William Chambers, "On the Sanitary Condition of the Old Town of Edinburgh," *LRS*, 153–55.

9 Charles Mott, "On the State of the Labouring Classes in the Manufacturing Districts of Lancashire, Cheshire, Derbyshire, and Staffordshire," *LREW*, 255–56.

10 Scott Alison added that if the state could claim a man for military service, it was "only right and proper" that it relieve his destitution ("Tranent," *LRS*, 118–19). Himmelfarb, *The Idea of Poverty: England in the Early Industrial Age* (New York: Random House, 1985), 55–56, quotes Adam Smith, "The patrimony which every man has in his own labour, as it is the original foundation of all other property, so it is the most sacred and inviolable. The patrimony of a poor man lies in the strength and dexterity of his hands."

the lower class of houses and cottages."[11] Medicine might have priority over property rights, but economics had priority over medicine, and economics effectively meant individualism. Convinced that anyone who "faithfully and charitably" studied "disease and the crushing weight of misery so extensively endured by the labouring classes" would recognize "that nearly all their afflictions, misfortunes, and maladies originate in the inveterate sources of ignorance, and improvidence or profligacy," Edward Senior and J. P. Kennedy, respectively assistant poor law commissioner and physician, would have the state teach and enforce a set of "Health Rules," posted in every mill or factory, taught in all schools, that would "protect our less fortunate brethren from the lamentable consequences of their own defects, faults, or errors." These "brethren" were to be taught "how to exercise a decent economy in the care of their persons, food, dress, labour, earnings, houses and families; how to apply rational means for the preservation of health, the prevention of epidemic inflictions, and the moral management of their sick, infirm, and disabled; and how, by the application of intellectual and religious knowledge, to avoid the evils which result from residence in unwholesome habitations, *from insufficient wages, and from excessively protracted or oppressive labour.*" That wages and work harmed health did not warrant state interference; at best the state could compensate, mainly by preaching that such conditions must be borne, though also by ensuring that landlords kept up cottages and tenants did not overcrowd "their sleeping-rooms, and especially their beds."[12]

In part, this habit of seeing health in terms of economics reflects the continuing, though waning, influence of Thomas Malthus. To some disciples, the principle of population implied that it was unhealthy to promote health: in a demographic sense, because promoting health might interfere with positive checks and permit the precarious survival of a squalid population too large for the region it occupied; and in a psychological sense because public guarantees of sustenance or medical care might encourage irresponsible reproduction. Philanthropic interference with natural laws must backfire. Mainly Malthusianism left its mark in what was unsaid. While there was little talk of "redundant" population, there was also little sense that a high mortality rate was itself a sufficient warrant for intervention: one had to explain why the population being protected was particularly valuable, or what social costs would be incurred by failure to protect it. As would Chadwick, most reporters concentrated on adult males, showing little interest in high mortality rates among infants, women, or Irish immigrants (who were seen as a health problem rather than as a population with its own health problems).[13] Like Chad-

---

11 Alfred Power, "On the Sanitary Inquiry in His Late District in Lancashire, etc.," *LREW*, 278; Power later (282) suggests that not all fever causes warrant public intervention.
12 J. P. Kennedy and Edward Senior, "Report on the Sanitary Condition of the Parish of Breadsall in the Shardlow Union," *LREW*, 191 (italics mine).
13 E.g., W. H. Duncan of Liverpool: "Among the causes of fever in Liverpool I might have enu-

wick, many tried to translate the lives lost from poor sanitation into monetary values. That such arguments were needed suggests the pervasiveness of the antithesis – that these deaths were social assets rather than debits.

Discussions about public health then were preoccupied with incentives: not just how to dissuade people from early marriage or indolence but how to persuade them to channel wages into savings banks or good food or to invest their hope in the established order rather than in revolutionary hysteria. No issue was straightforwardly medical; all had to be seen in terms of social, moral, and economic implications; fever was of significance as a cause of destitution, which was in turn a cause of revolution. The simple inference that illness is a problem whose solution is health is rare. Writers who appealed to humanity or to the duty of charity came closest to that view yet still found need for supplemental arguments. The exception is William Pulteney Alison. Rather than subordinating medicine to economics, he would reorder economic institutions in the name of health.[14]

## II

Any Malthus-inspired ambivalence notwithstanding, the medical reporters were in sympathy with Chadwick's project of sanitary reform. Conditions like those described in the metropolitan reports were widespread, harmed health, and led to pauperization, they agreed. The factors Chadwick highlighted – particularly decaying matter, exacerbated by poor drainage and ventilation – had long been deemed harmful. It should have been easy to collect a number of clear examples of that harm. Assistant Poor Law Commissioner W. J. Gilbert (willing enough to act as a medical authority on the occasion) offered one:

The diseases arising from malaria present themselves in many different forms . . . [and] frequently assume a character apparently not resulting from such causes. The inmates complain

merated the large proportion of poor Irish among the working population." In labeling them as causes, Duncan denies the Irish the status of victims of disease. They are also seen to constitute moral contagia: "By their example and intercourse with others they are rapidly lowering the standard of comfort among . . . their English neighbours, communicating their own vicious and apathetic habits, and fast extinguishing all sense of moral dignity, independence, and self-respect. No one interested in the welfare of his poorer brethren can contemplate the prospect without a feeling of melancholy foreboding; and I am persuaded that so long as the native inhabitants are exposed to the inroads of numerous hordes of uneducated Irish, spreading physical and moral contamination around them, it will be in vain to expect that any sanitary code can cause fever to disappear from Liverpool" (Duncan, "On the Sanitary State of Liverpool," *LREW*, 293–94). An exception is the report of the Birmingham committee, who, ignoring the London reports, organized their inquiry by leading causes of mortality and emphasized infant mortality and workplace accidents (A Committee of Physicians and Surgeons, "Report on the State of the Public Health in the Borough of Birmingham," *LREW*, 192–217).

14 W. P. Alison, *Observations on the Management of the Poor in Scotland, and Its Effects on the Health of Great Towns*, 2d ed. (Edinburgh: Blackwood, 1840), v–x, 20–22.

of fits, convulsions, paralysis, ulcers, indigestion, and various other diseases . . . and ascribe them to hereditary or personal infection, to low or unsuitable diet, hard work, exposure to cold, and other causes; but whenever such a regularly recurring complaint is found, almost invariably there is some open drain, some stagnant pool, or some long encouraged collection of decomposing animal or vegetable matter.[15]

Gilbert, one may say, loved his filth explanation well but not wisely. It was easy enough to find instances of physical causes, much harder to link them unequivocally with disease. As James Sym of Ayr complained, were it "a demonstrated truth that fever never originates from any other cause than from putrid miasmata . . . then there could be no difficulty in accounting for each individual case . . . because there is no instance in which some matter in a state of corruption may not be found sufficiently near to the patient to satisfy a theorist."[16] For such "theorists," Sym, and many others, had only contempt. They did not object to sanitary improvement, but only to the arbitrary elevation of one set of correlations to the status of *the cause*.

Even when they were not, like Sym, skeptical of Chadwick's claims, reporters sometimes complicated their explanations of disease outbreaks, recognizing a multiplicity of causes and of distinct causal questions. In their explanation of fever in the village of Breadsall (population 560, 76 cases, 5 deaths), Senior and Kennedy appealed to contagion to account for the beginning of the fever (it had been imported from nearby railroad workers), and to predisposing causes to account for the first case in the village, a fourteen-year-old girl, employed at fifteen pence/week at a mill several miles distant: "She would thus be exposed to great and frequent alternations of temperature, besides the fatigue of travelling to and from her daily occupation. These circumstances, in connexion with the deficient sustenance and clothing obtained by the miserable pittance of her wages, were causes quite sufficient to render this poor creature unusually liable to fever of the worst kind." To explain its propagation in the village they appealed to local miasms and bad living con-

---

15 W. J. Gilbert, "Report on the Sanitary State of the Labouring Classes in the Counties of Devon and Cornwall," *LREW*, 1.

16 James Sym, "Report on the Sanitary Condition of the Town of Ayr," *LRS*, 235. Sym presented a counterexample to the epidemiological examples Chadwick used. "Cross-street is inhabited by colliers as well as weavers, the houses of the two classes are intermingled, the stench around the doors and the filth of the interior are as great amongst the colliers as amongst the weavers; but the colliers and their families live on a more nutritious diet than the weavers; and . . . while fever rages amongst the weavers; it is not by any means a prevalent disease with the colliers, although small pox and other epidemics are equally severe with both trades. . . . This is not owing to the colliers being men of sounder constitutions than the weavers, for they are unhealthy looking, broken down by accidents, and whisky, generally affected with chronic bronchitis, and on the whole short-lived. Their blood, however, is of a better crasis than that of the half-famished weavers, in consequence of their superior diet. In short, I cannot, from the investigation I have made into the localities and progression of fever, connect its ravages with the nuisances which are exterior to the houses of the poor. It seems to me to be the offspring of their poverty itself, which renders their constitution susceptible of attacks, when exposed to contagion."

ditions: an "insalubrious position . . . the abundance of animal and vegetable matter in progress of decomposition . . . the bad state of the brooks, with morbific exhalations emitted from their margins . . . the large quantities of feculent water stagnating and evaporating on the adjacent meadows; the crowded state of the houses, and the great number of persons who sleep in the same room, and even in the same bed."[17] It is futile to try to categorize such an explanation as contagionist or miasmatist – the disease had no "simple exclusive cause."[18]

Some gave long lists of factors, seeing no need to spell out the relations among them yet inexplicably designating one as primary: for example, "in our opinion, anxiety of mind, penury, and starvation, and the depression of the bodily and mental powers which attends these conditions, are more frequent causes of fever than all the other sources to which it is attributed."[19] Or "the overcrowding and neglect of ventilation, the dissipated habits, and above all, the poverty and destitution which prevail amongst the inhabitants of the low and filthy quarters of large towns, are more powerful causes of fever than the malaria to which those people are exposed."[20] Some soberly warned against oversimplification: "The sources of disease, whether inherent in the human body or acting upon it as external causes, are so various in their numbers and mode of action, and even so mutually influential, that it is, under any circumstances, difficult to distinguish and define them."[21]

It was not a helpful response. However sympathetic, the local reporters were too disorganized to further the goal of sanitary improvement even as *one* means of improving health. Part of the problem was their unwillingness to give primary status to a malarial poison (or even to physical causes generally). Perhaps they were vexed at Chadwick's disregard of medical subtleties (and by implication his contempt for their professional competence). Some Scots were clearly using the Sanitary Inquiry to pursue Alison's agenda, even at the expense of Chadwick's (though the two were not necessarily incompatible).

In putting together the *Sanitary Report* Chadwick would largely ignore them. From his perspective they were woefully naive. Here was Edward de Vitre, physician to the Lancaster Dispensary and Fever Hospital, apologizing for including a section on poverty as a cause of disease:

17 Kennedy and Senior, "Breadsall," *LREW,* 182–91.
18 After all this Kennedy and Senior blamed the epidemic on the people themselves, whom they had nonetheless described as frugal, industrious, and sober ("Breadsall," *LREW,* 187–88, 191). Fry of Bodmin similarly gave a clear account of a contagious typhus "traceable from house to house in those exposed to it" but then noted the conditions "peculiarly favourable to its propagation" as clay soil, lack of ventilation, "eating and sleeping" in the same room, lack of privies, and speculation in dung. These were listed as "exciting causes" (in Gilbert, "Devon and Cornwall," *LREW,* 11–12).
19 "Birmingham Report," *LREW,* 206–7.
20 Richard Baron Howard, "On the Prevalence of Diseases Arising from Contagion, Malaria, and Certain Other Physical Causes amongst the Labouring Classes in Manchester," *LREW,* 317.
21 Adamson, "St. Andrews," *LRS,* 283.

The title . . . may at first strike you as supererogatory, but as I could not select a better term for the division, and as poverty does not imply destitution (which the Poor Laws of England under all circumstances relieve), and more especially as I consider it one of the most fruitful sources of disease, I think it advisable, in an inquiry like the present, not to omit anything having such a tendency, which is capable of being obviated, even however remotely, either by a sanitary police regulation, or by the due exercise of moral influence.[22]

Here was Richard Baron Howard of Manchester, writing that it made *no difference* whether the "destitution" that was "the most influential" cause of fever in Manchester was due to "the frequent want of employment, the disproportion between the rate of wages and the price of provisions and the necessaries of life, or to habits of reckless improvidence and dissipation," and claiming that it was government's duty "to devise means for insuring them these [common] necessaries [of life], whether their inability to procure them arises from causes which they themselves might be taught, by ordinary prudence and forethought, to avoid, or from circumstances which they cannot control."[23]

Maybe to the pathologist the origin of destitution made no difference, but it made a world of difference in preventing fever, Chadwick insisted, as anyone with a minimal acquaintance of political economy would know. People like Howard seemed not to appreciate that in discussing causes of disease they were seen to be making statements about responsibility and preventability, even culpability. In their fairy-tale world young doctors banished disease simply by declaring "the government shall feed," not for a moment understanding the economic, moral, and practical aspects of such a policy. Because those aspects were being ignored, Chadwick and Southwood Smith tended to see the destitution–fever claim as a fatalist view of disease.[24] If poverty were unavoidable even in the best economy, then to blame disease on poverty was like calling it an act of God, an event unfortunate but unpreventable.

De Vitre, Howard, and their colleagues were neither naive nor apolitical. Their apparent ingenuousness is usually a front. They were, however, operating in a very different political environment than was Chadwick. Theirs was a politics instantiated in medical practice, not in national legislation. Indeed, the very idea of a small town surgeon–general practitioner, a craftsman after all, having the audacity to dictate policy was a bit preposterous. Yet contemporary medical theory certainly could underwrite social criticism. Some, like

---

22 "Sanitary Condition of the Town of Lancaster," *LREW*, 345.
23 Howard, "Manchester," *LREW*, 330.
24 I find no one c. 1840 using the "destitution–fever" view to argue that there is no point spending public money to prevent disease, since it is due to inevitable poverty. A decade later, when there was a powerful and costly sanitary juggernaut to be derailed, some did make that argument (e.g., *Statements and Observations in Relation to the Report of William Lee C.E. to the General Board of Health on a Preliminary Enquiry into the Sanitary Condition of the Inhabitants of the City of Ely* [Ely: Thomas Hicks, 1850] in *Ely–GBH Correspondence*, PRO MH 13/68). In 1840 "public health" was still amorphous and such concerns are attempts to shape it, not block it.

Alison and his comrades in Scotland, the poor law medical officers in England and Wales, were using it in that way. Did those uses reflect a vision privileging health over capital, or were they only pragmatic observations of concerned medical men? We cannot say – those writing were too far from power to feel any need to espouse a coherent political philosophy.

Nonetheless the differences between their approach and Chadwick's were fundamental. Where he tended to treat health as an abstract state that people were automatically in when economic incentives were operating efficiently, they tended to define it concretely and see it as a prerequisite for economic and social efficiency. Some brought up occupational disease, a subject we have seen Chadwick avoiding. Sometimes they did so simply in identifying significant local causes of illness, yet to the degree that disease lowered efficiency they were also recognizing that work that harmed health was ultimately uneconomic. Essential to the work or not, industrial diseases and accidents were common.[25] In Birmingham, burns (mainly of children), manglings, and the chronic effects of exposure to lead, dry grinding, and great variations of temperature and humidity were the principal problems.[26] In the Lothian coal districts, Scott Alison and William Stevenson noted a "black spit," exclusive to colliers, "produced I should suppose by their inhaling small particles of coal."[27] Both Bakers, Robert of Leeds and William of Derby, saw factory work as a key public health problem. For the latter, "the factory system as a whole" was the most important general cause of disease remediable by legislation: it produced "the most extensive and the deepest rooted injury to the health of the labouring population . . . it breeds up puny parents of a future puny race, who, in their turn, perpetuate, and increase the evil."[28] Robert Baker echoed the Sadler witnesses of a decade earlier: long standing or sitting constrained the play of the lungs, distorted the growing legs, flattened the arch, inflamed the hemorrhoids, and led to the "plethorizing" of the digestion.[29]

Most forceful in arguing that the economists' imperative to work could as easily induce degradation as progress was Scott Alison of Tranent. He described the typical course of chronic industrial diseases among colliers: though unfit, the diseased father of young children would still work, pushing his

---

25 Directly countering Chadwick's claims of the inessentiality of occupational disease, Scott Alison compared mortality rates among dirty and disorderly Tranent colliers and clean and well-behaved Pencaitland colliers. He concluded that "the manifest shortness of life must be greatly owing to the unwholesome nature of their occupation" ("Tranent," *LRS*, 103).

26 "Birmingham Report," *LREW*, 208, 216–17.

27 William Stevenson, "On the Sanitary Condition amd [*sic*] General Economy of the Town of Musselburgh and Parish of Inveresk, in the County of Mid-Lothian," *LRS*, 145; Scott Alison, "Tranent," *LRS*, 103.

28 William Baker, "On the Sanitary Condition of Derby," *LREW*, 163.

29 Robert Baker, "On the State and Condition of the Town of Leeds in the West Riding of the County of York," *LREW*, 390–92. Baker did note that conditions of dwellings and habits complemented these factors.

disease into a fatal decline, during which his children would have to be re-moved from school to work. Such a scenario could not produce social or moral progress; work could not be a means of betterment and comfort if it led directly to poverty, death, and ignorance. In his view, the most serious effect of Chadwick's physical causes was not the acute fever that burdened society with widows and orphans, but the working person's normal chronic unhealthiness.[30] And the underlying cause of that unhealthiness was poverty. Even if nutrition were adequate, poverty operated in many other ways to produce degradation and disease. It left its victim in the cheapest and worst housing, crowded and exposed to Chadwick's physical causes, and usually without the education needed to move up in the world.[31]

As we saw earlier, diagnoses like these had been common, but more in regard to particular outbreaks than to a comprehensive health policy. In a constitutional medicine, however, to identify causes was not to identify remedies or preventives. With so many factors affecting vitality, there were many possibilities for intervention. One set of interventions might obviate the need for others: outdoor work, like fishing or farming, might counteract bad streets and houses. Good food and warm clothes might help one withstand malaria or carry on work that would otherwise cause illness; alternatively, a malaria-free environment might allow one better to tolerate cold, hunger, and hard work.[32] Even the broadest argument, that disease was a product of the totality of a laborer's life, had an inbuilt ambivalence, even in the hands of Sym, most radical of the Scots and star of *The Spectator*'s attack on Chadwick. Having railed against the comfortable belief that fever and "wretchedness" could be prevented by more scavenging or by "well meaning ladies distributing . . . religious tracts"; having asserted that something "more palpable" was needed – "better food and more of it, better clothes, better beds, better houses, and less incessant toil" – Sym concluded that "larger sums of money in proportion to the number of the poor must be distributed": either "assessments must be increased, or the number of poor must be curtailed."[33] In a climate in which the woes of the Scottish working class were being regularly blamed on surplus (Irish) population, a reader might as readily take Sym to be calling for some strong population restraint as for greater aid.

The chasm between cause and preventive is evident also in the frequent attributions of disease to trade cycles. Depressions hit Glasgow in 1816–17, 1819–20, 1826–27, 1829, 1837. On a smaller scale, they occurred every year to those whose trade was seasonal or dependent on good weather. "Even the most prudent and economical may be reduced to penury," Baird wrote, "from

30  Alison, "Tranent," *LRS*, 102, 106. See also Adamson, "St. Andrews," *LRS*, 283.
31  Baird, "Glasgow," *LRS*, 186. The strongest proponent of this view was Sym ("Ayr," *LRS*, 232).
32  Stevenson, "Musselburgh," *LRS*, 133; "Birmingham Report," *LREW*, 216–17; Jenks, "Brighton," *LREW*, 68.
33  Sym, "Ayr," *LRS*, 233, 237–38. See also Adamson, "St. Andrews," *LRS*, 281.

the inclemency of the weather, which almost every winter . . . interrupts the masons, slaters and out-door labourers; the sudden convulsions and fluctuations of trade . . . the high price of provisions; and, above all, their liability to diseases, especially of an epidemic nature."[34] One could not prevent snowstorms, perhaps not epidemics, but what of those spasms of overproduction so inherent to industrial capitalism, or food prices, artificially inflated by the corn laws?

As to how far diagnoses were to imply preventives, medical reporters were reticent. In contrast to Chadwick, however, they tended not to feel the constraining force of narrow and arbitrary conceptions of the politically possible. Nor, looking out on society from the traditions of their own profession, were they cowed by orthodox economics. By letting health be the starting point, not a hoped for outcome of economic policy, they were invoking quite different laws of human existence. Unapologetically, Sym noted that Ayr butchers regularly broke the laws of the market in the name of health (and social stability). They sold meat on a sliding scale: "beef . . . for which an opulent customer will pay 7d per lb., is readily purchased by a collier's wife at 5d."[35]

### III

If many of them recognized a pathogenic role for social and economic conditions, the medical informants were by no means working-class spokesmen: with the exception of William Pulteney Alison, they shared Chadwick's vision of an alien and dangerous population. Their reluctance to hold the poor responsible for their own situations originated less in the medical tradition of focusing on the disease rather than the acts that caused it than in their inability to see such people as fully human. Like Chadwick, they found it hard to distinguish innocent victims of circumstances beyond their control from a class so "demoralized" by circumstances as to have become irresponsible, or even dangerous. In such a climate of fear, the redefinitions of body and disease Chadwick offered, and the corresponding possibility of conducting medical and social relations through bricks and sewers, were attractive. No longer was the medical subject to be an individual with a unique history of encounters with health-modifying events. If not a cellar or a court, it became one of a class of interchangeable bodies generated in such places.

Both in Chadwick's report and in the *Local Reports* "demoralization" was widely seen as a concomitant of disease and misery. It is never defined, but refers both to a presumed subjective state characterized by a lack of hope and a feeling that further struggle is futile, as well as the abandonment of socially

34 Baird, "Glasgow," *LRS*, 166.
35 Sym, "Ayr," *LRS*, 217. Local citizens also intervened to stimulate the market during stagnant periods in the local weaving industry (227).

acceptable behavior. Demoralization was a function of "character," and the great question of the day was, as Assistant Poor Law Commissioner Tufnell put it, "whether the character of the labouring population depends on their circumstances, or their circumstances on their character?" Chadwick is credited with the former view, but his views were more complex, as were those of the medical reporters. Tufnell, and most poor law staffers, tended to stress the latter. While there were reciprocal effects, he still held that "the feelings, habits, and dispositions of the poor have an infinitely stronger influence on their comfort and condition than any of the natural evils that may surround them." While inadequate drainage was a significant cause of disease in his rural district, nonetheless "dirty habits, neglect of ventilation, and want of foresight have tended much to add force and frequency to those pestilential attacks."[36]

Tufnell did not object to sanitary improvement, but only to the determinism that underlay it: "the common doctrine" ignored "the fact that, they have minds as well as bodies to be taken care of, and implies that when the latter is attended to, and they have the means of material prosperity at command, all that is necessary for their welfare has been done." All this "making drains, building good cottages, increasing employment and increasing wages, may fail, may even end in a result precisely contrary to what was intended, unless . . . parallel endeavours are set on foot to improve the higher and nobler part of our natures."[37] What these were to be, Tufnell did not say: he spoke of "sound education," but his only specific example was economical cookery.

By contrast, numerous medical men asserted that the targeted classes had, in effect, lost or never possessed what Tufnell called "mind." The sort of environment he saw in Tranent would overwhelm a child, wrote Scott Alison: "If children so situated do not become vicious and abandoned . . . it will not be from the want of an atmosphere fitted for the growth of depravity. . . . When children so placed become vicious and commit crime, it occurs to me that they are themselves less to blame than those who possess the power to amend their condition, but neglect to exercise it."[38]

Adults succumbed too. In the tradition of Locke, the effects of dirt on the mind were seen as no less determinate than the effects of gravity on mass: "The eyes of the people, old and young, become familiarized with the spectacle of filth, and thus habits of uncleanliness and debased ideas of propriety and decency are ingrafted," wrote William Chambers, the prominent Edin-

---

36 E. C. Tufnell, "On the Dwellings and General Economy of the Labouring Classes of Kent and Sussex," *LREW*, 51–52; cf. Mott, "Lancashire, Cheshire, Derbyshire, and Staffordshire," *LREW*, 237: "It is unquestionably true that the deplorable state of destitution and wretchedness . . . might in most cases have been averted by common prudence and economy."
37 Tufnell, "Kent and Sussex," *LREW*, 56.
38 Alison, "Tranent," *LRS*, 115. See also Stevenson, "Musselburgh," *LRS*, 142.

burgh publisher.[39] Robert Baker of Leeds noted that just as public cattle slaughtering "has a tendency to brutalize the feelings, so the perpetual presentation of these uncleanly loci to the eye, dulls the energies of even the most willing housewives, and weakens in time the most cleanly original determinations." He urged newly married couples to leave such neighborhoods quickly. Those who stayed, "by repeated exhibitions of indecency and vulgarity," would "sink into . . . moral degradation."[40] Howard of Manchester noted "a most baneful *moral* effect" and "a want of self-respect and a disregard for decency of appearance" resulting "from long familiarity with all kinds of loathsome sights and stench."[41]

If demoralization were a physical process, so too might be recovery. Duncan of Liverpool noted that when a court had been "flagged and plentifully supplied with water, the inhabitants have appeared to feel a pride in keeping it in proper order." Brisco of Whitehaven held that better houses would make the poor more moral and more "frugal, cleanly, healthy and happy" (and "much better able to pay a somewhat higher rent").[42]

Such "But for a length of drain go I" arguments did not in fact reduce social distance between writer and subject. They reflected a double standard: a life that could be transformed by a simple sewer was surely very different from that of a free-willed social analyst able to see through such bread and circuses. Determinism was a way to understand others, not one's own kind. For the most part, the reporters relied on what they saw and smelled; they found themselves unable to imagine a *life* of labor. A few tried. Charles Mott, assistant commissioner for the industrial Northwest, acknowledged, as Kay had a decade earlier, that when workers were "pent up in a close, dusty atmosphere from half-past five or six o'clock in the morning till seven or eight at night, from week to week, without change, without intermission, it is not to be wondered at that they fly to the spirit and beer-shops . . . to seek those . . . pleasures and comforts which their own destitute and comfortless homes deny." Yet his only solution was public walks and other recreations, which might "relieve the tedium of . . . monotonous employment."[43]

A result of this failure of imagination was that the reporters tended to assume the demoralization that was to be explained. They had trouble conceiving that the very behavior that appalled them might be a free and prudent response in a different social, physical, and economic environment than they

---

39 Chambers, "Edinburgh," *LRS*, 154.
40 Baker, "Leeds," *LREW*, 354–55, 362.
41 Howard, "Manchester," *LREW*, 312.
42 Duncan, "Liverpool," *LREW*, 286; Brisco in Sir John Walsham, "Second Report on the State of the Dwellings of the Labouring Classes in Cumberland, Durham, Northumberland, and Westmoreland," *LREW*, 433.
43 Mott, "Lancashire, Cheshire, Derbyshire, and Staffordshire," *LREW*, 239.

were used to. "The people themselves are inert," complained the vice-chairman of the Cockermouth Union; "their thoughts are engrossed by the great business of finding daily food; and they will not listen to any lectures upon the theory of infection, or the connexion between dirt and disease."[44] But was this really "inertness"? Could lectures really substitute for food?

The prospect of a working class with its own agenda elicited the strongest dehumanizing declamations, the representation of the poor as animals or even as vegetables. Uniting the idea of the sinful, willful human with the image of the instinct-driven beast, several writers attributed overcrowdedness to the "herding" habit.[45] The minds of Tranent colliers were "scarcely . . . exercised," wrote Scott Alison; "they seldom reason more than . . . lower animals; they judge very precipitately and very erroneously, and they act upon the first impulse however violent." He went on: "Many may be said to vegetate, or, like aquatic plants, chiefly to imbibe, for they are excited by nothing; they are alive to no considerations such as engage or sustain the attention of other men." Having asserted that "political, social, religious, and all great and national questions are totally uninteresting to the majority of these degraded men," he noted a page later that they were all Chartists.[46]

Less dramatic than the Chartist horror were the perverse working-class "habits" of raising pigs and collecting (and often speculating in) dung. While James Sym thought pig keeping invited theft – "It is well known that a pig cannot be profitably fed by a poor person in a town by honest means"[47] – few felt a need to explain their condemnations; pig keeping transgressed implicit notions of cleanliness and decency (and, perhaps, dependence?).

While reporters agreed that dung heaps were objectionable, a great gulf separated those who objected to dung hoarding as a cause of disease, or an outrage to eye or nose, all the while acknowledging that it might be a sig-

---

44 Spedding in Sir John Walsham, "Second Report," *LREW*, 435.
45 Baker, "Derby," *LREW*, 162; Tippets in Tufnell, "Kent and Sussex," *LREW*, 47–48; George Robinson in Weale, "On Cottage Accommodation in Bedford, Northampton, and Stafford," *LREW*, 126–28.
46 Alison, "Tranent," *LRS*, 96–97. It is especially interesting to find Scott Alison making such remarks, for his report on Tranent was by far the most thorough and least doctrinaire. He had practiced in Tranent for six years and recognized several working-class cultures, distinct in occupation, neighborhood, and ethnicity. Writing from his new practice in London (he would become a tuberculosis specialist), he was, unlike most other reporters, free from local pressure. See also John Gibson on Lanark (*LRS*, 247), where people were "grossly ignorant and immoral; these desecrate the sabbath, employing it as a day of amusement and dissipation. . . . It is chiefly among these ignorant and careless people that profligacy prevails, and is followed by its usual attendants, poverty and disease. (Most of this class of people are Chartists, who are constantly declaiming against the extravagance of the government, and all who possess more property than themselves.)"
47 Sym, "Ayr," *LRS*, 237. William Stevenson was alone in maintaining that pigs were "a slight nuisance compared with many others, the odour arising from them being I should think delightful, compared with that of many of the nuisances to be found in the neighbourhood of their doors, and certainly not unconducive to health" ("Musselburgh," *LRS*, 138–39).

nificant source of income, and those who saw it as a transgression of social order. James Cameron of Tain reflects the former view:

There are various causes which render the collection of manure profitable to the inhabitants: their food principally consisting of potatoes . . . it requires all their ingenuity throughout the year to collect a sufficient supply [of manure] towards a succeeding crop; and the farmers in the neighbourhood are in the habit of purchasing cart-loads from them, for which they pay from 1s. 6d. to 2s. 6d. per load. Thus the greatest pains are taken by the inhabitants to procure and collect impurities of all descriptions; such as ashes, dirty water, decayed and decomposed matter, etc.: and this mass is husbanded with the greatest care and attention, and lies at their doors during most part of the year.

Cameron recognized the importance of this asset, though he worried about the "offensive and unwholesome effluvia" and dampness it generated.[48] From Cornwall, B. J. Ball wrote that "a pit of this sort is considered by almost every poor man . . . as a necessary appendage to his cottage; he even values it at half his living, and says that, if he is obliged to do away with the pit, he cannot grow his potatoes, etc: not thinking it is the very nursery of the fever which rages so on his children."[49]

Compare the tone of Chadwick's associate Arnott, describing the closes of Glasgow: "The dungheaps received all filth which the swarm of wretched inhabitants could give; and we learned that a considerable part of the rent of the houses was paid by the produce of the dungheaps. Thus, worse off than wild animals, many of which withdraw to a distance and conceal their ordure, the dwellers in these courts had converted their shame into a kind of money by which their lodging was to be paid."[50] In admitting that dung paid the rent, Arnott admitted it as a family asset, yet this could not be legitimate enterprise: such income was a corrupt currency – only "a kind of money" – used not by persons, but by a "swarm of wretched inhabitants." (Within a decade, as it became clear that human dung would be the property of middle-class ratepayers and would be recycled through the pipe sewers they owned,

---

48 Cameron, "Report on the Sanitary Condition and General Economy of the Town of Tain and the District of Easter Ross, Made to the Poor Law Commissioners," *LRS*, 315. See also Charles Simpson on Stamford: "In villages, the poor are in the habit of depositing filth in the immediate vicinity of their dwellings, and since this is done for the money (to them no trifling sum) they obtain for it, there is great difficulty in (as there ought to be much consideration in any enactment that may be contemplated) its prevention. . . . In . . . a village in the Ketton district . . . the committee for that purpose [ending a typhus epidemic] could only obtain the removal of those heaps of dirt by purchase. Since then they have accumulated again" (in Senior, "On the Causes of Disease Affecting the Labouring Classes in the Counties of Leicester, Lincoln, Nottingham, and Rutland," *LREW*, 158). W. J. Gilbert reported twenty-load dung heaps near Truro ("Devon and Cornwall," *LREW*, 1–15).
49 In Gilbert, "Devon and Cornwall," *LREW*, 7.
50 Arnott, "Edinburgh and Glasgow," *LRS*, 9. Chadwick quotes this passage in *Report on the Sanitary Condition of the Labouring Population of Great Britain*, ed. M. W. Flinn (Edinburgh: Edinburgh University Press, 1965), 98 [to be cited as *Sanitary Report*].

that shame would disappear.) Dehane of Wolverhampton tried to explain why classical economics failed to apply here: he claimed that dung hoarding could not be rational if some failed to engage in it.[51] It was not the dung heaps that differed but authors' attitudes. At Ayr, where children kept dung collections beneath their beds, Sym simply averted to the unhealthfulness of the practice; he saw no need to dehumanize.[52]

If dung hoarding revealed that the poor had their own form of capitalism, window-sealing showed the poor taking rational steps to protect their health. The refusal of the poor to appreciate the importance of ventilation was a long-standing complaint of medical men. Whether one saw the fever poison as a miasm or as a contagious effluvium, ventilation was crucial for prevention and cure. A snug, cozy, and weatherproof cottage was not an unmitigated good. Arnott (and Chadwick) noted that fever had not spread to the western Highlands until "benevolent" landlords had replaced their tenants' hovels with sound cottages.[53] "The science of ventilation has not made much progress in Scotland among the lower orders," wrote W. H. Forrest of Stirling, "and when its importance is stated to them, they . . . show a great contempt. . . . I am almost daily in the practice, when attending fever cases, of opening a window for the purpose of admitting fresh air, but as soon as I leave . . . the window is closed, and continues so till my next visit."[54] Fortunately windows in the dwellings of the poor were usually broken (sometimes by fever-fighting doctors); unfortunately the gaps were usually stuffed with rags.[55]

As with the response to dung keeping, this vexation at the unwillingness to be ventilated distinguishes those for whom the poor were objects whose diseases were a public problem from those who tried to see them as rational beings making (in their view) unwise choices. The few who inquired into this fear of air found that cold and damp (and the colds and respiratory diseases these produced) seemed more immediate threats than did a remote risk of fever. People blocked windows to conserve fuel and compensate for inadequate clothes, bedclothes, and sometimes, food.[56] In doing so they were taking

---

51 J. Dehane, "On the Sanitary Condition of the Town of Wolverhampton," *LREW*, 221.
52 Sym, "Ayr," *LRS*, 220–21.
53 *Sanitary Report*, 197; Arnott, "Edinburgh and Glasgow," *LRS*, 9.
54 Forrest, "Stirling," *LRS*, 264. De Vitre told much the same story: "It is almost a hopeless task endeavouring to convince them of the utility of what really appears to be beyond their comprehension, as they nearly unanimously object to the admission of fresh air into a sick-room, and if convinced at all, it is always against their own *judgment*" ("Lancaster," *LREW*, 343).
55 See Mr. Foreman, the Gateshead workhouse master, in Sir John Walsham, "Second Report," *LREW*, 418–19, 425–26; A. Kilgour and J. Galen, "On the Sanitary Condition of the Poor of Aberdeen," *LRS*, 296–97; Stevenson, "Musselburgh," *LRS*, 134. Breaking windows was reputedly the practice of James Gregory, Alison's predecessor in the Edinburgh medical practice chair (Robert Willis, in Royal Commission on the State of Large Towns and Populous Places, *First Report*, *P.P.*, 1844, 17, [572.], Evidence, qq 3290–3312).
56 See Mr. Watkinson, "the intelligent relieving officer of Chorlton-on-Medlock Union," in Mott, "Lancashire, Cheshire, Derbyshire, and Staffordshire," *LREW*, 236–37: "The greatest privation the inhabitants of cellars experience is want of fire; they deem it essential to have a fire by night

rational action against the most important predisposing factors. Before the ascendancy of political economy, supplying coal had been a common public response to fever epidemics and economic distress. Fever doctors had recognized the futility of preaching ventilation without providing heat.

## IV

As would Chadwick, most local reporters focused on men of working age. Their illness and death constituted the public health problem. Women, children, and the aged would surely benefit from sanitary improvement too, but their health did not constitute the *public* problem. In part, this orientation reflected the poor-law context of the report. As husbands, fathers, or the grown-up children of the elderly, healthy male adults were, through their employment, to be the guarantors of the health of their wives, children, and aged parents. Given wage differentials between the sexes, it was the husband's continued ability to work that usually determined whether a family would be forced onto the parish.

In practice this focus meant that a number of health problems were effectively marginalized in these formative years of British public health. Matters like infant and childhood mortality and infanticide arise occasionally but are not followed up. Puerperal fever is not mentioned, though it had been accommodated within the same etiological schema as other fevers. There is scant interest in women's work, even though women's wages were often less than half men's. Where women and children entered the discussions it was rarely in regard to their health problems per se, but rather to how these affected the health and morality of men. James Cameron saw unskilled midwives as a significant health problem in the sparsely populated north of Scotland. The members of the Birmingham Committee saw prostitution as a significant public health problem (they did not say how or why). They and Baker of Leeds (and Chadwick) attributed infant mortality chiefly to a lack of training for girls in domestic economy and child care. Poor housewifery also drove husbands to drink and disease.[57] Scott Alison, who examined a great range of social factors, did find domestic violence and desertion to be significant health problems in Tranent's collier families. Yet he too tended to see the significance of women's lives in terms of men's welfare. Chadwick would quote his description of the domestic bliss of the farm laborer: "A fire sheds its cheerful influence over the scene; the kettle never wants hot water; and the honest,

as well as by day; and when this cannot be obtained, the damp air is overpowering to the constitution, and this, added to the scantiness of bed-covering, brings on a variety of diseases." Also Stevenson, "Musselburgh," *LRS*, 135.

57 None of these, however, objected to women's working in factories as did some reformers. "Birmingham Report," *LREW*, 198, 210–11; Cameron, "Tain and Easter Ross," *LRS*, 329; Baker, "Leeds," *LREW*, 377, 390–95. But see Scott Alison, "Tranent," *LRS*, 126.

frugal housewife is ever discharging some household duty in a spirit of placid contentment, attending to her partner when present, or preparing his meals against his return from the fields."[58]

We have seen this sort of orientation in the *Sanitary Report* itself, but in his questionnaires Chadwick had not overtly steered the inquiry in this direction. Thus it is all the more remarkable how much the reporters shared his view, especially as (so far as one can tell from the examples they gave) the health problems of women and children formed a significant part of their practices. This lack of concern with women's lives does mark a change from earlier in the century, when the plight (and health) of women had been central in discussions of general health and welfare. Malthus himself had seen women's welfare as the keystone of social well-being – "Among those unfortunate females with which all great towns abound, more real distress and aggravated misery are perhaps to be found than in any other department of human life."[59] Yet in 1834, in the name of pragmatic administration, Chadwick's new poor law had effectively put responsibility for illegitimate children on the heads of those "unfortunate females" in absolving fathers of legal and financial burden. In a generally unpopular law, these bastardy clauses were the most hated.[60] Arnott's horror at the "half-dressed wretches" of Glasgow had replaced Malthus's concern.[61]

Again, the exception is William Pulteney Alison. Alison focused on those least visible in the "social conditions" debates of the day: elderly women, usually widows, without any obvious income. He did not approach these matters of health from the contexts of crime prevention or political economy or careful management of the parish purse. His long experience as a dispensary doctor was simply that children, women, and the elderly suffered illness disproportionately. He was also a Malthusian. To appreciate how people might act to check population one had to gauge how they viewed their own lives – what they hoped for, what they thought they could control, how they made choices. In his view, a quantum of human dignity, which it was society's duty to underwrite, was the key precondition of prudence. (Chadwick and Chalmers would have agreed but seen the sources of that dignity elsewhere.)[62]

This orientation toward the acute diseases of working age men would be

---

58 Alison, "Tranent," *LRS*, 87, 98–99, cf. 85. On domestic violence see also Stevenson, "Mussel-burgh," *LRS*, 141.

59 T. R. Malthus, *An Essay on the Principle of Population; or A View of Its Past and Present Effects on Human Happiness; With an Inquiry into our Prospects Respecting the Future Removal or Mitigation of the Evils Which It Occasions. The Version Published in 1803, with the Variora of 1806, 1807, 1817, and 1826*, 2 vols., ed. Patricia James (Cambridge: Cambridge University Press/Royal Economic Society, 1989), I, 18.

60 Lionel Rose, *Massacre of the Innocents: Infanticide in Great Britain 1800–1939* (London: Routledge and Kegan Paul, 1986), 22–34.

61 Arnott, "Edinburgh and Glasgow," *LRS*, 8–10.

62 W. P. Alison, *Observations*, v–vi, 49. See also Chambers, "Edinburgh," *LRS*, 153–55; de Vitre, "Lancaster," *LREW*, 342; Adamson, "St. Andrews," *LRS*, 279.

long-standing in British public health. When John Simon became medical officer to the Privy Council in 1858, sanitation, at least temporarily, ceased to dominate. Simon began with the intention of prioritizing inquiries and interventions by the most common causes of death and disease. Within that framework, infant mortality, nutrition, and various issues of women's health took a higher position in the public health agenda. Yet that approach could not be sustained: for social and political, as well as biological, reasons, some causes of diseases common in some populations were far more resistant to remediation than others.

## V

Arnott's revulsion at the "wretches" of Glasgow raises the last point of how far there was a "sanitary sensibility," a common visceral response to the conditions in which poor people lived. For the sanitary movement was not principally a product of mortality statistics or epidemiological demonstrations, but a spasm of revulsion. Ostensibly this was toward the physical environment – what could be seen or smelled, but in fact it was raw fear of unknown others of another class: revulsion was a vehicle that expressed and maintained social distance. Chadwick, as we have seen, was a master in its evocation.

Passage after passage in the *Local Reports* recounted the revulsion of the dispensary doctor called to a cellar or cottage. That doctors were disgusted was significant. After all, they were daily familiar with the unpleasant, the indecent, the unspeakable; surely what disgusted a dispensary doctor must be the apotheosis of pollution. Sometimes sensations are so dominant that we learn little of structure, even less of people. Wrote one: "The walls . . . were black, the sheets were black, and the patients themselves were blacker still; two of the children were absolutely sticking together. I have relished many a biscuit and a glass of wine in Mr. Grainger's dissecting-room when ten dead bodies were lying on the tables under dissection, but was entirely deprived of my appetite during these cases."[63]

Again with the signal exception of Alison, most local reporters shuddered at the same things that disgusted Chadwick. The range of things they shuddered at was broad. A medical officer of Sleaford Union attributed fever to an "intolerable" smell "arising" (in part) from "the dirty clothes of the children being allowed to accumulate."[64] W. H. Parker, an assistant commissioner,

---

63 J. F. Handley, in *Sanitary Report,* 316. Given working-class reaction to anatomical dissection and the great controversy over the Anatomy Act slightly over a decade earlier, this passage (and Chadwick's inclusion of it) reflects a particularly galling insensitivity, manifest in the claim that the dissecting room was in fact a much more sanitary and less disgusting place than the laborer's cottage (or even that working-class persons were more palatable dead than living). See also Joseph Childers, "Observation and Representation: Mr. Chadwick Writes the Poor," *Victorian Studies* 37 (1994): 405–32.

64 In Senior, "Leicester, Lincoln, Nottingham, and Rutland," *LREW,* 157.

reflected a distrust of things organic – a thatched cottage was an active morbid force:

The vegetable substances mixed with the mud, to make it bind, rapidly decompose, leaving the walls porous. The earth of the floor is full of vegetable matter, and from there being nothing to cut off contact with the surrounding mould, it is practically liable to damp. The floor is frequently charged with animal matter thrown on it by the inmates, and this rapidly decomposes by alternate action of heat and moisture. Thatch placed in contact with such walls speedily decays, yielding a gas of the most deleterious quality. Fever of every type and diarrhoea are endemic diseases in the parish and the neighbourhood.[65]

The Whitehaven Union chairman attributed typhus to a family's living "above a room filled with potatoes, which decay very fast from the place being so damp."[66] In later years this horror of life would strengthen as the urban environment became the site of a Manichean battle between the rival forces of vital organization and decomposition.

While we may want to ask how their noses (and eyes) were educated, the reporters give us little help in answering that question. Like Chadwick, they take refuge in empiricism; reactions parade as facts. A typical motif is the journey from the safe and familiar into a cellar or hovel, where the observer is struck by a full blow of condensed awfulness. In describing (his reaction to) Manchester, Richard Baron Howard began on the public street: "The filthy and disgraceful state of many of the streets in those densely populated and neglected parts of the town where the indigent poor chiefly reside, cannot fail to exercise a most baneful influence on their health." He found "whole streets . . . unpaved . . . worn into deep ruts and holes, in which water constantly stagnates, and . . . so covered with refuse and excrementitious matter as to be almost impassable from depth of mud, and intolerable from stench." Then one went to "the narrow lanes, confined courts, and alleys leading from those, [where] similar nuisances exist, if possible to a still greater extent; and, as ventilation is here more obstructed, their effects are still more pernicious." There one found secret marvels: "privies in the most disgusting state of filth, open cesspools, obstructed drains, ditches full of stagnant water, dunghills, pigsties, etc." One can almost see the lengthening shadows and thickening air.

Yet the inquiring visitor must go behind, off the street: "Dwellings perhaps even still more insalubrious are those cottages situated at the backs of the houses fronting the street, the only entrance to which is through some nameless narrow passage, converted generally, as if by common consent, into a receptacle for ordure and the most offensive kinds of filth and rubbish. . . . Surrounded on all sides by high walls, no current of air can gain access to

65 W. H. Parker, "On the Sanitary State of the Counties of Berkshire, Buckinghamshire, and Oxford," *LREW*, 91.
66 In Walsham, "Second Report," *LREW*, 425.

disperse and dilute the noxious effluvia, or disturb the reeking atmosphere of these areas." But until one went inside one had not reached the acme of foulness: "If the interior of the dwellings . . . be examined, they will be found . . . to correspond with the filthy condition of the exterior, and to present all the indications of negligence, slovenliness, and discomfort – of abject poverty and destitution, which the appearance from without would lead us to predict. . . . Dirty in an extreme degree, damp, shamefully out of repair, and barely furnished . . . a table, a chair, or a stool, a few, and very few, articles of culinary apparatus, some shavings, or a little straw in a corner, with a scanty piece or two of filthy bed-covering."

At this point Howard tells us that all we are seeing is unbelievable. He invites us to imagine as much as we can and then to amplify our image by some untold factor – something like trying to imagine infinity: "The wretched condition of many of the cellars will scarcely be credited by those who have not visited them – dark, damp, and filthy, incapable of ventilation, and constantly liable to be flooded – they present a most dismal appearance, and are quite unfit to be inhabited by civilized beings. . . . Windows neither keep out the wind nor rain, and the floors are sometimes not half covered with bricks or flags."

The allusion to "civilized beings" is the first indication that there may be humans about; given the high population density of the neighborhoods in which a Manchester dispensary doctor practiced, Howard would have been surrounded by people during such a tour, yet he has thus far given the impression of a place wholly depopulated. And the allusion to these "beings" is ambivalent: on one hand Howard wants us to agree that these housing conditions are unacceptable, but we may also decide that because this environment is "unfit" for "civilized beings," those beings are surely not civilized but belong to some other fearsome species.

Finally, Howard lets us know that after all, he has gone to these places to see people: "I have occasionally visited patients where the bedding or straw on which they lay was placed, without any protection, on a floor not only damp, but literally wet. The wretched occupants of these miserable abodes, as might be expected, are grossly negligent of personal cleanliness; they suffer from scantiness of clothing and bedding, too often from deficiency of food, from want of fuel and other necessaries of life, and have altogether a squalid and unhealthy appearance – the natural consequence of living amidst such fertile sources of diseases." The closest these "wretched occupants" come to possessing agency is in being negligent, and it is not clear whether Howard is accusing them of willful negligence or of ignorance, or simply describing the impossibility of keeping things clean in such a place. Otherwise, these people are simply silent sufferers of conditions.

In his peroration, Howard observed that it was "in these loathsome and pestiferous localities that disease rages in all its malignancy and power." But disease was a minor incident in the social explorer's journey into the inferno of insanitation.[67] It is significant that these views are Howard's. Of the English reporters, he was closest to Alison. Yet whatever his compassion, Howard could not get beyond relating to humans in terms of physical surroundings.

In some passages the human and the environment even merge into a compound horror. A Mr. Tippets, a Sussex medical officer, wrote of "families herding together in a small house, breathing an originally pestilential air, and rendering it more so by the hot, unwholesome, and confined effluvia of their own bodies, thereby rendering any case of fever that might arise . . . one of a most malignant, contagious, and dangerous character." Whether we are to blame the smallness of the house, the family's audacity in electing to live together in it, or their insistence on breathing and emitting effluvia is not clear and makes no difference. All these react upon one another, further lowering moral standards, thereby further increasing crowdedness and filth, and so on. The result is a force field of malignity that will produce a virulent fever in anyone who enters it. Remarkably, in treating the residents as part of an environmental cause of fever, Tippets dodges the fact that they, caught in this force field, will be its main victims; in his rendering they are not mainly ill people but components of a threatening system.[68]

A good deal of the subhumanness reporters attributed to their subjects resulted directly from their inability to imagine how people existed in such situations. W. H. Duncan tells us to protect our senses when we go into one of Liverpool's enclosed courts – "careful management of both eye and nose" is necessary for "the unpractised visitor" – yet it is somehow not a problem for those who live there. Indeed, he is surprised to meet "an intelligent Irishman" (as if this were an oxymoron) who actually agrees that conditions are deplorable: "The stench at night he said was enough to 'rise the roof off his skull as he lay in bed.' " William Stevenson noted that he had "sometimes found the smell insupportable, and yet these poor creatures will live as contentedly amidst all this dirt, as they would do in the cleanest place you might put them in." The Birmingham Committee told of privies "in a state which renders it impossible for us to conceive how they could be used; they were without doors and overflowing with filth," yet clearly they were used.[69]

Unable to communicate with those whose world they were briefly enter-

---

67  Howard, "Manchester," *LREW*, 305–6. Howard also took care to remind readers of the unique credibility (and courage) of dispensary doctors like him: "It is amidst such melancholy scenes that he, more than any other class of men, becomes acquainted with the hidden sufferings, miseries, and almost incredible destitution of his fellow-creatures."

68  In Tufnell, "Kent and Sussex," *LREW*, 48.

69  Yet not by all, the committee admitted. "The more decent females could not frequent them, but had recourse to utensils in their bed-rooms, which they emptied at night." The passage is one of the relatively few in which rational choice depictions displace brutalization-by-filth depictions ("Birmingham Report," *LREW*, 195). See also Duncan, "Liverpool," *LREW*, 287–88; Stevenson, "Musselburgh," *LRS*, 137.

ing, the medical reporters looked for physical signs of their mental/moral life. Reading furnishings was a chief method of inquiry of the Manchester Statistical Society, and in a less formal sense of Chadwick and many others. John Adamson, writing on St. Andrews, was confused by "a rather curious fact, that where there is the lowest notion of cleanliness, there is often exhibited an attempt at ornament, by gaudily-coloured prints pasted upon the walls."[70]

It is ironic that sanitary inquiry, apparently dedicated to making a set of common decencies universally available, should so strongly reinforce social distance. But that is what it did; the humans in the filth and not the filth itself was what fascinated the reporters, and it was those humans' minds, not their diseases, which especially intrigued them. The result was the construction of a species utterly alien and greatly to be feared.

## VI

With this review of Chadwick's reporters we can begin to make sense of how a constituency for the "sanitary solution" to the condition-of-England problem formed so quickly in the midforties. It was not that legions of worthy burghers read Chadwick and immediately experienced some transformative sanitary awakening. Quite the contrary. On the larger issues of the *Sanitary Report*, issues of the moralizing and management of a desperate and unruly people, Chadwick had gauged the mood of an influential segment of the public: professionals, the commercial classes, and those "fit and proper persons" who manned local government. That mood was fear. It fed upon visions of a dehumanized proletariat and in turn reinforced them. Given the prevailing level of animosity, illustrated for example in the *Northern Liberator* or J. R. Stephens's sermons, it would be unrealistic to expect a more moderate response.[71] Sanitation was, after all, the gentlest of policemen. One could promote drains and water in a spirit of pious benignity, without finger pointing or apoplectic rage. But the Chadwick of the sewers was no less the unrelenting disciplinarian than the Chadwick of the workhouse or the Chadwick who led an armed force to Lancashire to arrest Stephens.

Fear was not the only factor that pushed public health away from a more "social" agenda. At the time that agenda was also incoherent. It is quite true that many medical reporters dissented strongly from Chadwick's sanitary reductionism. Whether they did so to support Alison or to advance the interests

70 Adamson, "St. Andrews," *LRS*, 273; also Charles Barham, "On the Sanitary State of Truro," *LREW*, 18–19. See also A. P. Donajgrodzki, " 'Social Police' and the Bureaucratic Elite: A Vision of Order in the Age of Reform," *Social Control in Nineteenth Century Britain*, ed. A. P. Donajgrodzki (London: Croom Helm, 1977), 58.
71 See, for example, "The Rev. J. R. Stephens – Mr. Stephens' Sermon at Ashton," *Northern Liberator*, 12 January 1839; "[Speech Picked up near Morpeth]," *Northern Liberator*, 12 January 1839; "Suppressed Papers of the British Association. Left in Newcastle upon Tyne in August Last," *Northern Liberator*, 8 December 1838.

of poor law medical officers matters little; in pointing out that food, heat, clothing, and rest from work were quite as much desiderata of health as sound sewers they were drawing on long-standing conventions of medical thought, on their own experience practicing among the poor, and, one is tempted to add, on simple common sense. Yet despite *The Spectator*'s endorsement of their critique, and the fact that Delane's *Times* and Wakley's *Lancet* had been hammering the same message for years, the view that severe poverty caused disease was fading rapidly. A few years later, when the Irish famine arrived with typhus in tow, sanitarianism was so dominant that this new famine fever hardly made it onto the public health agenda, at least outside of Ireland. Alison, it is true, kept publishing tracts illustrating the link between poverty and fever, but at least in London few took notice.[72]

The most important reason for this rapid decline, I think, is that there was no clear way to go from the demonstrated truth that poverty causes disease to a public policy: cause did not imply remedy. Following a half century of declamations about the pauperizing tendencies of any relief, especially in the form of necessaries of life, there was little enthusiasm for making food a central and regular part of public health. Some who stressed the hunger-fever link found the Anti-Corn Law League a vehicle for their concern, though the league was committed less to ensuring that people were fed than to promoting an economic policy which would, it believed, make food cheaper and consequently more accessible.

The closest thing to a political principle that might have underwritten an Alisonian public health was Cobbett's argument, later modified by Marx, that the laborer's body was a form of property, which it was the state's duty to protect.[73] What Cobbett left out, of course, was that the state did not automatically protect the gentleman's estate; the gentry paid men of business to protect it from assaults in private bill committees or Chancery actions. Who would pay to protect the body of the free laborer? Possibly a kindly paternalist

---

72 See W. P. Alison, *Observations on the Epidemic Fever of 1843 in Scotland and Its Connection with the Destitute Condition of the Poor* (Edinburgh: Blackwood, 1844); idem, *Observations on the Famine of 1846–7 in the Highlands of Scotland and in Ireland as Illustrating the Connection of the Principle of Population with the Management of the Poor* (Edinburgh: Blackwood, 1847); Joseph Robins, *The Miasma: Epidemic and Panic in Nineteenth Century Ireland* (Dublin: Institute of Public Administration, 1995). Chadwick explained the association of fever with the Irish famine by observing that "want and causes of physical depression in Ireland were accompanied by removable causes, which aggravated their effects." The problem was that since potatoes wouldn't grow (and there was no seed for them), the manure that would otherwise fertilize them became a source of disease (Edwin Chadwick, *Health of Towns. Report of the Speeches . . . to Promote a Subscription in Behalf of the Widow and Children of Dr. J. R. Lynch* [London: Chapman, Elcoate, 1847], 8).

73 Slaney made this argument in the 1848 debates on the Public Health Act: Sanitation should be looked on "not as a matter of compassion, but as one of justice – whether the poor man's property – his health, his strength, his sinews, his power to labour – the poor man's only property – were not to be protected as well as the property of the rich"; the "poor man's property was his health, strength, and power to labour" (*Hansard's Parliamentary Debates, 3rd series, 96*, 1848, 412; *98*, 1848, 769). See also Himmelfarb, *The Idea of Poverty*, 55–56, 212.

employer or landlord or state, but in such a case the laborer could hardly be said to be free.[74] Once Cobbett and the radicals had set off on the road to liberty there would be no good place to stop until one had gotten well past Marx to a state in which free workers reordered society to protect the property of their bodies. At the time, however, bread and liberty did not mix well, as is evident in the much described conflict between northern and southern Chartism. One could not expect to have the government supply food and regulate work and yet claim that one was achieving liberty – unless of course the collective one was the state. And it wasn't. Alison was no Marx – he was more a medical Lord Ashley, quite as much a defender of the established order.

The only viable prospect for the state's protecting the laborer's embodied property (other than factory reform, which remained controversial) was Chadwick's sanitation. However much one might rage at Chadwick's heavy-handed rejection of social causes of disease, it was hard to oppose sanitation. Chadwick's was the only game in town, and as even Alison admitted, sanitation was unquestionably good. Chadwick, of course, had other reasons than protecting the worker's property for promoting it – undermining pesky medical officers, courting Peel, staking out an independent administrative domain, strengthening central government, even lowering poor rates.

This then is the beginning of the first great transformation in British public health – the metamorphosis of social into environmental problems. To be sure, earlier writers had been concerned with environmental quality. Yet they had focused on the effects of the environment on social and moral condition. After the transformation, the state of the environment would be problematic in its own right. One still assumed that environmental conditions affected human institutions and behaviors, yet focused so much on the dwelling, pipe, or drain that these effectively became proxies for the social and the subjective. It was a profound transformation, altering the deep structures of language. "Misery" in pre-Chadwickian literature often includes a subjective state of anxiety, sorrow, despair, sometimes triggered by real social conditions – exhausting work, cold and hunger, or the fear of losing one's employment. After 1845, it is increasingly a term to be applied to physical conditions: the dirt, stench, and damp, which presumably accompany the traditional misery are

---

74 The difficulty of squaring the circle did not prevent people from talking as if it could be done: "Where the situation of the labourer *is attended to in regard to his domestic comforts and conveniences*, it has a most decided effect upon his habits both as regards industry and the *fostering of a spirit of independence*" (James Gray in Walsham, "Second Report," *LREW*, 428 [italics mine]; cf. Sym, "Ayr," *LRS*, 224–25). Sym argues that a paternalist approach "tends to vitiate the morals, and degrade the spirit of independence." Alison took the view that once people were provided with "a certain degree of comfort, and the feeling of certain *artificial wants*," they would become sober citizens (W. P. Alison, *Reply to the Pamphlet Entitled "Proposed Alteration of the Scottish Poor Law Considered and Commented on," by David Monypenny, Esq. of Pitmilly* [Edinburgh: Blackwood, 1840], 42fn).

"miserable." Similarly, "depression," hitherto a pathological condition jointly physical and mental, disappears from the medical gaze until it reappears as a mental illness in the twentieth century. "Distress," hitherto used to describe both a state of the economy and the appropriate reaction to it, ceased on the whole to have this dual signification.

By no means was this transformation instantaneous, but it was rapid. The chief vehicle for confirming Chadwick's transformation was the Royal Commission on the Health of Towns and Populous Districts, which sat from spring 1843 to winter 1845. The ways of defining and habits of thinking it instantiated were not challenged, and within a decade, public health was something quite different from what it had been in the midthirties.

# 7

## Sanitation Triumphant: The Health of Towns Commission, 1843–1845

The view Chadwick had been fighting, that poverty caused disease, was finally buried in the work of the Royal Commission on the Health of Towns and Populous Districts. It went quietly, not in noisy controversy but in the silence of an agenda. The Health of Towns Commission was issued in May 1843, barely nine months after the *Sanitary Report*, and reported in June 1844 and February 1845. Historians have not known what to make of it. It is on the one hand Chadwick's vindication: doubt Chadwick if you must, but not a panel of independent experts. But it is seen also as a temporizing move of dithering Tories who would not see the obvious or do the necessary: as an unnecessary three year postponement of public health legislation.[1]

It is better to see the commission as an *extension* of Chadwick's work: the vindication was in its mission. Whether it was "necessary" begs the question of whether public health was striving toward some recognized destiny that would be embodied in the act of 1848. Chadwick thought it necessary, as did the Tory home secretary, Sir James Graham, and R. A. Slaney, convener of the 1840 Health of Towns Select Committee.[2] The main dissentient was Lord Normanby, author of three public health bills – for town drainage, building regulations, and "borough improvements" generally – the previous Whig government had introduced in 1841 on the recommendations of Slaney's com-

---

1 Lord Normanby in Health of Towns Association, *Abstract of the Proceedings of the Public Meeting Held at Exeter Hall, December 11, 1844* (London: Charles Knight, [1845]), 5; S. E. Finer, *The Life and Times of Sir Edwin Chadwick* (London: Methuen, 1952), cf. 228, 232–34; R. A. Lewis, *Edwin Chadwick and the Public Health Movement, 1832–1854* (London: Longmans, Green, 1952), 83, 89, 106–7; David Roberts, *Victorian Origins of the British Welfare State* (Hamden, Conn.: Archon Books, 1969), 140–41; Edward H. Gibson, "The Public Health Agitation in England, 1838–1848: A Newspaper and Parliamentary History" (Ph.D. diss., University of North Carolina, Chapel Hill, 1955), 161, 191–93, 198; Oliver MacDonagh, *Early Victorian Government, 1830–1870* (London: Weidenfeld and Nicolson, 1977), 142–43.

2 Slaney, now out of the House, repeatedly urged Peel to issue it, promising to fund the investigation himself (Shrewsbury Records Centre, Slaney Diaries, v. 7, October 1841, September 1842; v. 8, August 1843); on Chadwick, see Lewis, *Chadwick*, 106–7.

mittee. (Facing a flurry of amendments, the falling Whig government had passed none.)[3]

But each looked to the commission for something different: for Chadwick, it might lead to some public career free of his poor law masters; for Slaney and Graham, it offered comfort for the masses and social stability, with Slaney emphasizing the former, Graham the latter. All three were responding to a continuing crisis. The army had stopped the August insurrection but the riots went on sporadically through the winter of 1842–43, and there was still no sign of prosperity. Something, real or symbolic, was needed to offer hope: perhaps sanitary improvement. When we consider that no cholera epidemic threatened, that the hygienic principles were hardly novel, and that localities had already been obtaining improvement acts for sanitary purposes for nearly a century, the priority sanitation had achieved is remarkable.

The commission's achievements were mainly technical and political. It amassed vast data on how to build sewerage works and water supplies, and to recycle sewage; the proposals for high-pressure constant supplies of water and egg-shaped, graded, and regularly flushed sewers, covered in the *Sanitary Report* in a few paragraphs, were the subject of pages of testimony from sewers commission surveyors, water engineers, and architects. It is less clear, however, that the relevant technical communities actually used or learned from that accumulated knowledge. Politically, its investigations themselves awakened an interest in sanitation in several towns. It, much more than the *Sanitary Report*, launched the sanitary movement of the mid-1840s.[4] That its findings either made a case for public health or showed how public health institutions should best be organized is less clear.

Though he had no official link with the commission, Chadwick was involved in almost every aspect of it. He had drafted its charge, submitted a list of potential commissioners, produced the questionnaire for use in field investigations, identified and "precognised" several witnesses, attended all its meetings, chaired the subcommittee that digested the local evidence, accompanied some of the commissioners on their field investigations and badgered them about their reports, written substantial portions of its first report and drafted the recommendations in the second. Lyon Playfair, one of the com-

3 Chadwick opposed these bills, more vehemently than one might expect. His grounds were that they insulted medical men, in failing to make use of the experience of the poor law medical officers. He also objected to the machinery for implementation. Lewis attributes Chadwick's opposition to the Whigs' preemption of the Sanitary Inquiry. It is also worth noting that Normanby gratuitously attacked the Poor Law Commission [PLC], apparently in an effort to win the support of Tory radicals. See Gibson, "The Public Health Agitation in England," 88; *Hansard's Parliamentary Debates, 3rd series, 57*, 542–43; *58*, 892, 1317; Chadwick to Lord Normanby, 3 February 1841, University College London [UCL] Chadwick Papers, #1578; Lewis, *Chadwick*, 84.

4 Health of Towns Association, *Report of the Sub-Committee on the Answers Returned to Questions Addressed to the Principal Towns of England and Wales, and on the Objections from Corporate Bodies to the Public Health Bill* (London: Clowes, 1848), 22–24; *Hansard's Parliamentary Debates 3rd series 91*, 1847, 645.

missioners, treated him as supervisor-secretary, apprising Chadwick of his own investigations, asking him for commission work to take on his holiday. Chadwick's efforts were sufficiently well recognized that he was paid for his expenses.[5] But most important was the mission. Writing to Graham in March 1843, Chadwick listed matters that needed attention, in sanitary engineering, law, and medicine – everything from the best materials and modes of manufacture for water pipes, drains, and traps to the finance of sanitary works and the powers and duties of the new sanitary authorities.[6] Graham accepted this orientation, writing to would-be commissioners that their purpose was to determine "the best mode of preserving the Public Health *by an improved system of sewerage in large Cities, by a more abundant Supply of Water and by better construction of the dwellings of the Poor.*" In its first report the commission explained that while it was interested in all the causes of poor health, the only remedies it would consider were structural – drainage, water, building regulations – which would require minimal legislation.[7] In its second it held that the key question of the *Sanitary Report* of whether destitution was cause or consequence of fever was moot: one could endorse sanitary reform "without entering into any discussion of the influence which poverty and distress may occasion on the rates of mortality, which no sanatory improvements can entirely prevent."[8] For the most part witnesses and commissioners accepted these constraints. Thus Duncan of Liverpool, though unconvinced that fever could be explained solely by miasms, was willing to omit factors like poverty from his report.[9]

In accepting that the focus of the Health of Towns Commission would be

5 He did not however receive an honorarium as the commissioners did, perhaps because he was already on the public payroll (Buccleuch to Chadwick, 18 December 1845, UCL Chadwick Papers, #1771). Also Slaney Diaries, Shrewsbury Records Centre, v. 8, August 1843, 17 Jan 1844; *Minutes, Health of Towns Commission,* 25 January 1844, Public Record Office [PRO] MH 7/1, 64–65; Chadwick to Slaney, 21 December 1843, UCL Chadwick Papers #2181/2; Playfair to Chadwick, 30 September, 3 October 1843, 22 February 1844, UCL Chadwick Papers #1588; John Simon, *English Sanitary Institutions, Reviewed in Their Course of Development, and in Some of Their Political and Social Relations* (London: Cassell and Co., 1890), 198. On the list of questions see *Minutes, Health of Towns Commission,* 18, 20, 22 July 1843, PRO MH 7/1, 48, 50–53. Cf. Finer, *Chadwick,* 234; Gibson, "The Public Health Agitation," 195; Anthony Brundage, *England's "Prussian Minister": Edwin Chadwick and the Politics of Government Growth, 1832–1854* (University Park: Pennsylvania State University Press, 1988), 92–96.
6 Chadwick to Sir J. Graham, 15 March 1843, UCL Chadwick Papers #849.
7 Graham to Commissioners, 17 April 1843, *Register of Papers, Health of Towns Commission,* PRO HO 45/416 (italics mine); Royal Commission on the State of Large Towns and Populous Districts, *First Report, P.P., 1844, 17,* [572.] [to be cited as HOT, *First Report*], vii-viii.
8 Royal Commission on the State of Large Towns and Populous Districts, *Second Report, P.P., 1845, 18,* [602.] [to be cited as HOT, *Second Report*], 2. Cf. Playfair, "Report on the Sanitary Condition of Large Towns in Lancashire," HOT, *Second Report,* 68, and the Alison disciple John Roberton, "On the Causes and Amount of Death in Manchester," HOT, *Second Report,* Appendix, pt. 2, 112.
9 W. H. Duncan, "On the Physical Causes of the High Rate of Mortality in Liverpool," HOT, *First Report,* 13, 18, 25.

220 Public Health and Social Justice

structures, the transformation of "public health" was effectively accomplished. Chadwick had succeeded in what Bruno Latour holds out as every scientist's goal: to "black box" his own work.[10] Questions on which the *Sanitary Report* had reached conclusions (i.e., was destitution cause or consequence of fever?) need not be reopened. There could be no objection to the principles of the *Sanitary Report*, Chadwick told Graham: they derived from the law of gravity.[11]

In two other important ways – the exclusion of Scotland and the organization of the inquiry in terms of place (towns) rather than people (laboring classes) – the commission's mission differed from that of the Sanitary Inquiry. From Scotland had come the most emphatic assertions of destitution as a cause of disease. But that issue had arisen in regard to Scottish poor law reform, concurrently subject of another royal commission, so there was justification for omitting Scotland. (In fact that commission would pay little attention to Alison's concern that destitution was a medical problem.) As for the urban focus, the switch from wretched and revolutionary people to towns circumvented messy social and moral issues. Certainly sanitation would mitigate social problems, but it need not be held hostage to controversial arguments about environmental determinism or savings in poor rates. In focusing on towns, the commission was also drawing in a new constituency, middle-class municipal "improvers" who, since the mid-eighteenth century, had pressed Parliament for powers to widen, pave, drain, and light streets in their towns; to ban or regulate offensive trades. The improvement commissions they established at much expense were concerned less with the state of the masses than with the state of the streets on which the middle classes lived or worked.[12] Still, it was an ingenious political construct: the sanitary movement would unite widespread middle-class concerns with local amenities, central government concerns with economy and social order, and evangelical visions of a coming world of morality, decency, and cleanliness. Could anyone possibly object?


I


Because Chadwick's recommendations have often been portrayed as honest common sense, their confirmation by independent inquirers has not seemed particularly problematic to historians. Yet while they willingly involved themselves in a Chadwickian enterprise, the commissioners were neither placehunting yes-men nor dunces bamboozled by Chadwick's brilliance. There is

---

10 Bruno Latour, *Science in Action* (Cambridge, Mass.: Harvard University Press, 1987).
11 Chadwick to Graham, 15 March 1843, UCL Chadwick Papers #849.
12 Frederick H. Spencer, *Municipal Origins: An Account of English Private Bill Legislation Relating to Local Government, 1740–1835; with a Chapter on Private Bill Procedure* (London: Constable and Co., 1911); John Prest, *Liberty and Locality: Parliament, Permissive Legislation, and Ratepayers' Democracies in the Nineteenth Century* (Oxford: Clarendon Press, 1990).

a striking difference between the commission's reports, where Chadwick's hand was strong, and the reports of individual commissioners, some of whom raised issues that had either not been considered in the *Sanitary Report* – infant mortality rates – or had been suppressed, such as pulmonary consumption and ventilation. Nevertheless, whatever they found, when properly interpreted and presented, could be put to service in the sanitarian cause: the 1833 factory medical commissioners had been far more refractory, but Chadwick had made them do his work. After reviewing these "expansions" of sanitarianism, I shall return to the commission's central concerns: reform of local administration, sewer and waterworks design, and the hope that sewage farming would underwrite the costs of sanitary reform.

There were thirteen Health of Towns commissioners. Both the duke of Buccleuch, the chairman, and Lord Lincoln (heir of the duke of Newcastle) were astute Tory politicians and capable administrators, members of Peel's inner circle. Robert Slaney, Malthusian, Whig, evangelical, paternalist Shropshire landowner, was deeply concerned with the "condition of the people" and deeply fearful of revolution. We shall see more of him in the next chapter. As registrar general, George Graham, brother to Sir James Graham, was William Farr's boss. His was a political appointment; nonetheless he was an able administrator whose protection fostered Farr's sanitary activism.

The remaining commissioners were professional men and many of them were Chadwick's choices. Four were connected with medicine: D. B. Reid was an Edinburgh physician–chemist and ventilation consultant (working on the Houses of Parliament). James Ranald Martin had retired from an illustrious career as an Indian army surgeon to become an inspector of army hospitals; Richard Owen was a professor of anatomy at the Royal College of Surgeons. The Liebig-trained chemist Lyon Playfair (only twenty-five) had originally been educated as a doctor. He was in search of a gentleman's career, which he would find mainly in Liberal party politics rather than chemistry. Four others represented engineering. Robert Stephenson was at the height of his career as a railroad engineer and was (hardly surprisingly in the mid-1840s) really too busy to bother much with the commission. He and William Cubitt (later Tory M.P. and lord mayor of London) were members of the Great George Street elite: the cadre of civil engineers who got bills through Parliament, headed massive development and reclamation projects, and ran the Institution of Civil Engineers. By contrast, William Denison and James Smith of Deanston were marginal engineers. Denison's stellar career as a colonial administrator (he would serve a short time as governor-general of India) had not yet begun; he was but an obscure captain of Royal Engineers. Smith was a maverick capitalist and scientific farmer. He had run his Ayrshire cotton mill in a spirit of innovative paternalism reminiscent of his former neighbor Robert Owen, but Smith's utopianism had focused on clever devices rather than on socialism and new religions. No less eccentric than Owen, Smith was politically safer. He became enraptured with the prospect of profit from sewage and served as one of Chadwick's first group of engineering inspectors. The final commissioner was Sir Henry de la Beche, a geological bureaucrat (and first head of the Geological Survey).[13] Chadwick had nominated de la Beche, Stephenson, Denison, Owen, and Smith.[14]

A few observations on this group: The four politicians had much in common. They represented landed interests rather than the manufacturing towns and were far removed from any sort of radicalism. The professionals were independent of ties to existing institutions of sanitary engineering and local government, so much so, indeed, that (with the exception of Smith and Reid on certain issues) they hardly qualified as experts on the issues of inquiry. Indeed, their expertise was in some cases astonishingly remote. Owen, after all, was a comparative anatomist and vertebrate paleontologist (coiner of the term "dinosaur").[15] None of the other medical men had significant experience of urban practice or of medical practice at all, for that matter. De la Beche was a coal geologist. Stephenson and Cubitt were general practice civil engineers, much more involved with railroads than with water and sewers. None of them had experience in the important matters of local administration and finance.

But ignorance is no guarantee of tractability. The unanimity of the commissioners would be a key source of Chadwick's later credibility, and it is well to ask how it was achieved. Here were eight independent professionals, with varied backgrounds and training, studying complex and controversial social problems in different regions and reaching substantive consensus.

Chadwick's relations with the several commissioners were quite different. As nonprofessionals, Buccleuch, Lincoln, and Graham kept aloof from technical issues and did not take on any of the local investigations. Slaney was a long-standing (and rather naive and uncritical) friend of the new poor law. For him, to be doing good was enough. By the spring of 1845 Stephenson and Cubitt were taking no part in the deliberations. Stephenson did oppose

13  On Playfair and de la Beche see *A Biographical Dictionary of Scientists,* ed. T. I. Williams (New York: Wiley, 1969), 137–38, 420–21. On Slaney see Paul Richards, "R. A. Slaney, the Industrial Town, and Early Victorian Social Policy," *Social History* 4 (1979): 85–101. On Cubitt and Slaney see *Who's Who of British Members of Parliament,* Vol. 1, *1832–1885: A Biographical Dictionary of the House of Commons,* ed. Michael Stenton (Atlantic Highlands, N.J.: Harvester Press, 1976). On Graham, see John M. Eyler, *Victorian Social Medicine: The Ideas and Methods of William Farr* (Baltimore: Johns Hopkins University Press, 1979), 46. On Martin and Reid, see Frederick Boase, *Modern English Biography* (Truro: Netherton and Worth, 1892–1921). On Denison (1804–71) see *Minutes of Proceedings, Institution of Civil Engineers 33* (1871): 251–59; on Smith (1789–1850) see Thomas Ferguson, *The Dawn of Scottish Social Welfare: A Survey from Medieval Times to 1863* (Edinburgh: Thomas Nelson, 1948), 89.

14  Chadwick to Graham, 15 March 1843, UCL Chadwick Papers #849.

15  Cf. Finer, *Chadwick,* 234: "Now it is not at all surprising that the Commissioners should have confirmed all of Chadwick's views, for although they were the most creative brains of their time in their own particular fields of work, their work was just what made it likely that they would approve such views."

Chadwick's principles of water supply but did not force the issue.[16] Owen and de la Beche would remain allies in Chadwick's campaigns for several years. Neither claimed expertise in sanitary science, but the anatomist of the College of Surgeons, the chief of the Geological Survey, and the secretary to the Poor Law Commission held in common an administrator's abhorrence of all things radical and ad hoc. Each deferred to the other; they got along well. Smith of Deanston on the other hand was a kindred spirit. He and Chadwick shared a fascination with drains, liquid manure, and social discipline. The young Playfair was seeking patronage and, like Chadwick, willing to work devilishly hard to make science deliver political goods. Chadwick had less influence with Reid, Martin, and Denison. Denison was sufficiently occupied elsewhere to be innocuous, Reid and Martin less so.[17] In short, while we do not have records of deliberations on particular issues, it is pretty clear that Chadwick could usually count on strong support from Slaney, Owen, de la Beche, Smith of Deanston, and Playfair, and acquiescence from the others.[18]

Within a month of receiving its charge the commission was already hard at it, meeting three days a week for five hour sessions to hear from architects and engineers, sewers commission officials, and a few (surprisingly few) medical men. A first series of hearings lasted from June to mid-July 1843, a second set from February to March 1844.[19] Chadwick was also securing reports from selected individuals in a handful of towns: from W. H. Duncan, future medical officer of Liverpool; from two Lancashire clergymen-statists, the Reverends Clay of Preston and Coulthart of Ashton-under-Lyne; from P. H. Holland, a well connected young surgeon interested in sewage recycling, on Chorlton-on-Medlock; from Thomas Laycock, an aggressive and controversial doctor (ultimately successor to Alison's chair in Edinburgh) on York; and from an up-and-coming Nottingham water and gas engineer, Thomas Hawksley. This testimony and these reports formed the bulk of the commission's first report of June 1844.

A second report appeared in February 1845, consisting mainly of the investigations of individual commissioners. The commission had divided the country into sections for individual investigation: de la Beche took the Southwest and South Wales, Playfair took Lancashire, Reid the North, Owen the city of Lancaster, Denison Woolwich and Salisbury, while Martin investigated the East Midlands and Portsmouth, Slaney the West Midlands, and Smith the

---

16 "Budget for Expenses of Commissioners," *Register of Papers, Health of Towns Commission*, 31 May 1844, PRO HO 45/416. While active commissioners like Playfair and Reid devoted one hundred days or more to commission work, Stephenson and Cubitt devoted eight and six days, respectively.

17 For Chadwick's assessment of Martin see Chadwick to Lord Morpeth, 15 September 1848, UCL Chadwick Papers #1055.

18 Some of the work, for example, the digesting of the reports for the commission's first report, was also done in a subcommittee chaired by Chadwick (Slaney Diaries, Shrewsbury Records Centre, v. 8, 17 January 1844).

19 Ibid., August 1843.

West Riding of Yorkshire. A water report by Stephenson is said to have been suppressed by Chadwick.[20] Their reports were products of a process that began with the commissioner's asking the town's mayor to form a committee to respond to a long list of questions about sanitary facilities. A visit followed, featuring a tour of the worst districts (local assessments were often too positive, some commissioners noted) and a combination hearing-meeting to go over the responses. The commissioner would then write his report.[21]

Despite Chadwick's efforts to impose uniformity by using questionnaires there was considerable unevenness in the contributions. The fifty towns reported on were represented in very different levels of detail. Still, the results are impressive. Many writers had gone to great trouble to work up tables and figures, and the searcher after hard data will find the commission's reports much easier to use than the reports of Chadwick's inquiry.


II


On to substance: "Public health" could not pass from social policy to sewer design without some strong medical theory to carry it. While it received a few reports from regional practitioners like Duncan and Laycock, the few medical witnesses the commission heard were Londoners, most with close ties to Chadwick: his associates Southwood Smith and Neil Arnott; also Robert Willis, former surgeon of the Royal Infirmary for Children; Joseph Toynbee of the St. James's and St. George's Dispensary; C.J.B. Aldis of the Farringdon Dispensary; E. Rigby of the York Road Lying-In Hospital; and W. A. Guy, professor of forensic medicine at King's College.

The star was Southwood Smith, serving as one of four royal commissioners on the employment of children in mines and manufactories. His testimony was the first major airing of his views since the "Physical Causes" report of 1838. The criticisms of Tait, Cowan, Davidson, Alison, and Hudson had not shifted Smith: he ignored them. The dogma of 1838 remained intact: a filth poison caused fever and, indirectly, most other diseases and social problems.

Smith had decided that the filth poison could account for even more than he had supposed five years earlier. Fever was only the "most obvious and rapidly fatal" filth disease, and its incidence afforded only "a very inadequate view of the pernicious agency of the poison unceasingly generated in these filthy and neglected districts."[22] Most importantly, it could be seen as anterior

20  *Minutes, Health of Towns Commission*, 18 July 1843, PRO MH 7/1, 42. On the Stephenson report see Lewis, *Chadwick*, 85.

21  HOT, *First Report*, x; Slaney, "Report on the State of Birmingham and Other Towns," HOT, *Second Report*, Appendix, pt. 1, 1; Slaney Diaries, v. 8, 16–30 August–4 December 1843. The procedure would be the model for the engineering inspectors of the General Board of Health and its successor agencies.

22  HOT, *First Report*, Evidence, qq 929, 973, 977.

to inflammation and debility, the proximate causes identified by rival theorists. Most deaths, Smith admitted, resulted not from fever but from "diseases of digestive organs, inflammation of the air-passages and lungs, and by consumption." All these were inflammations, Smith argued, and all were the work of the poison. For example, pulmonary consumption: "By a disordered state of the digestive organs [caused by exposure to the filth poison] . . . the body is often so much enfeebled that it is wholly incapable of resisting the frequent and sudden changes in temperature . . . the consequence is that the person . . . perishes by inflammation set up in some vital organ . . . or by consumption, the consequence of that inflammation."[23] A sudden temperature change (like that experienced on emerging from a hot and humid cotton mill into a cold Lancashire night) was indeed a frequent explanation for consumption. It could be seen as constituting a sufficient cause, or as Smith presents it here, as affecting a suitably predisposed constitution. Yet others would have invoked the full range of predisposing factors to account for this systemic disorder (and many would see susceptibility to cold as a common effect of hunger).

Because filth was also "a sedative poison," Smith could subsume debilitationist pathologies, which emphasized the attrition of the constitution by forces that sapped vitality. He claimed that the filth poison had "depressing effects on both body and mind" and was "one of the main causes, not only of . . . mental apathy [but of] . . . physical listlessness." It induced "a feeling of depression . . . [that was] one of the chief inducements to the use of stimulants" (which for Smith included the opium given to soothe children). By enfeebling mothers, it was a key cause of excessive child mortality.[24] He did admit that the lower mortality rate of the wealthy West End of London than in the poor East End was "partly owing to the better food and clothing of the wealthier classes, to their more temperate habits, and less exhausting labour, and especially to the better care taken of their infants and children," yet filth removal remained the means to prevent disease among the poor.[25]

Far more comprehensively than had Chadwick, Smith would medicalize moral choice and social policy. People did not drink because they made wrong decisions or because inebriation was a valid response to ugliness, poverty, and exhausting work; the route from filth to apathy was as far beyond the realm of the will as any reflex action.[26] Likewise, to find that the filth poison was the primary sedative influence was to downplay what had previously been the important depressing factors. "Listlessness" need no longer be the result of exhaustion or hunger. Just as the reflex bypasses the consciousness, Smith's

23 Ibid., q 929.
24 Ibid., qq 931, 934–35, 945.
25 Ibid., q 923.
26 Smith does not deny moral choices, nor physiological effects that begin with psychological inputs – the lack of proper sanitary facilities must have "a debasing effect on the human mind" – but they play a subsidiary role in his explanations; see ibid., qq 951–54, 980, 989.

pathology bypassed the social and subjective. At the end of his examination, the commission offered him a chance to add anything he thought important. He chose the grand question of why Alison's agenda was impossible; why it was imperative to equate public health with sanitation: "No government can prevent the existence of poverty; no benevolence can reach the evils of extreme poverty under the circumstances which at present accompany it; but there is ground of hope and encouragement in the thought that the most painful and debasing of these circumstances are adventitious, and form no necessary and inevitable part of the condition of that large class of every community which must earn their daily bread by manual labour." The result of attending to these "adventitious" circumstances would be "an unmixed good."[27]

Testifying a month later, Arnott too renewed the attack on Alison, citing cases in which fever was not linked to economic distress (Alison had never claimed that the destitution–fever link was either determinate or exclusive). Mainly, however, Arnott was a bridge from medicine to engineering. He presented himself as a physicist specializing in ventilation and the bulk of his testimony was technical. Like Smith, Reid, and many later medically trained sanitarians, he was not shy about trespassing on architecture and engineering.[28]

In fact, ventilation received much more attention than decaying filth in the medical testimony. This was typical of discussions of fever etiology and it is therefore worth asking how ventilation (e.g., regulations on air flow or on volume per capita for houses and workshops, or codes for erecting buildings or laying out well-aired streets) so quickly became peripheral in sanitary legislation and administration.[29] Certainly it was easier to legislate new sewers than better air, yet there were precedents in local acts for such intervention and suitable technological solutions.

The answer is that Chadwick and his colleagues were able to impose an exclusive and narrow conception of what ventilation did and why it was important: mainly, it was a way to dilute and diffuse the filth poison. As such it was needed only where sewers were bad; if filth were continually carried off, it could never get into the streets and rooms where ventilation technologies operated. Conceived thus, poor ventilation was no longer linked to

27 Ibid., qq 920, 1027.
28 Ibid., qq 3893–98, 3902–19. The other medical men also focused on poor ventilation, particularly as a cause of consumption; ibid., qq 3290–3316 (Willis), 5526–5552 (Toynbee), 5558–5613 (Guy), 6003–7 (Aldis), 6020–27 (Rigby).
29 Even these issues did not address the crowdedness problem. Liverpool's 1842 improvement act required eviction of residents of substandard cellars. Since it did not provide additional housing, the effect was to increase overcrowding. Finding this outrageous, Graham asked Playfair to look into it. Playfair's recognition that in solving one public health problem Liverpool had created another may well have had much to do with making clear the intractability of the crowdedness problem and focusing attention on less paradoxical reforms ("Papers on Liverpool Cellars," *Register of Papers, Health of Towns Commission*, May 1844, PRO HO 45/416; James Aspinall, HOT, *Second Report*, Evidence, qq 30–34).

crowdedness. Within limits, a filth-free dwelling should be no less healthy when crowded than when uncrowded. In most other ventilation-related pathologies crowdedness was an issue. One we have seen: the idea that ventilation neutralizes person-to-person contagion. Or health might be harmed by a deficit of oxygen or an excess of combustion products (or in a workplace, an excess of dusts and vapors). In all but the last, calls for better ventilation could equally be calls for more room. In practice, air harmful in one of these ways would often be harmful in several, and the several pathological effects were rarely distinguishable. The Chadwickians did not deny other pathological mechanisms or claim that crowded dwellings were safe, but they did project the impression that they had the problem well in hand, and that the attack on filth was by far the best way to improve air.[30]

Within the commission, however, there were other views. Commissioner D. B. Reid, an Edinburgh trained physician, rivaled Arnott as a ventilation expert. Drawing on a different tradition of ventilation pathology, Reid arrived at quite different public health priorities.[31] Moving air was as important for Reid as moving water was for Chadwick and had as great a range of moral and social effects. Reid agreed that "noxious exhalations" were the exciting causes of fever but emphasized predisposition much more than Southwood Smith: fever affected only those whose "constitution[s] had been broken down by disease, poverty, dissipation, or the injurious influence of an oppressive atmosphere."[32] In Reid's view "oppressive," unfulfilling air was the chief predisposer: "The evils from defective ventilation are . . . great . . . and the continuity of their operation gives them a power . . . which cannot be too minutely investigated. Few pause to consider the necessary consequences of 20 respirations per minute, 1200 per hour, or 28,800 in a single day and night, where not only a noxious atmosphere is inhaled, and brought directly in contact with the blood, but where also the state of the air diminishes the amount of discharge of . . . noxious products." Such air affected the mind, causing "headache and apoplexy" and a tendency to "depression which leads at times to low spirits, or even to suicide."[33]

---

30 Cf. HOT, *Second Report*, 1–2. The commissioners first write that their major concern is with "vitiated air in the quarters occupied by the poor" and on the next page interpret this to mean the "effects produced by emanations from animal or vegetable matter in a state of decay." For their recommendations on ventilation see ibid., 59–64. As Anthony Wohl has noted, housing is marginalized as a public health problem in the same way as crowdedness (*The Eternal Slum: Housing and Social Policy in Victorian London* [London: Edward Arnold, 1977], 2–14).

31 D. B. Reid, "Report on the Sanatory Condition of Newcastle, Gateshead, North Shields, Sunderland, Durham, and Carlisle," HOT, *Second Report*, Appendix, pt. 2, 119–216. Reid's *Illustrations of the Theory and Practice of Ventilation* (London: Longman, Brown, Green, and Longmans, 1844) appeared during the commission's inquiries.

32 Reid, "Newcastle, Gateshead, etc.," 130; idem, *Theory and Practice of Ventilation*, 7–26. Reid's list of the effects of overbreathed air was quite as comprehensive as Smith's list of the effects of the filth poison.

33 Reid, "Newcastle, Gateshead, etc.," 138–39. Reid was aware of the gaseous diffusion experiments

Like Chadwick, Reid saw public structures as the way to prevent disease, but his ideas led in strikingly different directions in regard to such issues as how far working-class people could be seen as rational actors and what role economic distress played in producing disease. Reid's pathology was combustion-centered; it focused on the interrelations among fuel (food), oxygen, and the heat produced. Too much air and too little food might be actively dangerous. Under "low diet" people were unable to bear "that amount of air which would otherwise be agreeable." For them, "protection from cold is the first and greatest desideratum . . . and the less the supply of the air, where the chemistry of the system is not in high condition and amply supplied with materials for producing internal warmth . . . the less is the extent to which its [cold's] influence is felt." Thus, far from being irrational, sealing dwellings to maximize warmth was a survival mechanism; the poor intuitively knew that they must bank the physiological fire to make the fuel last.[34] Air that was rank to a middle-class outsider used to a richer mix was fine for the underfed slum dweller, though it left that person in a suboptimal and perhaps subhuman state. It followed that without warmth and food, ventilation was inadequate; the mind and morality of the poor would engage only when the flame was turned up.[35] Recognizing that people did respond rationally to their conditions

of Dalton and Graham. He regarded them as wonderful means of natural purification but as inadequate in the sorts of circumstances he had encountered. Others too struggled for ways to give visibility to matters of air quality in hopes of inducing their readers to be on guard against the dangers to which they were exposing themselves; e.g., Duncan, "Liverpool," 12: "By the mere action of the lungs of the inhabitants of Liverpool, for instance, a stratum of air sufficient to cover the entire surface of the town, to a depth of three feet, is daily rendered unfit for the purposes of respiration. If to this we add the changes caused by the products of the combustion from forges, furnaces, and other fires, mingling with the atmosphere (to say nothing of the enormous quantity of gas, oil, and candles nightly consumed in large towns), and by the escape of gaseous effluvia from manufactories of different kinds, we shall have enumerated the principal sources of the unavoidable vitiation of the air of towns."

34 Reid, "Newcastle, Gateshead, etc.," 136–37. He made the point more directly in his book: "Ventilation need not be expected where food, fuel, and clothing are deficient. Heat is still more essential to the human frame than fresh air, which consumes the body by slow combustion or oxygenation, when food is not supplied. Defective ventilation reduces the oxygenation, preserves warmth, stupefies the feelings, and allays the pangs of hunger" (Reid, *Theory and Practice of Ventilation*, 38, 174, 182). Arnott (*On Warming and Ventilating; with Directions for Making and Using the Thermometer-Stove or Self-Regulating Fire* [London: Longman, Orme, Brown, Green, and Longmans, 1838], 58) saw the same response as ignorance rather than as an adaptation. He tells of Buckinghamshire lace makers, who, "to save the expense of fire . . . were wont, in winter, to choose, among the rooms belonging to their families, the smallest, which would contain to the number of twenty or thirty of them, and there to congregate, and keep themselves warm by their breathing. The odour of their breaths, although unperceived by themselves, soon became, to a stranger entering, exceedingly offensive. The pale faces, broken health, and early deaths, of many of the ignorant self-destroyers, told . . . what they had been doing."

35 During the factory hearings of 1832 the same argument was made with regard to the need to ventilate the houses of Parliament. Debate in an airless chamber led to as much irrationality and unhealth as did long work in a poorly ventilated mill (Charles Wing, *Evils of the Factory System Demonstrated by Parliamentary Evidence* [London: Saunders and Otley, 1837], cvii). To study such

of life, Reid proposed ventilation devices they could adjust, in contrast with the fixed structures – chimneys, windows, and doors – advocated by others.[36] In making these suggestions Reid was not trying to be politically provocative. He accepted that some industries were unavoidably dusty (all the more necessary then to have good household ventilation).[37] This image of the vital flame was ancient, as was the hunger–fresh air link. Witnesses to Sadler's 1832 Factory Committee had reported that workers demanded extra pay if windows were kept open.[38] Yet in the Health of Towns Commission, Reid's ideas were apostasy – they implied that poverty was a health problem in its own right. But, having spent over thirty pages illustrating his ventilation pathology with complicated charts of air flow, even the heterodox Reid at the beginning of his local reports accepted the mission of documenting defective sewerage, drainage, and cleaning. Ventilation got little attention thereafter.

## III

While the commissioners highlighted different points, their conclusions were largely those of the *Sanitary Report*. The evangelical Slaney gave much attention to the institutional bases of decency and civility, which he found to be cleanliness and decent housing. De la Beche took great interest in medical climatology and differential mortality rates. Owen focused on bad sewerage and fever, taking it as established that the former caused the latter. Denison, the army engineer, concerned himself with public works; Smith of Deanston with recycling. Martin, the Indian army surgeon, found much evidence of

effects Reid had a habit of producing subtle alterations in the atmosphere during his dinner parties and watching the reaction of guests (*Theory and Practice of Ventilation*, 180).

36 Reid's views were echoed by the only working-class witness the commission heard, John Brooks, a Leicestershire weaver. Brooks, who had worked sixteen-hour days in a small and poorly ventilated room and himself had consumption, which he attributed in part to bad air, nonetheless preferred warm stale air to fresh cold air: "We become accustomed to this vitiated air [and] do not perceive it; it is only annoying in the morning when we leave another air and come into it" (HOT, *First Report*, Evidence, qq 537–42, 583–93). For Arnott and Guy (HOT, *Second Report*, Evidence, q 5612) coercion might be necessary to enforce ventilation. Among medical witnesses only Robert Willis took coldness seriously as a cause of disease; Willis's examiners tried to suggest that it was not the cold itself, but only change of temperature that was the problem (HOT, *First Report*, Evidence, qq 3290–3312).

37 Reid, "Newcastle, Gateshead, etc.," 121, 137, 142.

38 Wing, *Evils of the Factory System*, cvii; Wakley also raised the issue in criticizing the 1848 Public Health Bill *(Hansard's Parliamentary Debates, 3rd series, 96*, 1848, 414–18). Among Health of Towns Commission witnesses, Willis and Aldis appealed to such concepts, the latter noting that "the vitiated atmosphere, and the close state in which the patients live produces first physical depression, then functional disorder, and ultimately organic change," and observing that those he treated were "emaciated, pale and thin, and in a low condition, the cases of asthenia being of common occurrence. They complain of sinking, depression of the strength and spirits, loss of appetite." HOT, *First Report*, Evidence, qq 6003–4. Another medical witness, Rigby, used Reid's ventilation schemes, ibid., q 6020.

illness caused by inadequate diet among artisans in the East Midlands, but his conclusions were thoroughly Chadwickian: water, sewerage, scavenging, boards of health staffed with specialist engineers, and medical policemen.[39]

Of them all, Playfair was the most virulent, more Chadwickian even than Chadwick himself. His district was militant Lancashire, surely the most sensitive, and his report was the most comprehensive and detailed. Playfair raised the most contentious issues of the *Sanitary Report* and gratuitously renewed the attack on Chadwick's opponents. He castigated amateur government, even the relatively ambitious and well-heeled governments in Liverpool and Manchester; expounded on the vast value of sewage; dismissed debates on the causes of fever as the irrelevant indulgences of theorists; brandished statistics; was eloquent in his shock at the habits and "propensities" of working-class people, whom he simultaneously represented as victims of conditions and as willfully bad.

There were a few novelties in the Health of Towns reports, however, issues that had either not arisen or been suppressed in the *Sanitary Report*: consumption, high infant mortality (purportedly due to use of sedatives), and the effects on health of inadequate toilet facilities. All were assimilated into Chadwick's emerging sanitarianism, becoming part of the evidence on which it was founded.

In many places consumption, including scrofula (seen as a precursor), and often lumped with other respiratory diseases, was the leading cause of death. It caused about a third of the deaths in Reid's district, about 18 percent in Liverpool, 40 percent of deaths in the twenty to sixty age group in Bath (fever accounted only for 2 percent). In Clifton, consumption deaths clearly demarcated the gentry from the working classes.[40] But what did all this death signify? Such factors as cold, flimsy clothing, overwork, and poor diet were too central to traditional consumption etiology to be ignored, but one could deemphasize them. It would not do to admit that this leading killer was the simple manifestation of exhausting poverty.

There were three alternative emphases. One could appeal to other parts of the causal network. William Kay, the Clifton dispensary doctor who demonstrated the class specificity of consumption, attributed it to heredity. De la Beche stressed differences in climate and medical care to explain differential consumption rates.[41] Or one could follow Southwood Smith and list con-

39  Slaney, "Birmingham," 8–19; Owen, "Report on the Sanatory Condition of Lancaster," HOT, *Second Report*, Appendix, pt. 2, 222; J. R. Martin, "Report on the Sanatory Condition of Nottingham, Coventry, Leicester, Derby, Norwich, and Portsmouth," HOT, ibid., 250–55, 262–64, 269.

40  Reid, "Newcastle, Gateshead, etc.," 123; Duncan, "Liverpool," 21; H. T. De la Beche, "Report on the City of Bath and Its Sanitary Condition," HOT, *Second Report*, Appendix, pt. 1, 118; William Kay, "Report on the Sanitary Condition of Clifton," ibid., 80.

41  Kay, "Clifton," 80; De la Beche, "Report on the Sanitary Condition of Swansea," HOT, *Second Report*, Appendix, pt. 1, 139–40; idem, "Report on the Sanitary Condition of Frome," ibid., 129.

sumption among the innumerable filth diseases. Playfair, for example, spoke of "that large class of pulmonary diseases formerly exclusively ascribed to climatical influences . . . scrofulous affections, or other diseases having their origin in the bad physical or moral conditions of our large towns."[42] Finally, one could show that consumption rates reflected acceptable factors (ventilation) more than unacceptable factors (work). W. A. Guy, who devoted most of his testimony to the disease, claimed the greater mortality rate among sedentary indoor workers than outdoor workers indicated the importance of ventilation. De la Beche found consumption slightly more frequent among tradesmen than artisans, who would be subject to dusts.[43]

While the Health of Towns commissioners took a greater interest in infant mortality than Chadwick had in the *Sanitary Report*, the status of infant mortality remained ambiguous. It was not the welfare of infants that prompted the interest so much as the hope that the infant mortality rate might be the best proxy for physical conditions (infants, after all, could not suffer occupational diseases). It would certainly have been more used had not others seen it as a better proxy for poverty.[44]

In fact, most of the discussion of infant mortality in the commission's reports dealt with the inescapably social problem of child doping, which proved to be the sensation of the investigation. Working parents left small children with irresponsible child minders who simplified their work by dosing their charges with narcotic "quietners" like "Godfrey's Cordial." The consequent addiction led to an often fatal decline. Most of the evidence came from the Northwest. The Reverend J. R. Coulthart of Ashton-under-Lyne estimated that half the local children were being dosed and plaintively noted that they were "excessively fond of such mixtures, many of them preferring compositions of this kind to their mothers' milk." He told of infants "a few months old," able to identify "these 'Godfrey' bottles on the shelves of frequented druggists." Reverend Clay found the practice widespread at Preston; Martin called it "infanticide" in Nottingham. Mainly, however, it was Playfair, with access to Peel, who made a sensation of this "universal practice." Leaving statistics aside he

---

42 Playfair, "Lancashire," 48; see also HOT, *First Report*, vii; Duncan, "Liverpool," 20–22; John Leigh, "On the Injurious Effects of Coal Smoke," HOT, *Second Report*, Appendix, pt. 2, 117–18; W. A. Guy, HOT, *First Report*, Evidence, q 5603. Duncan cited Clark as having induced consumption in rabbits through providing a "cold, dark, damp close situation, and supplying them with innutritious food." But as he explicitly excluded food from consideration in his report, the former structural causes were emphasized.

43 Guy, HOT, *First Report*, Evidence, qq 5558–5568, 5581, 5590–92; De la Beche, "Frome," 129. The commission endorsed De la Beche's point (HOT, *Second Report*, 2).

44 Thomas Hawksley, "Nottingham," HOT, *First Report*, Appendix, 140–42; Martin, "Nottingham, Coventry, etc.," 278; Duncan, "Liverpool," 20. Playfair went so far as to suggest that the infant mortality rate was inverse to destitution, since mothers were without work they would be unable to afford Godfrey's Cordial and would take better care of their children (Playfair, "Lancashire," 70, also 53). But see William Kay, "Report on the Sanitary Condition of the City of Bristol," HOT, *Second Report*, Appendix, pt. 1, 93.

rolled out testimonial after testimonial, confessing that it was "difficult to write calmly on facts such as these."[45]

But what kind of problem was this? Who or what was culpable; what remediable social error was in play? Opinions differed. The Malthusian Clay saw these deaths as the outcome of too many births, and in turn of too many youthful and imprudent marriages. Martin absolved parents and blamed political economy: "Owing to the hard labour and reduced wages of the working classes, the mothers are unable to nurse or take care of their infants . . . therefore, to keep them quiet, opiates are given, and . . . doses are increased till life is passed away." It was a question not of "innate vice" but of "poverty."[46] After "laborious inquiry," Playfair proposed a sanitarian explanation: "The custom of administering narcotics to children originated primarily in, and is upheld by, the physical causes of disease acting upon the younger portion of the community. On the removal of these causes, the general inducement to the continuance of this system would cease, for the irritability and difficulty of management of children would diminish with their increased health." In short, babies cried because they needed good sewers. The inescapably social turned out after all to be a matter of structures.[47]

The commission endorsed Playfair: "As soon as the physical causes producing irritation and constitutional disturbance, or disease, are removed, one of the great inducements to the use of opiates will be diminished, and the moral evils lessened which now tend to the extension of the practice." It congratulated itself for mentioning the matter at all. "Although an inquiry into this subject may not be . . . strictly within the terms of our Commission . . . we should be remiss . . . if we did not draw attention to the facts . . . laid before us."[48]

Last is the issue of "sanitary conveniences." Some of Chadwick's informants had casually noted that privies in the neighborhoods of the poor were few and dirty. The investigating commissioners had far more to say about privy accommodation. Constipation and urine retention must be great health problems, a number of them insisted (without offering evidence that they were).

---

45 The Reverend J. R. Coulthart, "Ashton-under-Lyne," HOT, *First Report*, Appendix, 77. The Reverend William Clay, "Borough of Preston," HOT, *First Report*, Appendix, 46–47, 54; Martin, "Nottingham, Coventry, etc.," 256; Playfair, "Lancashire," 61–62, 66–67. Cf. W. Fleming, "Report on the Schools in Manchester and Salford," HOT, *Second Report*, Appendix, pt. 2, 104. On Playfair and Peel see Playfair to Chadwick, 15 December 1844, UCL Chadwick Papers #1588. In general see Elia Vallone Chepaitis, "The Opium of the Children: Domestic Opium and Infant Drugging in Early Victorian England" (Ph.D diss., University of Connecticut, Storrs, 1985); Terry M. Parssinen, *Secret Passions, Secret Remedies: Narcotic Drugs in British Society, 1820–1930* (Manchester: Manchester University Press, 1983), 42–46; Virginia Berridge and Griffith Edwards, *Opium and the People: Opiate Use in Nineteenth-Century England* (London: Allen Lane, 1981), 97–104.

46 Martin, "Nottingham, Coventry, etc.," 256.

47 Playfair, "Lancashire," 67.

48 HOT, *Second Report*, 2, 5.

Worse yet, the unavailability of places to relieve oneself discreetly surely led to brutalization and even "licentiousness."[49]

These concerns tell us more about the commissioners than those they were investigating. They suggest too how much the transformation of public health involved a transformation of the medical role from "attorney for the poor" to defender of middle-class sensibilities. For surely these commissioners were projecting their own revulsion and discomfort. Unable to appreciate hunger, weariness, and despair, they located the key threat to health in their own contracted sphincters and the key threat to social order in the confused reactions (combined revulsion and erotic arousal) to the idea of women being so necessarily public in their private acts (and it is clear their concern for morality is more with women than with men).[50] Such concerns were not unprecedented; factory investigators had worried that mixed or insufficiently private toilet facilities might cause moral or physical harm. By and large Chadwick's informants (and local medical men who gave evidence to the commission) simply had not seen the circumstances of excretion as worth singling out from the totality of conditions of life. Somehow people made do; doubtless they had lower standards than the commissioners could conceive of, but the lack of private places for elimination was not the great threat to working-class health.

## IV

Mainly what characterizes the Health of Towns Commission reports is a descent into the pit of technical minutiae. While Chadwick had argued that the social and moral were grounded in the physical, his "sanitary idea" – the system of water, drains, recycling of wastes – had been only one of several matters to which he had called attention at the end of the *Sanitary Report*. Yet the generals of policy (with Chadwick's counsel) had plucked from the report this idea and determined that it would be the front on which social advance would take place. For most of the rest of the century Chadwick's sanitary idea would serve as the primary axiom of public health policy. Institutions – social, legal, administrative – would be judged by their compatibility with it. Even as late as the 1890s Local Government Board epidemiologists investigating a

49 Slaney, "Birmingham," 8; De la Beche, "Report on the Sanitary Condition of Merthyr Tydvil," HOT, *Second Report*, Appendix, pt. 1, 145. Also see Hawksley, "Nottingham," 131; Playfair, "Lancashire," 16; Reid, "Newcastle, Gateshead, etc.," 134.

50 These observations are certainly of a piece with the interminable coy allusions to the moral effects of bed or bedroom sharing considered earlier. For the voyeurism of sanitary investigation see Playfair to Chadwick, undated, autumn 1843, UCL Chadwick Papers #1588: "Last night I spent entirely in going through all the *lodging houses* and *brothels* in this town. I began at 12 and finished at half past 4 – so I saw a prodigious quantity – such sights! frequently 14 in a room, women and men lying stark naked together!"

broad range of diseases tended to attribute good health to good drainage, and so on, and disease to inadequacies in sanitary technologies (however impalpable those inadequacies might be).

Aside from the medical witnesses, most of those testifying to the commission during its first year dealt with five issues. Three were matters of the feasibility of new technologies: high-pressure, constant, water supplies; water-carriage waste removal; and profit-making approaches to recycling sewage. The fourth issue was that of the powers and practices of the existing institutions that provided sanitary services; the fifth was the availability of expertise. The first three are developed here; the latter two in later chapters.

Common to the treatment of the three technologies was an attempt to redefine the criteria of success. To make the case for reform it was necessary to represent what existed as inadequate; the complacent public had to be made to see the present as pathological. Thus a water supply was to be inadequate if water were not always available within every home; sewers were no good if they did not rapidly carry off household wastes. And while in many places town refuse was already being carted off to fertilize farmland, this recycling was unacceptable because the refuse was not being automatically and immediately removed by water. Recognizing that Chadwick and the commissioners were imposing new standards as well as new technologies is key to understanding the great "centralization" issue, the antipathy that arose between Chadwick's General Board of Health and local authorities. As we shall see, those municipal corporations, improvement commissions, and sewers commissions which had been "improving" in preceding decades were stunned by these new standards. They were being charged with wasting money and endangering health, and not even credited with good intentions.

With regard to water the commission's main concern was that it be always available, ideally within the home.[51] In most British towns public water supply was initially undertaken by companies of investors, often local people concerned more with the development of their town or with provision of water to their own homes or works than with modest dividends or the prospect of great rises of share prices.[52] A waterworks was not a risk-free investment; for

51  HOT, *First Report*, xii.
52  HOT, *Second Report*, 46–57. J. A. Hassan finds 102 companies being established between 1821 and 1851; after 1866 many of these would be taken over by local authorities; by 1914 80 percent of 1130 boroughs and urban district councils had publicly owned water supplies ("The Growth and Impact of the British Water Industry in the Nineteenth Century," *Economic History Review*, 2nd series *38* [1985]: 531–47). These generalizations about the motives of capitalists do not so clearly apply to investors in large markets like London or Liverpool (Bernard Rudden, *The New River: A Legal History* [Oxford: Clarendon Press, 1985]; J. Aspinall, HOT, *Second Report*, Evidence, qq 150–52). On this "social overhead capital" see Phyllis Deane, *The First Industrial Revolution* (Cambridge: Cambridge University Press, 1965), 77–80; Christopher Hamlin, "Muddling in Bumbledom: Local Governments and Large Sanitary Improvements: The Cases of Four British Towns, 1855–1885," *Victorian Studies 32* (1988): 55–83. To my knowledge no study of shareholding

that reason, Chadwick himself had argued that water was often better left to investors rather than public bodies. One might face legal problems in securing access to water or routing mains across the land. Making water flow through pipes may seem so simple that we find it hard to conceive of things going wrong, but there were innumerable technical problems as well. Just as James Watt had thought it unwise to trust high-pressure steam engines, though possible to build them, many water engineers preferred a low-pressure intermittent system in which water was directed to one district at a time. Once every few days the subscriber filled a cistern (or a bucket), which was to serve the household until the next fill. Engineers could make do with smaller reservoir and pumping capacity and need not worry so much about bursting fittings. Chadwick and the commission, on the other hand, called for constant high pressure throughout a system of mains, an approach which would have required extensive retrofitting with plumbing fixtures able to withstand that pressure.

It was easy enough to show the benefits of constant water. The commission's main argument was that constant availability was essential for cleanliness.[53] But there were also advantages in hosing down streets, fighting fires. In-home water would prevent all the bad things that happened in standpipe queues.[54] The commission gave little attention to water for cooking and drinking. Though many medical men believed foul water harmed health in some way – not necessarily by causing acute disease – the commissioners were unconcerned with quality; to the chemist–commissioner Lyon Playfair, impurity meant hardness, which impeded the cleaning power of soap.[55]

Proof of the feasibility of a constant water supply was given by Thomas Hawksley, who would become the most influential water engineer of the Victorian era and one of Chadwick's principal nemeses. When he became engineer to a new water company that would supply eight thousand houses in Nottingham, Hawksley was already experienced as a gas engineer, where a constant-service, pressurized network was essential. This Trent Company was a great success, the maintenance and control of its mains requiring only one man and one boy.[56] The technology could be applied anywhere, Chad-

among provincial water companies exists, but for the analogous gas industry see John F. Wilson, *Lighting the Town: A Study of Management in the North West Gas Industry, 1805–1880* (London: Chapman, 1991).

53 HOT, *Second Report*, 5.

54 R. Thom, HOT, *First Report*, Evidence, qq 108–10; Hawksley, ibid., qq 5352–70, 5381–403.

55 Playfair, "Lancashire," 32–39; see also Thomas Clarke, HOT, *First Report*, Evidence, qq 39–104; Christopher Hamlin, *A Science of Impurity: Water Analysis in Nineteenth Century Britain* (Berkeley: University of California Press, 1990).

56 Hawksley, HOT, *First Report*, Evidence, 5215–66. On Hawksley (1807–93) see "Memoir of Thomas Hawksley," *Minutes of Proceedings, Institution of Civil Engineers* 117 (1893): 364–76; G. M. Binnie, *Early Victorian Water Engineers* (London: Thomas Telford, 1981), ch. 1–2.

wick and the commission insisted, a conclusion Hawksley, invoking the professional's prerogative of judging each case independently, would subsequently reject.

It was not enough, however, to show that constant high-pressure water was good and practical; it had to be shown to be imperative. Increasingly, the source of this imperative was the idea of coordinated works: every component was to be finely tuned to every other component. Constant water was as necessary to service the drains as the drains were to service the water: a certain flow had to pass from mains to drains whether or not people used it along the way. One had to be careful, however, to downplay this "drainage" argument lest the poor sewers of most towns become an excuse for rejecting constant water – where the sewers led nowhere it was no advantage to have copious water to flush them.

To enforce this coordinated works imperative the commission appealed to two stratagems: science and vilification. Constant service was to be equated with high science; intermittent service was to be depicted as antiquated and atheoretical, the alternative of the ignorant. Fundamental principles like those embodied in Hawksley's many formulae (e.g., for relating pipe thickness to diameter or estimating friction or water consumption) must replace so-called experience. (Though they were in fact more often rules of thumb than deductions from theory, formulae were the sign of science.)[57] Moreover, argued Chadwick and the commission, companies providing intermittent water were not serving the public interest, as indicated by the waste of capital manifest in rival companies competing to serve the same area. If profit not service dictated the companies' policies, then whatever they favored, consumers should oppose. The companies' opposition to constant water was thus its strongest endorsement.[58]

While the water campaign required undermining confidence in existing

---

57  HOT, *First Report*, Evidence, qq 5215–5345. In sharp contrast with Hawksley's testimony is that of Thomas Wicksteed, who, after a long career as engineer to three of the London water companies, had gone into private practice. When he testified in July 1843, Wicksteed had just finished constant-service high-pressure waterworks for Cork, yet far from endorsing high-pressure water service, he listed advantages and disadvantages. From experience he found constant service problematic, however appropriate it might be theoretically (HOT, *First Report*, Evidence, qq 4433–528). See also the evidence of Joseph Quick, the Southwark company engineer, ibid., q 5866.

58  Hawksley, HOT, *First Report*, Evidence, q 5473. Another way to enforce the coordinated works imperative was a "bootstrapping" approach in marketing sanitation. Get a town to buy one component of the finely tuned system, say a water supply or a full network of drains, and it would quickly feel the need for the others: the water would require drains, the drains water, and the sewage would have to go somewhere. Since the idea of simultaneously adopting three novel and costly technologies was terrifying, each might be presented as warranted in its own right, even though the representer knew full well that each necessitated the others. The full "sanitary idea" could then emerge as the independent discovery of each local authority rather than an axiom to be forced on them. See Roe, HOT, *Second Report*, Evidence, q 5959; Morpeth to Chadwick, 23 August 1847, UCL Chadwick Papers #1055.

institutions, that for sewage recycling required building a new institution. That town wastes had value was uncontroversial; that sewage irrigation on a grand scale would vastly increase agricultural production, repaying the costs of sanitary improvement and overthrowing the Malthusian principle of population, seemed too much a political economist's bedtime fantasy. It is in the commission's report that we first see the full range of arguments that would be used to establish the unquestionable practicality, astonishing profitability, and moral necessity of this technology. Recycling was "one of those measures which science and observation have called so forcibly into notice as to render it almost imperative as a question of rational economy," as the military engineer James Vetch put it.[59]

One way to do this was by publicizing the recycling industry that already existed. Manchester exported 647 barge loads of manure per week. At Ashton-under-Lyne 110 carts of night soil per week were sold to farmers at thirteen pence/cart. Playfair surveyed the scavenging economies of towns throughout Britain, finding the best returns in Scotland. Slaney and Smith of Deanston were both experimental agriculturalists, fascinated with liquid manures and tile drainage. The latter delighted in describing the York "muck" trade in which four hundred people worked ("gatherers" earned fourteen shillings/week). Each entrepreneur mixed "the dung to suit his customers," selling it on to a "larger muck merchant or agent" for shipment to Lincolnshire, where it commanded three shillings/ton. Each privy and ashpit was cleaned at least every second day, and an occupation of "snatchers" scavenged the leavings of the scavengers. Other wastes were recycled too: ash for bricks, shells and broken crockery for road paving, bones, rags.[60]

As important as it was to show that recycling was profitable, it was equally important to contrast the inefficiencies and dangers of cart or barge removal with Chadwick's water carriage. Much was at stake here. Chadwick's sewage irrigation was not "scale-neutral": town manure would no longer be accessible to a variety of customers at various distances and directions, but only to well-capitalized landowners near an outfall.[61] A redefinition of property was re-

59 HOT, *First Report*, Evidence, q 5777.
60 P. H. Holland, "Chorlton-upon-Medlock," HOT, *First Report*, Appendix, 68; Coulthart, "Ashton-under-Lyne," 73; Playfair, "Lancashire," 13; James Smith, "Report on the Sanatory Condition of York, Kingston-upon-Hull, Huddersfield, Leeds, Bradford, Sheffield," HOT, *Second Report*, Appendix, pt. 2, 308–10; Slaney Diaries, Shrewsbury Records Centre, v. 7, December 1838, January 1841, April 1842, July 1842. On other materials see HOT, *First Report*, Evidence, qq 4585–86, 4591. See also W. Thorn, HOT, *First Report*, Evidence, q 4631, on "flying dustmen" stealing ash.
61 Reid, "Newcastle, Gateshead, etc.," 133, noted opposition to sewage irrigation in Carlisle on these grounds. This was a live issue in the early 1850s and again in the mid-1860s, when the Metropolitan Board of Works was determining how to dispose of Greater London's sewage. It was faced with a choice between radial distribution systems which would make the sewage available to a larger number of farmers and intercepting systems that would concentrate it in one place, where it would be dealt with by the local authority or by a single contractor.

quired. In many places wastes belonged to the occupier or owner, not the local authority. As we have seen, for some it was a significant portion of household income. Thus along with allusions to profit came condemnations of dung hoarding, of the great cost of cartage or canal transport (especially in sprawling London), and of obnoxious and drunken night soil men. Liverpool's private act permitting householders to retain wastes for sale caused more sickness and death than "any other cause," insisted Playfair.[62] By contrast Chadwick's witnesses made great claims for sewage irrigation, a technology most had probably never seen in operation. Hawksley maintained that water-carried sewage would be more valuable than night soil because the fertilizing salts would be in solution.[63] Several were willing to state the exact profit that was going unclaimed. Vetch pegged the value of sewage at five shillings/head/year (more prudent than the eighteen shillings estimated by some agricultural chemists, he noted) and claimed that within seventeen years Leeds could be making a profit of £9000/year. The surgeon P. H. Holland claimed that for a £40,000 investment Manchester sewers could return at least £12,000/year – pure profit in four years. Smith of Deanston predicted a clear profit of £1/year per person.[64] Playfair, whose mentor Liebig was a great recycling enthusiast, was most rhapsodic: a pound of urine was a pound of wheat; the excretions of each adult male yielded an acre of turnips. The impediment to sanitary improvement had always been cost, and the only solution, higher rates. But sewage promised a "supply of money . . . for carrying out . . . all the necessary works for promoting the health and comfort of the people altogether independent of rates," noted Smith. There would even be a surplus for "architectural and other improvements." The nation was losing about two million pounds per year, Playfair told Peel.[65]

62  HOT, *First Report*, Evidence, qq 4547, 4454, 4566, 4596, 4607–8, 4614, 4629, 4636–38, 4642, 4651–52, 4673, 4681–82; Slaney, "Birmingham, etc.," 3; Playfair, "Lancashire," 14, 44; Reid, "Newcastle, Gateshead, etc.," 191; Owen, "Lancaster," 224.

63  HOT, *First Report*, Evidence, q 5432; Cresy, ibid., qq 2261–62. An exception was John Dean, an agricultural engineer from Devon, where there was a sewage irrigation project at Ashburton (HOT, *First Report*, Evidence, qq 6059–69). Surprisingly, Dean was not a major witness. Edinburgh, the most successful example, was little talked of because of its ambivalent status as both profitable and objectionable. But see Smith of Deanston, "Report on the Application of Sewer Water to the Purposes of Agriculture, with a View to the Establishment of an Independent Income for the Improvement of Towns," HOT, *Second Report*, Appendix, pt. 2, 326.

64  Vetch, HOT, *First Report*, Evidence, qq 5771–74, 5786. Playfair, for example, claimed that the annual worth of human excreta in Flanders was one pound, seven shillings/head, and felt he was being cautious in counting on only ten shillings/head ("Lancashire," 47); Smith, "Sewer Water," 326; Holland, "Chorlton-upon-Medlock," 69.

65  Justus Liebig, *Familiar Letters on Chemistry, and Its Relation to Commerce, Physiology, and Agriculture,* ed. John Gardner (Philadelphia: Campbell and Co., 1843), 36–46; Smith, "Sewer Water," 325; Playfair, "Lancashire," 46–47; Lyon Playfair to Chadwick, 19 April 1842, UCL Chadwick Papers #1588. Privately there was skepticism, not so much about whether the figures were correct as whether they were credible (Chadwick to Buccleuch, 11 January 1845, UCL Chadwick Papers #2181/6).

Such calculations and promises pervade the sanitary literature for the next three decades. Accompanying them were appeals to Providence. Southwood Smith (Unitarian minister and natural theologian as well as fever doctor) told of the great complementarity between the needs of plants and the needs of animals, which was "the foundation of all rational and efficient sanatory regulations." If only the refuse which tainted the air "of the crowded city . . . [were] promptly removed and spread out on the surface of the surrounding country, [it would] not only give it healthfulness, but clothe it with verdure, and endue it with inexhaustible fertility. These are great laws of nature . . . a due conformity with which would bring us health, plenty, and happiness, but which we cannot disregard any more than we disregard any other physical law."[66] Playfair appealed to "a recognized principle of agriculture, that the excreta of those animals which subsist on a certain kind of food form the manure best adapted to the production of the same food; and hence the refuse of a town is the best productive manure for the food of the residents of that town."[67]

Of the trinity of technologies making up the "sanitary idea," sewerage was primary, however. As with water, sewers would be assessed against an increasingly rigorous set of criteria in the coming years, effectively redefining the term "sewer" itself. In the *Sanitary Report* Chadwick had been concerned that there simply was no adequate drainage in many places – sewers were needed as much to dry the soil as to remove wastes. By the mid-1840s, however, efficient discharge was clearly primary. In part the shift reflected the new focus: when one focused on the residences of the poor as in Chadwick's class-based inquiry, one found dampness and standing water as immediate impediments to comfort and health. When one focused on the town and included wealthy and middle-class districts one often found sewers, but all too often they were "sewers of vicious construction," as Chadwick would put it. They did not belong to any system, were not uniformly connected with buildings, did not conduct sewage rapidly to an outfall. All were central to the sanitary idea. However successfully a sewer removed runoff – its traditional task – if it did not also quickly conduct water closet discharges and other house and street wastes to a place of recycling it was a failure. "Conduits, not reservoirs," proclaimed Southwood Smith.[68] Old sewers were worse than none, Chadwick would assert frequently in the next decade.

Giving immediacy to this new sewerage agenda was a threat to health that had received little attention in the *Sanitary Report*: a "sewer gas" generated

66 HOT, *First Report*, Evidence, q 1002. Among the odder witnesses was Nathaniel Bagshaw Ward, inventor of the self-sustaining terrarium, in which, as in a miniature town, "vegetable respiration counterbalances animal respiration by purifying the air which animals vitiate." HOT, *First Report*, Evidence, qq 1061–64.
67 Playfair, "Lancashire," 46; see also Smith, "Sewer Water," 325–26.
68 HOT, *First Report*, ix–x; Evidence, qq 992–93.

when organic matter in sewers decayed, and then rose back through the network into the houses and streets whence the sewage had come to cause disease. As Southwood Smith himself explained it:

Without . . . regular and abundant . . . water, drains . . . become positively injurious. They generate and diffuse the very poison . . . which it is their object to prevent. When the animal and vegetable matters . . . are not . . . washed away, they become stagnant [in] . . . circumstances highly favourable to their decomposition . . . along all the great thoroughfares, close to the pavement, and opposite the doors of dwelling-houses, are placed gully holes, most conveniently situated for the regular escape of the poison. . . . In this manner a drain may become at once a laboratory in which poison is generated on an immense scale, and a conduit, by which it is effectually spread abroad.

Poison was steadily rising from "every inch of drain which is not regularly washed by a good stream of water," he warned.[69]

This "sewer gas" would remain a flexible explanation for disease for the rest of the century. It was not a new idea and had been a central concern of an 1834 select committee on London's sewers, but it did make clear that any sewer in which sewage stagnated was not only inefficient, but deadly – to precisely those middle-class people living in the best sewered districts whose consent would be necessary to implement the sanitary idea.[70]

In focusing attention on an unpopular institution, the seven Greater London sewers commissions, the commission's campaign for better sewers paralleled its call for better water. Many of the sad band of sewers commission officers who testified in the summer of 1843 had already undergone a similar inquisition before Slaney's Health of Towns Committee in 1840; some were veterans of select committees in 1834 and even 1823, and many would be grilled again by Chadwick's Metropolitan Sanitary Commission in 1847. Relatively powerless and easily available as witnesses, sewers commission staffers were ideal scapegoats.[71] On each occasion, the questions were much the same: progress of sewerage in their districts, designs of sewers, modes of planning and financing construction, explanations for anything that could be found amiss (no excuses accepted). They were taxed for tolerating poorly drained areas, for ignoring the filth–disease relationship, and for rewarding themselves with lavish dinners. Indeed, to confront a sewers commission surveyor with a description of foul conditions in his district became a standard motif of sanitarian political theater.

Even more than with constant water, and much more than with recycling,

---

69 HOT, *First Report*, x; Evidence, q 995.

70 William Dyce Guthrie, HOT, *First Report*, Evidence, q 1113; J. S. Gaskoin and W. H. Walker, in "Select Committee on Metropolis Sewers," *P.P.*, 1834, 15 [584.], qq 960–84.

71 Note the hurt and bewildered tone in Kelsey to Chadwick, 2 September 1842, in "General Sanitary," UCL Chadwick Papers #45. Also see City of London Sewers Commission to PLC, 10 November 1842, *PLC Registers of Correspondence*, PRO MH 20/1.

this scapegoating helped politicize sanitation. What was at stake was not simply a technical matter of getting sewers built and streets cleaned, but a moral revolution in government. Bad people and bad institutions were to be rejected for good ones. Since bad technology resulted from bad institutions, better institutions would automatically generate better technology. Correspondingly, the belief that there *was* a vastly better technology, only kept in check by corruption and sloth, highlighted the failures of those institutions all the more clearly. Nurturing this belief were Chadwick's sewerage theorists. In general, with the exception of John Roe, surveyor of the Holborn and Finsbury Commission, they had little experience implementing their ideas. As we shall see, Chadwick's experts would come to power in 1847 when a Chadwick-dominated Metropolitan Sewers Commission consolidated most duties of the old commissions. That success would only be temporary: slick technology did not drive politics out of transforming the urban landscape.

The attack on the sewers commissions is remarkable in indicating how quickly Chadwick had pressed his agenda on the Tories – here was a Tory royal commission forsaking tradition, constitution, and property in the name of efficiency. In fact, the sewers commissions were not so obstinate as the sanitarians pretended. Slowly and unevenly, they were responding to the sanitarians' critique. They were building new sewers. The City of London had built thirteen miles of sewers in the previous decade; the Westminster Commission, forty; the Surrey and Kent, eleven; and the Tower Hamlets Commission, thirteen. Roe's Holborn and Finsbury had built twenty-one miles in four years. Both the Surrey and the Tower Hamlets commissions used Roe's new flushing technique.[72] The City Commission's surveyor, Richard Kelsey, singled out for ridicule in the *Sanitary Report*, maintained that sewer building must reflect health needs, and that he took the advice of poor law medical officers in deciding where next to build sewers.[73]

The sewers commissions, like many ancient institutions that were attracting the reformers' ardor at the time, were not designed to deal with modern problems. Henry VIII had established them as juridical institutions, and not for sewer building or administration, or public health (they were still sometimes known as "sewers courts" though "sewers juries" had generally been abandoned). Usually sewers were built by landowners, only occasionally for "public benefit." Since a sewer changed drainage patterns to the benefit of

---

72 HOT, *First Report*, Evidence, qq 1428, 1613, 2480–90, 3498, 3500, 3503, 3397, 3406, 5840, 5822. By contrast the City Commission had built only ten miles of sewer between 1756 and 1832 (qq 3325–27). Many other towns had been active, too. Liverpool had spent £100,000 on nineteen miles of sewers in the early 1840s (Duncan, "Liverpool," 15; Aspinall, HOT, *Second Report*, Evidence, qq 98, 103, 106).

73 HOT, *First Report*, Evidence, qq 3334–35 (Kelsey), 2806–10 (Leslie); cf. Nottridge and Drew, of the Ravensbourne commission, who explicitly rejected the concern with health (qq 2668, 2699–2708, 2736–49).

some properties and the detriment of others, a public body was necessary to award damages and to divide costs, and this was what the commissions mainly did.[74] Hence the large number of commissioners (over two hundred in some cases), the inclusion of landowners, and the involvement of builders and architects, there precisely because they were "interested."[75] The projects they were taking on in the 1830s were still usually financed by assessing beneficiaries, but several of the commissions, despite Chadwick's opposition, were going to Parliament for increased powers, including powers for debt financing and for compelling connection of house drains to sewers.[76] Yet longstanding caution still prevented them from thinking in terms of comprehensive drainage plans and large capital outlay.[77]

But the royal commission's tone was not one of facilitating the modernization of antiquated institutions; it was one of denunciation. There was little said of the achievements of the sewers commissions and of other local authorities; much of their failings.[78] All were assessed on novel and only barely articulated criteria: how well had they constructed municipal infrastructure that was still on the drawing board; how efficiently had they administered and delivered services that were not yet unambiguously public; what were they doing about the death rate? Partly this denunciation was rhetorical convenience. To have represented this new local government agenda and these new technical criteria as recent inventions would have been to open a long debate of political philosophy. Better to present them as obvious, eternal, and unquestionable – not *a* way to go forward but *the* way. But, especially for Chadwick, it also reflected a style of thinking in which the human creations of the past had no standing. Using whatever means were necessary, the rubble of the past was to be swept away in the name of rational, coordinated administration. It is scarcely surprising that the responses of local governments to such a representation would be skepticism, hostility, and opposition to "centralization." And the stratagem would backfire. His attack on local government, certainly intemperate, in many cases unnecessary, would contribute significantly to Chadwick's downfall.

74  "Select Committee on Metropolis Sewers," *P.P.*, 1823, 5 [542.], 6–17; HOT, *Second Report*, 7–10; Simon, *English Sanitary Institutions*, 70–71; Lewis, *Chadwick*, 55–57; HOT, *First Report*, Evidence, qq 1327, 1440–44.
75  HOT, *First Report*, Evidence, q 2318; HOT, *Second Report*, Evidence, qq 184, 208–9, 226, 234–37. None of this is to deny that some of their practices were corrupt by any standards.
76  HOT, *First Report*, Evidence, qq 1564, 1624, 2327, 3331–32, p. 248; Beriah Drew, "First Report of the Metropolitan Sanitary Commission, Evidence," *P.P.*, 1847, 32, [888.], 29–31, 91–92.
77  HOT, *First Report*, Evidence, qq 2922, 3072–73, 3105–6.
78  W. T. Denison, "Report on the Sanatory Condition of the Town of Woolwich (also Salisbury)," HOT, *Second Report*, Appendix, pt. 2, 231; but see Southwood Smith, HOT, *First Report*, Evidence, q 920.

## V

In broad form the Health of Towns Commission's recommendations outlined the framework of public health legislation in Britain for the next half century. Sanitary undertakings were to involve central government (to ensure "uniformity of practice"), yet their execution and management were to be mainly in the hands of local authorities "properly constituted." Central government might intervene if works were not carried out in timely fashion or where public health problems were particularly severe. A skilled surveyor, whose appointment would be subject to central approval, would be the chief local executive officer. Local authorities were to enforce regulations on new building and street width as well as on sewerage, and to ensure that every dwelling had its own "necessary." They were not required to supply water but were to be able to acquire company-owned waterworks. The local authority was to own sewage, dust, and other recyclable rubbish, and it was to prevent smoke nuisances. Finally, almost as an afterthought, the commission recommended the appointment, again subject to central approval, of a local medical officer of health "to inspect and report upon the sanatory conditions . . . to enquire into the nature and prevalence of epidemic and other diseases affecting the rate of mortality, and the circumstances which originate and maintain such diseases."[79]

In this way, an easily justifiable and relatively uncontentious restriction in scope of a single inquiry shifted the focus of public health to municipal engineering and local government. The commission freed public health from the messy issues of poor law administration and the insoluble problem of guiding the ship of policy between political economy and medicine. It did so not by denying that food, fever, and exhaustion were real health problems, but simply by dropping them. The commissioners were not philosophers of social medicine; they were just dealing pragmatically with mundane matters of civil engineering and municipal administration. If this seems tantamount to pushing on with the solution whether or not it solves the problem, it should not, at least not entirely, for the dirt, poor drainage, and decomposing filth were real enough. That they harmed health was almost as uncontroversial then as it would be now.[80]

---

79 The commission determined most of these recommendations in June 1844. The antismoke clause and the call for medical officers were determined only in January 1845 *Minutes, Health of Towns Commission*, 18, 20, 22, 25, 27 June, 7 July 1844; 18, 21 January 1845, PRO MH 7/1. The recommendation for a medical officer was particularly controversial; Chadwick probably drafted the description of the post (Lewis, *Chadwick*, 80, also 96). For opinions on medical officers see HOT, *Second Report*, 66–67; "Memos and Drafts, 1842–46," UCL Chadwick Papers #47; Chadwick to Buccleuch, 11, 23 January, 31 March 1845, UCL Chadwick Papers #2181/6, #2181/7, #2181/9; to W. P. Alison, 16 April 1845, ibid., #2181/9; to Southwood Smith, 15, 22 April 1845, ibid., #2181/8, #2181/9; to Sir Benjamin Brodie, 31 March 1845, ibid., #2181/9.
80 Gibson, "The Public Health Agitation," 161.

But because we come to the history of public health familiar with local governments that involve themselves in everything from pot to potholes, it may be hard to appreciate how great a transformation this was. Chadwick orchestrated it. He was making a career jump, leaving poor law for urban improvement. He meant to take public health with him. Perhaps the move is implicit in the *Sanitary Report*, with its preoccupation with sanitary engineering and local government, but it is one thing to say that with better infrastructure will come better health, quite another to sever health from its connections with poverty and assume that it will be adequately addressed by an institution for road making, street sweeping, and dung collecting.[81]

The effects of this pragmatism would be far-reaching. "Public health" would come to be equated with "sanitary improvement," and "sanitary" to refer chiefly to municipal and household technologies that preserved the body from subversion by decomposing matter. Having made that equation, one need no longer inquire seriously into the incidence and etiology of disease – Chadwick's impatience with medicine is well known; progress on these fronts was from men like John Snow and William Budd, unattached to official public health.

Yet inquiries, agendas, recommendations are one thing. We have not yet seen a public ready to endorse these changes. In the next few years sanitary reform found a constituency, mainly through the propagandizing efforts of the Health of Towns Association, begun in December 1844. Chadwick was not much involved. In the *Sanitary Report* he had recognized cases where the risk-taking speculator must lead.[82] In early 1844 he had begun to organize a Towns Improvement Company to supply coordinated sanitary works at a healthy profit. This would occupy him for almost two years. It would fail, partly because there were more attractive uses for capital, perhaps also because there was a widely shared unwillingness to be coordinated by any system proposed by the hated Chadwick.

81  In the 1847 version of the bill, which failed to pass, these had been called "Boards of Health and Public Works" (ibid., 284). Chadwick's hybrid institution, the "Local Board of Health," survived only until 1858. From 1858 to 1871, "Local Boards," administered by the Local Government Act Office, would administer governmental and infrastructural affairs, with John Simon's Privy Council Medical Department overseeing matters of health and disease. The Local Government Board, established in 1872, concerned itself with the three separate functions of poor relief, health, and municipal engineering, but in a manner that generated ambiguity and conflict.

82  The case in question was water supply. Chadwick recognized that where urban water supplies had been obtained, hope of profit had been indispensable. His concern in 1842 was for places too small to attract capitalists (*Sanitary Report*, 143–47).

# 8

# The Politics of Public Health, 1841–1848

The years between the final report of the Health of Towns Commission in February 1845 and passage of the Public Health Act in August 1848 have usually been seen as a time of struggle, with cleanliness slowly pushing back the host of dirt, who complained of costly works and central control – surely national imposition of the means of health violated the Englishman's right to be as dirty as he chose. The story is that of small children forced to take baths: Chadwick would have them clean and healthy; they were content, even interested in, staying dirty and diseased.[1] What the story fails to explain is how the Public Health Act ever passed. Who supported it? Why? Were there so many enlightened Benthamites patiently warming the back benches of the House of Commons?

At least in principle, sanitation was an easy sell. It was redolent with Providence and progress. One could commit oneself to it without having to endorse anything in particular. With no pauperizing effects, it was an unobjectionable domain for philanthropy. The rights it interfered with – such as ownership of dung – were low on anyone's list of freedoms. It was to be not only free but profitable. The sanitarians promised to flush away every complicated social issue; they circumvented the squabbling anti–corn law leaguers and ten hours' champions, and stayed far back from the Chartist abyss.[2] One might say things were sanitary enough, or quibble about details, or complain about "centralization" (which meant many things), but one could no more object to the idea than we can to the idea of environmental sustainability.[3] One can even argue that this holy cause was not simply a good but the ideal to which all goods must measure up.[4]

---

1 S. E. Finer, *The Life and Times of Sir Edwin Chadwick* (London: Methuen, 1952), 294–95, characterizes the opposition as "spiteful . . . and most inane." See also R. A. Lewis, *Edwin Chadwick and the Public Health Movement, 1832–1854* (London: Longmans, Green, 1952), 62.

2 Diana Olien, *Morpeth: A Victorian Public Career* (Washington, D.C.: University Press of America, 1983), 294–95, 305–8.

3 See the statements of opponents to the Public Health Bills, *Hansard's Parliamentary Debates, 3rd series*, 94, 1847, 33–34, 37.

4 Lord Campbell in ibid., 99, 1848, 1402. This is not the place to indulge this argument, only to

It took Parliament far less time to pass a public health act than to regulate child labor, fix the poor law, repeal corn tariffs, emancipate Catholics, or reform itself. But for crises (like the Irish potato famine or the Tory schism of 1846) it would have taken less time.[5] In no sense was the act that Lord Morpeth passed in 1848 an exemplar of public health, even before it was mutilated by compromise. Like many legislative concoctions, it was a hash of interests and precedents mixed up by too many overworked and mediocre chefs. It is not clear that what passed was the only or best public health Parliament would have approved.

Public health legislation in the late 1840s had three political identities. Rhetorically and ideologically, it was a moral reform movement orchestrated mainly by the Health of Towns Association. Substantively, it belonged to urban improvement legislation, part of the system of laws developed mainly in the eighteenth century to empower towns to build not just waterworks and sewers, but docks and streets, markets and town halls. Last, it drew on technocratic precedents – Benthamite rationalization, Napoleonic coordination, but most importantly, Parliament's own practice, in the first third of the century, of commissioning engineers (notably Thomas Telford) to undertake capital-intensive public works projects for the development of parts of Scotland, Ireland, and Wales. Disease and death did not animate sanitary politics. In introducing (and defending) the public health bills of 1847 and 1848, Lord Morpeth (and Lord Normanby in 1841) alluded to preventable deaths and to the savings that would result from their prevention, but disease prevention per se had no constituency. Perhaps few believed the sanitarians' claims of lives and money saved (23 million pounds per year, said Playfair); perhaps few really cared.[6]

I

To comprehend the sanitarian passion we can do no better than to revisit the Shropshire barrister-landowner and Whig M.P. Robert Slaney. On everything from the morality-inducing effects of water and sewers to details of sewer design, Slaney independently reached the same conclusions as Chadwick. But

point out that many social analysts and critics have contrasted the modern preoccupation with health and length of life with the attitudes of an earlier time, when one's preoccupations might be with salvation, or enlightenment, or heightened experience. Ivan Illich has done perhaps the best job in helping us understand how illness and death may, as parts of natural conditions, be understood as fully compatible with a notion of "good" (*Medical Nemesis: The Expropriation of Health* [New York: Bantam, 1976], pt. III).

5 Cf. David Roberts, *Victorian Origins of the British Welfare State* (Hamden, Conn.: Archon Books, 1969), 68–70, 140–42; Olien, *Morpeth*, 294–97; Finer, *Chadwick*, 294–95; "Health of Towns Bill," *Civil Engineer and Architects Journal* 11 (1848): 120.

6 Playfair quoted by Lord Morpeth, *Hansard's Parliamentary Debates 3rd series, 91*, 1847, 619–20, 634; *98*, 1848, 738; *99*, 1848, 1401–3; "The Sanitary Question," *Fraser's Magazine 36* (1847): 368.

unlike Chadwick, propelled by problems of administration and career concerns (or Southwood Smith, driven by necessarian theology), Slaney arrived by a much broader road.

The young Slaney was an ardent Malthusian. His *Essay on the Employment of the Poor* (1819, 1822) denounced poor laws. Wages were insufficient for survival; by glutting the labor market with unneeded humans, poor laws were the cause. Charity and education were but palliatives; public employment was at the expense of private employment. With the population at its maximum, there was no avoiding the deadly effects of economic depressions. "As the employment slacken . . . death, in the common course of events, soon carries off the superfluous population. . . . Being before at the lowest allowance, they must now starve: fevers and other diseases, influenced by insufficient food, will rapidly thin the wretched sufferers." Whether this adjustment occurred "with more or less misery" was a function of wages, and in turn of prudential marriages. Slaney's solution was expanded agricultural employment, through scientific farming, easy enclosure, and game laws (which encouraged the gentry to stay in the country).[7]

For Slaney as for Alison, Malthusianism was not incompatible with activism. Locally, he was active in poor law matters and cottage building; nationally he preached self-help through the *Penny Magazine* of the Society for the Promotion of Useful Knowledge.[8] On industrialization, Slaney was no apologist. It and its cycles were inevitable; workers must cope, through self-help institutions like savings banks and medical clubs. Yet Slaney knew that such institutions were not keeping pace. Without "considerable improvements in the education and morality of the working classes" there would be "great evil and suffering." In 1838 he secured a select committee on education, which led to James Kay-Shuttleworth's appointment as Privy Council education secretary and ultimately to universal primary education in England.[9] Recognizing the great "discontent" in towns, he moved in January 1840 for a select committee to investigate its causes: "Neglect of the vast changes in our populous towns – no regulations of a *sanatory* nature as to the dwellings of the working classes, no adequate provisions agnst [sic] want of employment, no religious instruction, no education." Asked to narrow its focus, he concentrated on "neglect of the building, sewage, or sanatory regulations and the mass of misery, wretchedness, and disease and discontent thence arising." This was

---

7 Robert Slaney, *An Essay on the Employment of the Poor* (London: Hatchard, 1819), 2–4; in a second edition Slaney treated health as capital. Disease – a product of "poverty, and its direct consequence, want of cleanliness" – was a social cost of excess population. Every day of illness was lost wealth. Sickly workers could only do 40 percent as much as healthy workers, yet cost as much to maintain. Death before maturity was unrecouped investment (*An Essay on the Employment of the Poor, 2nd ed, with Additions, with a Letter by James Scarlett, M.P.* [London: Hatchard, 1822], 41–42).
8 Slaney Diaries, Shrewsbury Records Centre, v. 7, 2, 23 April 1837; June 1837; January 1839.
9 Ibid., 23 April 1837; November 1837; July 1838; January 1839.

the Health of Towns Committee. Its premise was that without sanitation, education and crime prevention were futile.[10]

Throughout the early 1840s Slaney repeatedly urged the government to take up sanitation, build parks, even swimming facilities. He published cheap editions of the education and health reports. Unwilling to be a part of electoral corruption, he left Parliament in 1841 and redoubled his sanitary efforts. In early 1842 he visited the "worst parts" of Wolverhampton and Bilston. As for Chadwick, what stood out were the bad drains; like Chadwick he took up drainage experiments. The Plug Plot riots of 1842 showed the urgent need for "improvements in the social conditions of the masses," he told Peel. In Shropshire he persuaded workers not to take to the streets by raising a subscription to keep a colliery working. Appointment to the Health of Towns Commission was a consummation long sought: "I shall not hesitate to give up my Hunting Shooting and other rural amusements for this better employment."[11]

To those who see early Victorian social reform through Dickensian eyes a "humanitarian advocate of the workhouse test" will be an oxymoron, and Slaney will make no sense. Well into the 1840s he continued to call for a "more stern working of the poor laws" and to worry at the "rapidly increasing" numbers of the very poor. But his was a descriptive not a vindictive Malthusianism. "Discontent" should trigger concern in "humane and thinking men" not the "starve, damn you" declamations of some Malthusians. Slaney the agriculturalist opposed the corn laws; though a champion of state sanitation he allied himself with Chadwick's Towns Improvement Company. And the Shrewsbury hunt was as central in his life as the welfare of the working classes.[12]

Slaney said what he saw and thought; he was neither subtle nor eloquent. He saw himself as a rich man trying to do good in a world of disorientation and inequality. He had the gift of seeing pretty clearly what was going on, of feeling strongly that conditions were dangerous and unjust, and of managing for most of his life to avoid complacency, cynicism, and self-interested self-delusion. He fits David Roberts's model of the early Victorian paternalist even down to his fascination with liquid manure: lots of Oxford, Coleridge, "duty of property," sense of sin, trust in markets and in capitalism, but also a strong sense of obligation to act.[13] There were many more or less like him. Some,

---

10  Ibid., January, February 1840.
11  Ibid., September, December 1840, April, October 1841, February, March, July, September 1842; v. 8, May 1843. Thus in Wolverhampton Slaney finds "total neglect of all due regulations as to building drainage and cleansing – no underground drains except in main streets – filth and wretchedness dreadful. No supply of water no scavengers."
12  Ibid., v. 7, June, October 1842; v. 8, August 1843; September, November 1845.
13  See Slaney's resolutions "to be diligently and beneficially employed" (ibid., v. 7, June 1837; also November 1837, April 1838). David Roberts, *Paternalism in Early Victorian England* (New Brunswick, N.J.: Rutgers University Press, 1979), 73–74, 136. Cf. R. A. Soloway, *Prelates and People:*

like the mercurial Lord Shaftesbury, were driven by grander passions of sin and outrage. Others saw conditions in a fuzzier way and dimly perceived sanitation as an unobjectionable, even mildly amusing, way to be publicly good.

The organization that would market sanitation, the Health of Towns Association, was full of these shallower Slaneys, men of state, the church, or the professions who gave their guineas to good causes and got their names on lists of patrons (and sometimes took care that the societies they joined endorsed policies that might put a bit of money in their pockets). The association was launched at Exeter Hall, the evangelicals' headquarters, in December 1844, two months before the final report of the Health of Towns Commission. Modeled on the Anti–Corn Law League, it had as its main purpose lobbying for comprehensive public health legislation, in particular for an act with certain provisions beneficial to doctors, landowners, and capitalists. To this end it was also concerned with gathering data and with spreading the sanitary gospel. By early 1848 there were chapters in Liverpool, Manchester, Edinburgh, York, Halifax, Bath, Derby, Walsall, Marlborough, Plymouth, Worcester, Rugby, and Newcastle. The Liverpool and Plymouth chapters published journals; the association also published the national *Journal of Public Health and Monthly Record of Sanitary Improvement*, which appeared from the end of 1847 through the middle of the next year.[14] Though it was to be an all party group, it was mainly Whig and coalesced around Lord Normanby and Southwood Smith. Chadwick was not involved, yet on some key and controversial matters there was an uncanny "ventriloquism" between the association's positions and his own.[15] It has been seen as the keeper of the flame of sanitary reform, nurturing it until the Whigs could return to pass the Public Health Act of 1848.

As understood by the association, sanitation was a broad church, the solution, somehow, to all social problems, no matter how distant they might seem from water and sewers. It is this theme of unity among those who did not normally share a common cause that marks the association's founding meeting. Like most Victorian public meetings, it was highly orchestrated –

*Ecclesiastical Social Thought in England, 1783–1852* (London: Routledge and Kegan Paul, 1969); David Roberts, *Paternalism in Early Victorian England* (New Brunswick, N.J.: Rutgers University Press, 1979); G. Kitson Clark, *Churchmen and the Condition of England, 1832–1885: A Study in the Development of Social Ideas and Practice from the Old Regime to the Modern State* (London: Methuen, 1973); Boyd Hilton, *The Age of Atonement: The Influence of Evangelicalism on Social and Economic Thought, 1785–1865* (Oxford: Clarendon Press, 1988).

14 Robert G. Paterson, "The Health of Towns Association in Great Britain, 1844–1849," *Bulletin of the History of Medicine* 22 (1948): 373–402; Lewis, *Chadwick*, 115; "Sanitary Intelligence," *Journal of Public Health and Monthly Record of Sanitary Improvement* 1 (1847): 28.

15 For "ventriloquism" see Lewis, *Chadwick*, 111–13; also see Finer, *Chadwick*, 239. Chadwick's letters suggest little direct involvement with the association. See Chadwick to Thomas Hawksley, 5 December 1844, University College London [UCL] Chadwick Papers #2181/6; Chadwick to Smith, 9 December 1844, UCL Chadwick Papers #2181/6; Chadwick to Morpeth, 24 August 1847, UCL Chadwick Papers #1055.

nothing contentious or critical. Some told sad stories of the sorry poor, but there was little of substance on the core issues of sewers and water. Choking on one's own virtue was the only sanitary hazard in sight. Wasn't it grand, began one, to find "subjects intimately connected with the public good in which men of all parties, widely dissenting from each other in politics and in religion, can happily and virtuously agree, and that in the meeting of their minds – in the confluence of their emotions – none but objects which it is a moral pleasure to contemplate should be serenely reflected!"[16]

Lord Normanby's opening remarks made clear the wide range of "health of towns" matters. He spoke first of the deterioration of "physical well-being" in those capital had assembled to do the nation's work. Anticipating Marx, he condemned an industrial system that wore out bodies and even claimed the little time between work and sleep needed to cultivate the "affections" and "faculties" of "a rational being." Such overwork led mothers to neglect infants and to infant mortality – or was that due to a "moral state" reflected in the "appalling" opiate use so vividly described by Playfair? Normanby asked his hearers, who had surely found it hard to leave their own firesides, to think of the "half-starved, half-clothed" poor in "crowded cellars" forced to choose between the "cutting blast and pestilential closeness." He himself would choose a slave (or Irish) cabin over a Liverpool cellar. And how was a competent army and navy to be recruited from a decrepit population? Normanby did get to the virtues of sewers, the advantages of defraying their cost by long loans, and the likely savings from sanitation, but never made it to disease prevention.[17]

Sir R. H. Inglis, antiquarian and Tory M.P. for Oxford University, followed, with details (square sewers in Lancaster) and statistics (correlation of mortality to ventilation in Nottingham). He alluded to an unmentionable problem of females that better drainage would remedy and to the need for a comprehensive system "under one superintending and responsible authority." (This concern with "physical condition" was far beneath the "diffusion of the light of Scripture," he added.)[18] Unlike Inglis, who had cribbed from blue books, Sir Benjamin Hawes, Whig M.P. for Lambeth, had toured with Alison. What he had seen, "no language could describe": "So degrading, so humiliating" – "darkness, filth, disease – an atmosphere scarcely endurable"; dwellings "rather fit for brutes than human beings." Hawes noted that destitution was "a fruitful cause enough" for disease, but their business was "physical causes." Social order and defense of property were his main concerns. They would be safe only when "the great mass of the people feel their material

16 Health of Towns Association, *Abstract of the Public Meeting Held at Exeter Hall, December 11, 1844* (London: Charles Knight [1845]), 20. Ironically, the example that occasioned that remark was the sanitation of Rome, which had already been decried by another speaker.
17 Ibid., 4–13.
18 Ibid., 13–16.

comforts and enjoyments increase in a reasonable and just proportion with property itself."[19]

Another Whig M.P., R. L. Sheil, focused on "moral wholesomeness": "How often are those who are encompassed by the effluvia of ordure enveloped in a miasma of the mind." Next, the Reverend W. E. Champneys, vicar of Whitechapel, explained how clergymen would support sanitary reform when they realized "how many souls were . . . hurried every year unprepared into eternity." How, he asked, could a small child, shivering through its third bout of fever, ever grow into a moral adult? Even more than Hawes, Champneys offered authenticity. Unable to alter burial customs, he disinfected corpses. He attacked "improvement." Beautifying the streets of the rich worsened conditions for the poor. The urban landscape became like the consumptive – beautiful surface, "havoc" within.[20]

For Champneys and a few others sanitation was less a means of preventing disease than a minimum criterion of liberty. In his parish were laborers who could not work because they were "so enfeebled . . . so exhausted, by the close, stifling, and poisonous atmosphere." Sir William Clay, Champneys's M.P., argued that sanitary conditions were the one thing the diligent, honest worker could not change. Bad sanitation could "neutralize his best exertions." Even those opposed to state meddling would recognize, argued William Cowper, Whig M.P. for Hertford (and later president of the General Board of Health), that "the owner of a court or alley could not claim the right of generating his own fever, because he could not pretend to confine it to his own tenants." In housing, laissez faire was "not humane," "not safe."[21] And so it went.

Some of this, perhaps, hints at Cobbett's view of health as a form of property. But not very strongly. It was hardly an occasion for radical talk; more a mix of hand-wringing and back-slapping. Sober reflection on the plight of the poor alternated with affirmation of the good fellows' commitment finally to do something for them. Most of the speeches were facile and reflected little firsthand knowledge. But that didn't matter. Chadwick had made sanitary condition the paradigm of social analysis and new facts were redundant. In creating the *Sanitary Report*, Chadwick (and his informants) had reduced and disempowered their subjects; in creating a political movement, the Health of

19 Ibid., 17–19.
20 Ibid., 21–25. On Champneys see Roberts, *Paternalism*, 159.
21 Health of Towns Association, *Abstract of the Public Meeting*, 26–27, 30–31. The professional speakers added little – it was not, after all, mainly their evening. Southwood Smith brought up the Waterloo analogy: The yearly toll of preventable diseases should be looked on as equivalent to the slaughter in a great and unnecessary battle. R. D. Grainger, a well-known anatomist, compared typhoid in Birmingham and Liverpool. The difference was housing: cellars in Liverpool, single-family houses in Birmingham. Grainger did not ask whether modes of housing might reflect modes of employment (35, 28). In presenting the resolutions of the meeting to Parliament, Normanby focused on opiates and burial clubs (*Hansard's Parliamentary Debates 3rd series*, 77, 1845, 449–52).

Towns Association was simply abstracting their abstraction. Sanitation was to be synonymous with doing good. The "poor," a particularly nebulous entity in this midway point between the great Chartist eruptions of 1838–42 and 1848, were to be objects of benevolence: whatever was most wrong in their lives, that was what sanitation fixed. This was the "poor man's bill," intoned speaker after speaker in the debates on public health bills in 1847 and 1848. Why then such concern to keep power "in the hands of the rich" by allowing plural voting, asked critics? And why no repeal of the window tax, the most direct threat to health and comfort?[22]

It took hold, this ethos of sanitary saintliness. Sanitation became the simple good cause. The belief that one was endowing the poor with bliss was what gave the banal business of sewer building such immediacy. On the hustings in 1847, Benjamin Disraeli found that it paid to have been a founding member of the Health of Towns Association: he could profess himself a sanitarian. (He'd done little to act on that profession, noted *Fraser's*.)[23]

How different the smug security of late 1844 from the crisis of early 1842, during which Chadwick had written the *Sanitary Report*. Now all was easy unanimity, for nothing was really at stake. Nothing challenged Chadwick's all-embracing paradigm of betterment. The "poor" were, temporarily, quiet, neither a problem nor a threat. Conditions were better, revolution less imminent. The Health of Towns Commission had successfully linked sanitary reform with urban improvement. Henceforth, "the poor" would be a rhetorical device used in a middle-class campaign. The middle classes would benefit from sanitation in simple ways: by being protected from smells, and thus from disease (smell *was* disease, Southwood Smith was now maintaining); by being set free of nonaccountable local government; and by gaining power to "improve" the urban environment.[24]

How much the meaning of sanitation had shifted is evident in Chadwick's 1847 address to a meeting to raise a fund for the widow of Jordan Lynch, a City of London medical officer who had died of fever caught attending the poor. Chadwick used the occasion to call the roll of fallen sanitary heroes: not only Lynch, but Dyce Guthrie and Butler Williams, drainage experts who had testified to the Health of Towns Commission, and the Liverpool social missionary the Reverend John Johns. In Liverpool and Leeds deaths and illnesses among those who visited the poor were prodigious, Chadwick told the meeting. Lynch had been engaged in a "service against ravages greater than

22 *Hansard's Parliamentary Debates 3rd series, 93*, 1847, 1282; *96*, 1848, 404–6, 409–10, 414–18; *98*, 1848, 735, 766, 1213–15; *99*, 1848, 691, 1401.

23 "The Sanitary Question," *Fraser's Magazine 36* (1847): 366; Roberts, *Paternalism*, 252.

24 Finer, *Chadwick*, 297–98. Lewis (*Chadwick*, 115) argues that "the weapons of the Anti–Corn Law League, though they were sharpened and given their cutting edge by the misery of the lower classes, were forged out of the solid core of middle-class interests." I would argue (he does not) that the same was true with sanitation. See also M. Sigsworth and M. Worboys, "The Public's View of Public Health in mid-Victorian Britain," *Urban History 21* (1994): 237–50.

the ravages of war . . . but without the glory, the excitement, and the support." To Chadwick, Lynch had admitted "a sense of the personal danger, but said cheerfully there was no avoiding it." Indeed, in working among the poor day after day, Lynch had committed martyrdom: sooner or later serious harm was inevitable.

If Lynch were the soldier volunteering for extra missions in hostile territory, who was the enemy and what was the cause? What Chadwick failed to mention is that those with whom Lynch worked constantly faced these causes of fever. Yet because the problem was Lynch's fever and not theirs, they were, in effect, the enemy, directly responsible for his death. When Chadwick came to the special importance of Lynch's work, his *cause* as it were, it was not numbers cured but science, greater "knowledge of the true causes of these epidemics, and the means of prevention." Thanks to Lynch we now knew "that we could place *even well-conditioned persons* under such circumstances . . . [and] produce typhus. Low and insufficient diet, amidst filth, spread and aggravate it, by depressing the system . . . cleanliness and ventilation will diminish it, even against mental depression and . . . low diet." (Ironically, what Lynch had discovered was that even he could get fever.) And since only cleanliness and air, and not food, could prevent it, well then, there was really no need to worry about those who lacked that food – at least not as a medical matter.[25]

At the end of the 1845 parliamentary session, Lord Lincoln, former Health of Towns Commission member and Peel's chief commissioner of woods and forests, introduced a "health of towns" bill based on the commission's reports. It was too late for passage; Lincoln simply wanted the bill considered in the recess. In most respects, Lincoln's bill was stronger than the bill Lord Morpeth would pass in 1848. Lincoln would have the districts of sanitary authorities coincide with drainage basins, a principle for which public health reformers would be fighting for the next half century. He proposed to put the sanitary needs of towns in the hands of a Home Office inspector who would formulate plans to be carried out by locally elected commissioners. Responsibility for initiating and completing projects would be shared by central and local units

25 Edwin Chadwick, *Health of Towns. Report of the Speeches . . . to Promote a Subscription in Behalf of the Widow and Children of Dr. J. R. Lynch* (London: Chapman, Elcoate, 1847), 4–7 (italics mine); also Southwood Smith, in ibid., 11; Finer, *Chadwick*, 294–95. In a letter to Morpeth he listed others: Dr. James Mitchell, assistant hand loom weaver commissioner and statistician, who had helped with the *Sanitary Report,* and the assistant poor law commissioner William Gilbert. Among Health of Towns Commissioners Playfair, De la Beche, Vetch, and Smith of Deanston had suffered significant illnesses. Southwood Smith had come down with fever three times (once almost fatally), he himself twice (Chadwick to Morpeth, 30 June 1847, UCL Chadwick Papers #1055). Lord Morpeth contrasted the "martyrs to . . . the causes of suffering humanity" with "the unofficial victims, those herds of sufferers" (*Hansard's Parliamentary Debates 3rd series, 96,* 1848, 396–97). Nor is the enemy metaphor facile: Lynch blamed the Irish poor for a great part of the city's poor health ("The Sanitary Question," *Fraser's Magazine 36* [1847]: 370).

of government. Political crises prevented further consideration in 1846.[26] The bill did, however, elicit a lengthy critique from a committee of the Health of Towns Association. Calling it an "excellent basis" for legislation, the committee went on to reject many of its provisions. [27] Its views shed much light on what was at stake in sanitary politics.

Capital accumulation for one thing. Lincoln's bill was objectionable in that "no facilities are afforded for the formation and no guarantee given for the protection, of Joint Stock companies." Naively, Lincoln had put his trust in local democracy and in general practice contractors and engineers. But companies, particularly Chadwick's struggling Towns Improvement Company – "an association including some of the largest capitalists in Europe," noted the committee – would do the work better, for a modest 6 percent guaranteed return. (For an additional fee they would even run the works.) Here the committee was emphatic: "The object of the legislature should be to ENGAGE AND REGULATE THE SPIRIT OF COMMERCIAL ENTERPRISE IN THE EXECUTION OF THE MEASURES OF SANATORY IMPROVEMENT." There would be plenty for these capitalists to do, the committee added: "scarcely a city or town in the kingdom" did not need "extensive works" of drainage, sewerage, or water, "and in the great majority it is necessary that such works should be commenced almost entirely anew."[28] In light of Chadwick's later attacks on the London water companies and his claim that he became involved in the Towns Improvement Company only when it seemed that public authorities would not undertake sanitation, the argument is intriguing.[29] Lincoln clearly saw sanita-

---

26 Health of Towns Association, *Report of the Committee to the Members of the Association on Lord Lincoln's Sewerage, Drainage, etc., of Towns' Bill* (London: Charles Knight, 1846), 5, 14–16, 22–24. Lincoln was following recommendations of the Health of Towns Commission (Royal Commission on the Health of Towns and Populous Districts, *Second Report, Parliamentary Papers [P.P.]*, 1845, *18*, [610.], 6, 16, 21 [to be cited as HOT, *Second Report*]). There were sixty members of the committee, including three bishops, fifteen members of the House of Commons, and ten medical men. Lewis *(Chadwick*, 125–29) sees the views in the report as Chadwick's. On its introduction see *Hansard's Parliamentary Debates 3rd series, 82*, 1845, 1077.

27 A great deal of the report is the usual sanitarian boilerplate – heartrending or horrifying examples of mothers living in unwatered tenements or driven by cesspools to amoral wretchedness – which did not directly address provisions in the bill. The committee went out of its way to denounce the destitution–disease view: "During the last year full employment has been given to the manufacturing population in certain manufacturing towns, at higher wages than were ever known in these places; yet the Registration Returns show that full employment at high wages has not been sufficient to preserve the population from an increased ratio of sickness and mortality; not that high wages can be supposed to increase sickness and mortality; but the returns clearly show that a high degree of prosperity is incapable of affording protection from disease, suffering, and premature death, arising from the neglect of efficient drainage, proper cleansing, a due supply of water, and other sanitary measures, which are actually extended to the inmates of well-regulated prisons, and which science might secure to the whole of the population" (Health of Towns Association, *Report of the Committee on Lord Lincoln's Bill*, 7).

28 Ibid., 26–30.

29 See Chadwick to Lord Morpeth, 23 April 1847, UCL Chadwick Papers #1055; Chadwick to Arthur Helps, 12 March 1845, UCL Chadwick Papers #2181/9; "The Public Health Bill: Its

tion as a duty of the state; it is not so clear that Chadwick and the Health of Towns Association did.

Who would pay for all this? Thanks to Chadwick's proposal that sanitary works be amortized over the life of the works, no one need suffer much burden. But what burden there was must fall on occupiers, not owners, the committee held: it was easier to identify the occupier. Thus blithely it dispatched one of the most contentious land issues of the century: whether tenants had a real interest in the capital improvements they paid for. In effect, the committee was treating sanitary works as services, not capital improvements. Yet, at the same time it was urging Parliament to legislate a huge gift to owners of property. But surely the poor would willingly pay – water would be worth six to nine pence/week, said one, so as not to have to go out for morning coffee.[30]

Last, the committee raised the issue of local medical officers of health, an office which, to some, has seemed the key achievement of Victorian public health. In the mid-1840s there was little agreement whether such an officer was needed or what one would do. Chadwick was ambivalent. He had advocated regional medical officers in the *Sanitary Report* but been more concerned with a local engineering officer. He had been more enthusiastic in the supplemental *Interment Report* of late 1843, seeing a role for medical officers in determining causes of death and ensuring safe burial.[31] He was, at that time, trying both to rein in the mutton-prescribing poor law medical officers and to discipline causes-of-death reporting. Coroners' juries and the public had a bad habit of attributing the deaths of the poor to poverty and of blaming the

Letter and Its Spirit," *Fraser's Magazine 38* (1848): 444–46; cf. Lewis, *Chadwick*, 307; Oliver MacDonagh, *Early Victorian Government, 1830–1870* (London: Weidenfeld and Nicolson, 1977), 143.

30 Health of Towns Association, *Report of the Committee on Lord Lincoln's Bill*, 28–33, 58. In this the committee was departing from traditions of local improvement legislation which assigned costs to owners and usually collected the entire fee up front rather than utilize long-term borrowing. Such fees would clearly have been beyond the means of many occupiers, and it would moreover have been unfair to assess a temporary resident for a permanent improvement (though, in effect, that is what the committee was recommending). Thus, part of the attraction of the loan scheme is that payments could be made low enough to be passed on to occupiers. Chadwick himself had objected to Normanby's bill on the grounds that costs would fall on "the most wretched occupiers" (Chadwick to Normanby, 3 February 1841, UCL Chadwick Papers #1578). By 1848 he was convinced that charging owners was politically impossible (Chadwick to Morpeth, 8 January 1848, UCL Chadwick Papers #1055). For a discussion of the implications of modes of taxation on sewer building see Lyon Playfair, "Report on the Sanitary Condition of Large Towns in Lancashire," HOT, *Second Report*, Appendix, pt. 2, 3–7. The public health bill of 1848 compromised on the question; occupiers were to be charged except in the cases of dwellings valued at less than ten pounds annual rental (*Hansard's Parliamentary Debates 3rd series, 98*, 1848, 1247). For Chadwick's later views see "Report by the General Board of Health on the Measures Adopted for the Execution of the Nuisances Removal and Diseases Prevention Act, and the Public Health Act up to July 1849," *P.P.*, 1849, *24*, [1115.], 58–59.

31 Edwin Chadwick, *Report on the Sanitary Condition of the Labouring Population of Great Britain. A Supplementary Report on the Results of a Special Inquiry into the Practice of Interment in Towns* (London: Clowes, 1843), 171–78; Lewis, *Chadwick*, 75, 80–81.

poor law. A trained medical officer might be relied on to see deaths in terms of insanitary places.[32] At the last minute the Health of Towns Commission had endorsed the idea of the local medical officer, but early drafts of the 1848 bill would not include such a provision. The pressure was mainly from medical men. In an overstocked market a new form of employment was important indeed.[33]

Lincoln's bill would have allowed the local commissions to appoint such officers, who would be charged with the general duties of keeping track of disease, identifying nuisances, and advising on ventilation. Following Chadwick, whose *Interments Report* it quoted at length, the committee thought Lincoln had missed "the primary and fundamental duties of the officer": "the verification of the fact as well as of the cause of death . . . and the personal examination on the spot of the sanatory circumstances under which death takes place."[34]

Beyond providing the intelligence needed to plan a sanitary offensive, the medical officer's visit to the bereaved family would have miraculous effects in quelling class conflict. Imagine how honored the bereaved would be by a visit from one "at the highest rank of his profession," representing the pinnacle of "science." While the medical officer was discovering social truths, the poor would learn that society, through the medical officer's redeeming love, had a stake in their well-being.

The effect . . . would be to place the most ignorant, forsaken, and helpless being in the community, in the moment of his utmost bewilderment and desolation, under the direction of an instructed mind; it would be to secure universally and invariably, the presence of knowledge and science in the abode into which death follows the footstep of disease. . . . With the visits of the policeman, the rent-collector, and the tax-gatherer, the poor are familiar; they see also the union surgeon, and the officer for administering parochial relief; occasionally the agent of some charitable society, and sometimes the clergyman, but there is no responsible officer whose proper duty it is to visit them in the season of distress and sorrow, for the express purpose of affording them protection, counsel, and help. The medical officer . . . would be such an officer; his mission would be one purely of benevolence, and most healing and beneficent would be . . . the appointment by the state of such a public servant.

To be sure, that purely benevolent visitor was also a policeman: the officer might be armed with "summary powers" – to dispose of corpses or "enforce

32 C. Hamlin, "Could You Starve to Death in England in 1839? The Chadwick–Farr Controversy and the Loss of the 'Social' in Public Health," *American Journal of Public Health 85* (1995): 856–66.
33 On the 1848 bill see John Sutherland to Chadwick, 17 February 1848, UCL Chadwick Papers #1920. See also Southwood Smith in Royal Commission on the Health of Towns and Populous Districts, *First Report*, P.P., 1844, 17, [542.], Evidence, qq 1025–26 [to be cited as HOT, *First Report*]; Wakley in *Hansard's Parliamentary Debates 3rd series, 96*, 1848, 1022–23.
34 Health of Towns Association, *Report of the Committee on Lord Lincoln's Bill*, 90–91.

ventilation . . . and . . . remove nuisances which originate and maintain disease," for example. But the poor would cooperate.[35]

I call attention to the particular issues of capital, rating, and medical officers because the Health of Towns Association has sometimes been taken to exemplify a process in which benevolent people of all parties simultaneously see that conditions are unacceptable and unite to change them. Yet the association's chief characteristic was not benevolence but class – for all the talk of sanitation as the good cause that united factions, on the most important matters its members were already united. Nonetheless, it would be unduly cynical to see benevolence as merely a front to advance the interests of the owners of capital and of land, and of a medical profession on the make. The faith in sanitary salvation was genuine enough, as was the benevolence, but neither called for forsaking the pursuit of legitimate interests.

## II

Under the name of "improvement" middle-class "sanitary reform" had been under way for well over a century. The value of ready water, of well drained and easily cleaned streets, of ventilation, is clear in the Georgian squares in many British and Irish towns and cities. Indeed, some historians speak of an "urban renaissance" paid for by India, the slave trade, and the industrial revolution.[36] The high importance put on these amenities is evident in the trouble Georgian town dwellers took to get them. A central tenet of the unwritten English constitution was the inability of local government to act without explicit legislative sanction, the doctrine of *ultra vires*.[37] Trivial matters that might seem only to require a nod from a midlevel administrator – installing

35  Ibid., 91, 98; cf. Chadwick, *Supplementary Report*, 201. If this sounds like medical officer-as-clergyman, that is no accident. With a divided church undecided about its social role, a combined medical–dissenter–evangelical coalition looked to take over some of the unoccupied territory. The interment question was a key site of interprofessional conflict. Who was to control the dead? The church, with its bulging graveyards (or worse the Irish Catholics with their wakes and watchings), or some representative of science, compassion, and moral order? See Ruth Richardson, *Death, Dissection, and the Destitute* (London: Penguin, 1988). On tractarian opposition see Playfair to Chadwick, 15 January 1844, UCL Chadwick Papers #1588.
36  C. W. Chalkin, *The Provincial Towns of Georgian England: A Study in the Building Process, 1740–1820* (Montreal: McGill-Queen's University Press, 1974), 49–105; P. J. Corfield, *The Impact of English Towns, 1700–1800* (Oxford: Oxford University Press, 1982); Peter Borsay, *The English Urban Renaissance: Culture and Society in the Provincial Town, 1660–1770* (Oxford: Clarendon Press, 1989), 80–114. In part the skepticism that Chadwick's sanitary proposals met reflected fear that they were not sanitary enough: Water closets seemed to invite river pollution; suburban meadows soaked in sewage seemed likely to create a fearsome fever-causing miasm (M. C. Buer, *Health, Wealth, and Population in the Early Days of the Industrial Revolution* [London: Routledge, 1926], 106–8, also 87, 110).
37  American readers may find this confusing. While the American constitution works from the assumption that governments may do anything not constitutionally proscribed, the English Constitution proceeds from the opposite assumption, that governments may do nothing without specific sanction.

lamps on streets or laying down pavement – required Parliament's permission through a local act.

Well into the nineteenth century, the obtaining of such permission was not clearly the responsibility of any particular unit of local government. Roads and poor law were parish responsibilities, while the counties maintained bridges and jails. Most older towns had municipal corporations, but these were less city governments than corporate entities with privileges for regulating commerce and often for administering particular kinds of justice. Prior to the Municipal Corporations Act of 1835, most were not accountable to an electorate. Their members – often masters in certain trades – were more akin to a town's owners than its governors or managers. Some municipal corporations administered charitable institutions, but in no sense did they see themselves as responsible for social welfare.[38] Liverpool corporation's interest in environmental services and economic development was rare.

Thus, the great age of improvement from 1750 to 1835 was not mainly a matter of town governments undertaking new responsibilities. Often it meant creating new institutions, usually called "improvement," paving, or police commissions, from scratch. More than thirty of these were created each decade between 1760 and 1800, and by the midnineteenth century they oversaw public services in three hundred towns. They were especially important in industrial towns like Birmingham and Manchester that had developed too recently to have corporations.[39]

What is most remarkable is that such commissions and the urban improvement they brought about were the result of genuine local initiative and remarkable perseverance – in getting organized, raising money, drafting a bill, hiring parliamentary agents and barristers, negotiating with opponents, waiting on and perhaps testifying before select committees. By the end of the eighteenth century a "normal act" had evolved, with a core set of proven clauses that a town trimmed to its particular needs. This normal act gave powers for paving, cleaning, and lighting specific streets; for a night watch; and for re-

---

38  Brian Keith-Lucas, *The Unreformed Local Government System* (London: Croom Helm, 1980), 51, 89; Josef Redlich and Francis Hirst, *The History of Local Government in England, Being a Reissue of Book I of Local Government in England*, 2d ed., Introduction and Epilogue by Bryan Keith-Lucas (New York: Augustus M. Kelley, 1970).

39  E. D. Jones and M. E. Falkus, "Urban Improvement and the English Economy in the 17th and 18th Centuries," *Research in Economic History* 4 (1979): 193–233. Jones and Falkus (220) trace the movement of improvement from the market towns of the south to the industrialized north. Beyond London, improvement commissions were established in 15 industrial places and 110 market towns between 1739 and 1799. For a different breakdown see Lord Morpeth in *Hansard's Parliamentary Debates 3rd series, 98*, 1848, 735–36. See also F. H. Spencer, *Municipal Origins: An Account of English Private Bill Legislation Relating to Local Government, 1740–1835; with a Chapter on Private Bill Procedure* (London: Constable, 1911), 42; Keith-Lucas, *Unreformed Local Government*, 30, 113, 152; Beatrice Webb and Sidney Webb, *English Local Government from the Revolution to the Municipal Corporations Act: Statutory Authorities for Special Purposes* (London: Longmans, Green, 1922), 242, 254–55 (Birmingham), 258–65 (Manchester).

moval of nuisances. Usually these latter were not threats to health, but impediments to free movement (like trades carried on in the street) or to comfort (pig keeping). "Improvement" clauses laid out procedures for the compulsory purchase of property to widen streets and standards for new construction.[40]

Where such commissions remained active they tended to evolve into comprehensive institutions of local government. Many returned to Parliament for further powers.[41] They sought more general authority to undertake improvements, regulate nuisances and new construction through bylaws, and take on capital debt. Some experimented with social services: a 1768 Devonshire act included a comprehensive social insurance plan; a Birmingham act of 1831 authorized a public day-care center. Indeed, much social legislation that would one day appear in a general act appeared first in local acts.[42] There was also growing interest in drains, water, and gas. Although the latter two were mainly the sphere of joint stock companies, these too were products of local initiative, and the line between private and public was fuzzy. Shareholders might also be commissioners; their investment in improvement might be in local authority debt as well as company shares.[43]

Though towns were acquiring sewers and water through these acts, rarely was "public health" prominent in these initiatives. A Dorchester bill called for improvement in the name of the "health, safety, and advantage" of the public, and public health was a central concern in an 1802 Liverpool bill that failed to pass.[44] But usually other motives dominated: commerce (the need for wide, well paved, well drained streets to handle the growing flow of goods and persons, or for water to fight warehouse fires), aesthetics (the keeping up of the new Georgian garden town), and security (streetlights and watchmen).[45] And however splendid, the works of the improvement commissions were usually restricted to main streets.[46] There was no pretense that "improvement" was for the poor. In Devonport, the poor had opposed a lighting and watching act on the grounds that they slept at night and hadn't anything worth stealing.[47] Still, the hygienic perspective suggested that every improvement of en-

---

40 Costs depended on the complexity of the bill, the number of rates it involved, and the amount of opposition generated (Spencer, *Municipal Origins*, 79–92).

41 From 1785 to 1800, while roughly sixty new commissions were established, 211 improvement acts were passed (Buer, *Health, Wealth, and Population*, 83).

42 Keith-Lucas, *Unreformed Local Government*, 131; Spencer, *Municipal Origins*, 295.

43 Spencer, *Municipal Origins*, 268–69, 275. On water incorporations see J. A. Hassan, "The Growth and Impact of the British Water Industry in the Nineteenth Century," *Economic History Review*, 2d series, *38* (1985): 534; on gas see John F. Wilson, *Lighting the Town: A Study of Management in the North West Gas Industry, 1805–1880* (London: Paul Chapman, 1991). See also Buer, *Health, Wealth, and Population*, 42.

44 Quoted in Spencer, *Municipal Origins*, 176; also see Buer, *Health, Wealth, and Population*, 85.

45 Webb and Webb, *Statutory Authorities*, 274; John Prest, *Liberty and Locality: Parliament, Permissive Legislation, and Ratepayers' Democracies in the Nineteenth Century* (Oxford: Clarendon Press, 1990), 66; Jones and Falkus, "Urban Improvement," 216–19.

46 Keith-Lucas, *Unreformed Local Government*, 118–20; Prest, *Liberty and Locality*, 178.

47 Spencer, *Municipal Origins*, 34. Indeed, working people might be the very problems the acts were

vironment would improve health and some historians have given these commissions a central role in public health: Keith-Lucas writes that "it was . . . through the development of local acts that real and permanent progress was made in sanitary matters."[48]

Here then was a vanguard of self-mobilized sanitarians who had gone to great trouble and expense to obtain powers to take control of their urban environment. Clearly they would be the main constituency for the better technology, broader powers, and simpler procedures that Chadwick and the Health of Towns Commission were developing. But while on the one hand they were needed to press for sanitary legislation, could they be trusted to carry out sanitary reform?

By the mid-1840s they were being much criticized. With the act of 1835 reforming municipal corporations, these leapfrogged over the improvement commissions, which were in many cases still self-appointing, as exemplars of progressive local government. Institutions that had hitherto exemplified reform, as expressions of popular will, now themselves needed reform. Along with local authorities generally, they also fell victim to the crisis mongering of Chadwick and his followers. Chadwick was unrelenting in his vilification; for him English local government was an accident of history, a monster badly needing to be replaced by a rational system. But sanitation was a moral crusade too, and righteousness was hard to summon unless there was some wickedness to attack. Girding their loins for the coming struggle, sanitarians portrayed these institutions not as honest makers of errors, but as willfully evil entities. One lecturer called for war on "the parochial primates, the corporation con-

---

to solve. A metropolitan act of 1690 explained the need for cleansing by complaining of the "dirt, filth, and coal ashes" that "the poorer sort of people" were throwing into residential squares (quoted in ibid., 197–98).

48   Keith-Lucas, *Unreformed Local Government*, 117, 120–21, 150; cf. idem, "Some Influences Affecting the Development of Sanitary Legislation in England," *Economic History Review*, 2d series, 6 (1953): 290–96; E. P. Hennock, "Urban Sanitary Reform a Generation Before Chadwick?" *Economic History Review*, 2d series, 10 (1957): 113–20; Spencer, *Municipal Origins*, 309; Buer, *Health, Wealth, and Population*, 86–87, 138; A. Sutcliffe, "Introduction: British Town Planning and the Historian," *British Town Planning: The Formative Years*, ed. A. Sutcliffe, 2–14 (Leicester: Leicester University Press, 1981); Gerry Kearns, "Cholera, Nuisances, and Environmental Management in Islington, 1830–1855," *Living and Dying in London*, eds. W. F. Bynum and Roy Porter, 94–125 (London: Wellcome Institute for the History of Medicine, 1991). The Webbs, however, write that "right down to the cholera epidemic of 1831–1832 we find practically no suggestion that any work of town improvement should be undertaken on the ground that it would promote the public health" (*Statutory Authorities*, 274). Prest, focusing on the continuation of adoptive and private bill legislation in the nineteenth century, is strongest in condemnation of the marginalization of this activity in most histories of public health: "In the twentieth century . . . biographers [of Chadwick and John Simon], sympathizing with their subjects, have been tempted to write as though the local Acts passed in the late eighteenth and early nineteenth centuries were worse than useless, that progress was made under the Public Health Act of 1848 (though less than there would have been had the Act been still more rigorous), and that the passage of the Local Government Act in 1858 was a retrograde step." "The overall picture presented in this study is almost exactly the opposite" (Prest, *Liberty and Locality*, 166–67).

claves, and the whole bray of beadledom."[49] Bad government was readily interchangeable with bad sanitation; after all, in a rational polity someone had to be responsible for everything. Thus, the air was thick with assertions and denials. Was Lincoln, or Stafford, or Exeter really the cleanest town in England or the acme of filth and irresponsibility?[50] Often there was little agreement even on the facts, much less on responsibility.

Probably the most sober appraisal of the capacities of local authorities is that of the Health of Towns commissioners. Evaluating local government was not an explicit part of their mission and they did not share a common view. They were relatively open minded on the question, however, and most of them visited several towns. We find four kinds of responses from them.[51] The first was that at least some local governments did a good job. In Chorlton-upon-Medlock, P. H. Holland reported considerable paving and cleaning under the police act. Reverend Coulthart told of the coordinated administration of Ashton-under-Lyne by police commission and court leet. Meeting twice yearly, the court indicated where privies, drains, and street repairs were needed, while the police commission supplied it with information and enforced its dictates. Reid found that the Newcastle-on-Tyne corporation had built more sewers in the past eight years than in the previous fifty. The Woolwich and Salisbury commissions were active but overwhelmed with mundane matters like road maintenance, Denison reported.[52] Holland, Reid, and Denison agreed that with more powers – such as powers for enforcing connection with sewers or for debt financing – there might be even more activity, but basically they were pleased with what they saw.[53]

49 The Reverend J. B. Owen, "Homes for the People," *Journal of Public Health and Monthly Record of Sanitary Improvement* 1 (1847): 28.

50 To adjudicate this question retrospectively is nearly impossible: One would need to know whether the descriptions of unremoved filth or corrupt government are accurate, are typical, and violated contemporary standards. In fact, most historians have been more impressed with the obtaining of the acts than with their use. Often only a tiny fraction of the commission attended meetings. Either loopholes inhibited action or the commissioners saw improvement as a one-time matter and failed to keep up with the needs of growing towns. Sometimes they failed to supervise those they entrusted with the watching, or lighting, or scavenging of streets (Webb and Webb, *Statutory Authorities*, 248–51; Finer, *Chadwick*, 213–15).

51 I also include the authors of invited local reports. The generalizations do not apply to their assessments of highly politicized authorities such as the City of London Corporation or the commissions of sewers.

52 P. H. Holland, "Chorlton-upon-Medlock," HOT, *First Report*, Appendix, 59–60, 69; the Reverend J. R. Coulthart, "Ashton-under-Lyne," ibid., 70–72; Reid, "Report on the Sanitary Condition of Newcastle, Gateshead, North Shields, Sunderland, Durham, and Carlisle," HOT, *Second Report*, Appendix, pt. 2, 157–59; W. T. Denison, "Report on the Sanatory Condition of the Town of Woolwich (also Salisbury)," ibid., 232, 235, 240.

53 Where things seemed to be working, that was not always the local authority's doing. In Huddersfield and Birkenhead and Ashton-under-Lyne large landowners tended to ensure orderly development and a reasonable level of services, unlike in places like Halifax, where most of the housing was being put up by small builders and speculators (James Smith, "Report on the Sanatory Condition of York, Kingston-upon-Hull, Huddersfield, Leeds, Bradford, and Sheffield," HOT, *Second Report*, Appendix, pt. 2, 317; Coulthart, "Ashton-under-Lyne," 70).

The second view was that limited powers, incompetence, and antiquated procedure overwhelmed good intentions; attend to these, and local government would provide adequate services. Courts leet, for example, the ancient manorial institution for identifying nuisances, often seemed oblivious to their sanitary responsibilities, perhaps because their findings were often ignored. Even where local acts required the provision of certain services, there were no enforcement mechanisms. Greater borrowing power was immensely important: it was impossible to build systems of sanitary works without long mortgages. So was expertise, if good laws and adequate borrowing capacity were not to be just an invitation to jobbery.[54]

The third view was that even when the members and officers of local authorities were honest men committed to sanitary reform (as they often were), and even when they had funds, powers, and expertise, local government was nonetheless inherently unsuited to comprehensive sanitation. For example, if sanitary districts were to coincide with drainage basins as Chadwick and the Health of Towns Commission recommended, existing local authorities were useless. But even if that were not done, some felt that local government was too much subject to short-term interests. Hawksley thought it so full of "mischievous diversion" and "petty hostility" that any increase in local powers would require a corresponding expansion of central oversight. Local government lacked the "sustained attention" sanitary projects demanded, Smith felt. Having heard the Leeds Town Council debate sewerage, he decided that despite its strong local act it was not up to the task. It needed reliable officers, more distance from the "popular clamour," and expert supervision, both to prod it and to restrain it.[55] Where party politics dominated, sanitary works might fall hostage, as with the Hull waterworks.[56] In Smith's view "general supervision of the public economy of large towns" was essential. It would allow comparison of "the cost and results of one town with those of another, thereby leading to a knowledge of the best system."[57] Finally, a few were unabashed centralizers, admiring the order of France.[58]

With the railway boom on top of a steady stream of municipal improvements, Parliament was overwhelmed with local and private legislation by the mid-1840s. Partly to lighten its own work, it began in 1845 to pass "clauses" acts, first for railroads and then in 1847 for gasworks, harbors, waterworks, fairs and markets, cemeteries, police, and, most importantly, a Towns Im-

54  Thomas Hawksley, "Nottingham," HOT, *First Report,* Appendix, 132, 136; Samuel Holme, "Liverpool," ibid., 194. In general see HOT, *Second Report,* 32–34, 42–43.
55  James Smith, "York, Kingston-upon-Hull, etc," HOT, *Second Report,* Appendix, pt. 2, 313.
56  HOT, *First Report,* Evidence, qq 5480–88 (Hawksley); 6129 (John Dean); James Smith, "General Observations on the Present Condition of Large Towns and the Comfort of the Inhabitants, and the Means of Improvement," HOT, *Second Report,* Appendix, pt. 2, 319, 321.
57  James Smith, "General Observations," HOT, *Second Report,* Appendix, pt. 2, 319.
58  W. H. Duncan, "On the Physical Causes of the High Rate of Mortality in Liverpool," HOT, *First Report,* Appendix, 32.

provement Clauses Act and a Public Commissions Act. These were collections of model clauses adapted from prior local acts that towns or companies could use in their bills. Their use would ease its work by focusing Parliament's scrutiny on those parts of a bill that were novel. For the bills' promoters, the result was cheaper, surer, loophole-free legislation. Using standard clauses did not guarantee passage, but they did represent what Parliament deemed appropriate powers for local authorities to possess.[59]

In addition, in 1846 the Whigs, following a Tory initiative, revised private bill procedure to include expert assessment of a proposed project. It had been recognized that the adversarial format of the select committee was unsatisfactory for adjudicating disputes between promoters and opponents or for judging the viability and prudence of a plan. Thus there was to be an inspection stage. Consulting engineers appointed by the Office of Woods and Forests would report to Parliament on the project for which a bill was sought.[60] The same session of 1846 also produced the first Nuisances Removal and Diseases Prevention Act. Passed in expectation of the return of cholera, this allowed a local authority to take action against "nuisances" on the statement of two "duly qualified medical practitioners" that these were harmful to health.

The clauses acts and the procedural revisions passed without controversy, but their most enthusiastic champions were radicals and Benthamites, including Edwin Chadwick: they reflected the radical concerns of accountability and cheapness, the Benthamite concerns for standardization and optimization.[61] Together, they and the Nuisances Removal Act would seem to accomplish most of what the 1848 Public Health Act would attempt.

These perspectives and initiatives make clear that it was by no means obvious, even among Chadwick's followers, that local governments were incapable of meeting the sanitarians' challenge – depending on what one understood that to be. How local and central complemented one another was a topic of much discussion. Perhaps there was need for a medical establishment

---

59 Cf. 10 & 11 Victoria c. 14 (markets and fairs), c. 15 (gasworks), c. 16 (Bodies of Commissioners), c. 17 (waterworks), c. 27 (docks and harbors), c. 34 (towns improvement – paving, draining, cleansing, lighting), c. 65 (cemeteries), and c. 89 (police). There was also a lands clauses act of 1845 of procedures for compulsory purchase of land by public bodies. See also John Simon, *English Sanitary Institutions, Reviewed in Their Course of Development, and in Some of Their Political and Social Relations* (London: Cassell and Co., 1890), 202.

60 Frederick Clifford, *A History of Private Bill Legislation*, 2 vols. (1887; reprint, New York: Augustus M. Kelley, 1972), II, 890–96; *Select Committee on Private Bills, P.P.*, 1846, *12*, (556.), iii–vii. See also Henry Parris, *The Government and the Railways in the Nineteenth Century* (London: Routledge and Kegan Paul, 1965).

61 Lewis *(Chadwick*, 134–37) sees Chadwick's concerns with standardizing private bill legislation as arising out of his experience in the Towns Improvement Company. Standardization would neutralize special interests and do away with trading witnesses. The preliminary inquiries would give voice to those not heard in select committee hearings. See also Finer, *Chadwick* 294–95; Simon, *English Sanitary Institutions*, 202; Edward Gibson, "The Public Health Agitation in England, 1838–1848: A Newspaper and Parliamentary History" (Ph.D. diss., University of North Carolina, Chapel Hill, 1955), 278; *Select Committee on Private Bills*, qq 274–324.

or for access to experienced and trustworthy engineers, or legislative or financial advice. That might imply state growth, but not state control. Many champions of sanitation were members (or would-be members) of local governments and had no wish to become junior bureaucrats. Chadwick himself was ambivalent about a sanitary dictatorship, only becoming enthusiastic as it became clearer that he would hold the post.[62]

### III

Sanitation's third political identity was that of a massive state investment in a coordinated system of infrastructure. Here it was not a constituency that mattered, but precedent. Belying its reputation for minimal state intervention and in defiance of the dominant ethos of laissez faire, the British government had orchestrated a vast series of public works projects in the first third of the nineteenth century, mainly in the north and west of Scotland, and in Ireland, the former directed by Thomas Telford, the latter mainly by Richard Griffith of the Irish Board of Works. In large part revolution-in-government historians have ignored this activity, partly because, however massive, it was undertaken relatively quietly and not as a manifestation of any philosophy of government growth, and partly because it did not have a permanent bureaucratic presence. Nonetheless, though hardly a philosophical radical, Telford was quietly practicing the scientific public administration of the Benthamites.

Initially the concern had been military: the vision of French fleets in remote Hibernian or Caledonian anchorages underwrote attempts to settle northwest Scotland and the building of a ship canal across the Great Glen. After the war, projects were undertaken in the hope that development might mitigate famine and economic dislocation. Ireland suffered periodic famines; in Scotland a demographic crisis followed collapse of the kelp industry and conversion of the Highlands from crofting to sheep raising.

In 1801, thanks to the patronage of the fabulously wealthy Tory politician Sir William Pulteney (on whose mansion he had worked as a mason), Thomas Telford, the Shropshire county surveyor, had been invited to plan development of the Highlands. Two years later he was authorized to build the Caledonian Canal and to undertake road, bridge, harbor, and even town building throughout the region. During his Scottish career Telford would produce roughly one thousand bridges, twelve hundred miles of road, forty-three harbors, and numerous churches and manses, advancing the development of Scotland by a century, he boasted.[63] In 1810 he was commissioned to build a fast

62 Cf. Chadwick to Buccleuch, early December and 17 December 1844, UCL Chadwick Papers #2181/6; Chadwick to Morpeth, 30 December 1846, 31 May 1848, UCL Chadwick Papers #1055.

63 J. B. Lawson, "Thomas Telford in Shrewsbury: The Metamorphosis of an Architect into a Civil Engineer," *Thomas Telford, Engineer*, ed. A. Penfold, 1–22 (London: Thomas Telford, 1980); A. R. G. Griffiths, *The Irish Board of Works, 1831–1878* (New York: Garland, 1987), 9; Sir Alexander

coach road from London to Holyhead, a project that required a series of new roads in North Wales, a bridge across the Menai Straits, and consolidation of existing turnpikes.[64] In 1817 he was appointed technical adviser to the Exchequer Bill Loan Commissioners (otherwise known as the Commissioners for Giving Employment to the Poor), which in succeeding years financed public works, mainly canals, to the extent of one and three quarter million pounds. In 1832 he was a one-man royal commission considering alternative water supplies for London.[65]

Thus for three decades Telford was chief engineer of a huge public works program that was never acknowledged as a public *policy*. All this time he was ostensibly in private practice and took other commissions, yet these too were often from public bodies – the kingdom of Sweden, the city of Edinburgh – seeking to foster commerce or health. That all this was incompatible with prevailing notions of government was sometimes noted but quickly passed over. Telford downplayed any political philosophy, presenting himself as a practical problem solver. His work was "improvement" – what towns were doing through private acts was what the state was doing in the wilds of Scotland, Ireland, and Wales. There could be no markets without transportation.[66] But the approach could equally be seen as colonial development: Charles Shaw, private secretary to the Irish lord lieutenant from 1821 to 1828, used the precedent of India to urge appointment of an inspector to superintend public works projects.[67]

What Chadwick hoped for in 1848 was to bring to the sewers, waterworks, and streets of English towns the scientific engineering Telford had brought to Scotland. Telford died in 1834, leaving no successor as unofficial public engineer; indeed, most engineers were leaving public business for the new railway frenzy. In many ways that heir was Chadwick. Telford had ruled the sort of empire Chadwick dreamed of. When, in the *Sanitary Report*, he railed against tiny and amateur units of government or urged the consolidation of

Gibb, *The Story of Telford: The Rise of Civil Engineering* (London: Maclehose, 1935), 60–87, 111; A. D. Cameron, *The Caledonian Canal* (Lavenham, Suffolk: Terence Dalton, 1972); Jean Lindsay, *The Canals of Scotland* (Newton Abbot: David and Charles, 1968), 142–77.

64 Gibb, *Telford*, 137; Barrie Trinder, "The Holyhead Road: An Engineering Project in Its Social Context," in Penfold, *Thomas Telford, Engineer*, 41–62.

65 Gibb, *Telford*, 163, 285.

66 It sounds like mercantilism: "The transportation of raw materials and manufactured goods, and, what is more important, of fuel and manure for agricultural purposes, and the circulating of its produce with facility and cheapness, if so limited, or rather rendered unpracticable on a large scale, would infallibly and speedily lessen the prosperity of the state" (Gibb, *Telford*, 146–47). Cf. Griffiths, *Irish Board of Works*, 9–15. One could appeal to Adam Smith himself for support for this view (see Sir Henry Parnell, *A Treatise on Roads; Wherein the Principles on Which Roads Should Be Made Are Explained and Illustrated by the Plans, Specifications, and Contracts Made Use of by Thomas Telford, Esq. on the Holyhead Road* [London: Longman, Rees, Orme, Brown, Green, and Longman, 1833], 1–4).

67 Griffiths, *Irish Board of Works*, 13–14. On Ireland as a laboratory for administrative experimentation, see MacDonagh, *Early Victorian Government*, 181–86.

power in the hands of a few truly scientific regional engineers, it was Telford he was echoing more than his mentor Bentham. How much better, Telford and Chadwick agreed, to invest substantial capital and hire a few scientifically trained road engineers to build a truly "permanent way" than to leave the matter to the parishes, which needed constantly to be cajoled into hiring ignorant labor to repair incompetently roads poorly designed to begin with. In building the Holyhead road, Telford had confronted and vanquished that wasteful amateurism, winning the turnpike trusts over to the side of science and coordination.[68] Both championed uniform practice based in experiment. For Telford, all was order: at every niche in his vast empire responsibilities and procedures were clearly specified. He revolutionized relations between engineers and contractors and methods of materials accounting. Like Bentham, he looked for "collateral" benefits: not only would smooth pavements shorten travel times, but "as roads are level and hard, there will be a saving of horse labour; fewer horses will be required; they will last longer, and a cheaper description of horse may be employed; less food will be consumed, and fewer servants will be wanted."[69]

In the mid-1840s then, public health had three identities: moral reform, with its joint concern for lowering poor rates and for disciplining the revolutionary poor; municipal improvement, with its vision of a middle-class space in which water closets smoothly flushed all cares away; and Telford's quiet revolution of centralized, scientific public works. They did not readily coexist. Telfordianism and moral reform implied central coordination and sweeping change, while municipal improvement was driven by a town's unique needs and privileged the status quo. The Telfordian engineer or the municipal improver could trust to the laws of physics; the moral reformer had to plumb the mysteries of "character." Cutting relief costs was central to moral reform; large expenditure characterized municipal improvement and Telfordianism. Improvement and moral reform tended to reify local class relations, matters to which the Telfordian engineer with his economies of scale was oblivious. For the next several years conflict in public health would reflect these tensions.[70]

## IV

We can look now at the passage of the Public Health Act of 1848. Historians have seen that act as a key step in the growth of the central state, even as part of the triumph of collectivism over individualism. In fact it was a relatively

68  Webb and Webb, *Statutory Authorities*, 135–65, 186–89, 209; MacDonagh, *Early Victorian Government*, 128; Keith-Lucas, *Unreformed Local Government*, 127.
69  Parnell, *A Treatise on Roads,* 1–4. Chadwick would use this example in the *Sanitary Report.*
70  Cf. E. P. Hennock, "Central/Local Government Relations in England, an Outline," *Urban History Yearbook* (1982): 38–47.

modest piece of legislation, giving to towns the powers needed to undertake sanitary improvements, and setting up the General Board of Health to facilitate and to supervise (loosely) those improvements. I will suggest here that while centralization (by which speakers usually meant something akin to French public administration) was the bogeyman in the debate, the issue was not so much state power as accountability in its exercise. Whether the act represented a collectivist move, on the other hand, will depend on what (or who) one takes the collective to be and how one feels about Chadwick as its embodiment. If one sees accountability as part of collectivism, it is possible to see the act as a (small) step away from collectivism and toward autocracy.

Public health bills focusing on sanitary improvement were introduced in 1841 by the Whig home secretary Lord Normanby, in 1845 and 1846 by the Tories (by Lord Lincoln, chief commissioner of woods and forests), and in 1847 and 1848 by the Whigs (by Lord Morpeth, Lincoln's successor). As a matter of state public health was uncontroversial – and uninteresting. The great orators did not speak; debate descended quickly into niggling minutiae. The problem was not so much winning support for a law as finding clauses that would not waste vast amounts of parliamentary time.[71] Sanitation was not a party matter; there was no obvious model to be lauded or condemned. Tory and Whig cabinets drew on different precedents but debate was unusually open, with the managers of bills willing to consider significant changes if they would facilitate passage.

The first attempt at general sanitary legislation were Lord Normanby's 1841 bills. Most who spoke on them favored them: much needed, they agreed – should be even stronger; essential to any advance in "social comfort," "moral condition," "religious improvement" (disease prevention was peripheral).[72] But not in their towns, they also insisted, which already had sanitary improvement well in hand. Such a case was made for Oxford, Cambridge, Birmingham, Bolton, Derby. Most brazen was the marquis of Salisbury's amendment protecting the Edinburgh sewage irrigators.[73] The bills trod on too many interests. They were abandoned and the government soon fell.

In 1845–48 there was again broad agreement that government must be a guarantor of health.[74] The great issue was how to enforce that guarantee. The approaches of Lord Lincoln and his Whig successor Lord Morpeth may appear to differ only in details of implementation, but at the time they seemed to imply different notions, both of government and of the nature of the sanitary problem. Using the model of prison administration, Lincoln proposed that

71 "The Sanitary Question," *Fraser's Magazine* 36 (1847): 367; Lewis, *Chadwick*, 349.
72 *Hansard's Parliamentary Debates* 3rd series, 56, 1841, 138, 536–37.
73 "Borough Improvements Bill," ibid., 57, 1841, 1293, 1451; "Drainage of Towns," ibid., 56, 1841, 541; 57, 1841, 1018–20, 1290, 1292, 1447–51.
74 On the passage of the public health bill see Finer, *Chadwick*, 322–24; for exemption claims see *Hansard's Parliamentary Debates* 3rd series, 98, 1848, 802.

local authorities would build and manage sanitary works but be held account-able to the Home Office and expected to follow plans issued by that office. Morpeth thought the Home Office was already too busy and envisioned an independent board with its own inspectors, who would supervise the sanitary efforts of existing municipal corporations. In equipping corporations with a vast range of powers, the act would complete the rationalization that the Municipal Corporations Act of 1835 had begun.[75]

This issue of the local unit of sanitary administration was the source of much acrimony. Taking the view that topography must dictate the boundaries of an entity concerned with drainage, Lincoln saw need for a new local au-thority exclusively concerned with sanitation. Morpeth, who considered san-itation inherent to municipal government, would assign it to the newly reformed municipal councils (or to a board of appointed and elected members in noncorporate towns). Where drainage was problematic, suburban or rural areas might be placed under municipal control for drainage purposes only. Neither solution seemed particularly attractive and much of the complaint about "centralization" arose in connection with them. Centralization in public health had little in common with centralization in education and policing, where civil or religious liberty was at stake.[76] Doubtful that they would get fair treatment from municipal corporations, suburban and rural interests saw themselves being sacrificed by some sanitary star chamber to the territorial lusts of nearby towns. Defenders of improvement commissions, especially in towns that also had municipal corporations, resented that these creations of the people were to be superseded regardless of how well they had performed. (Morpeth could say only that the reformed corporations were more demo-cratic than most improvement commissions.)[77] Thus the objection was less to state rule than to Parliament's abandonment of its children: Morpeth would leave them in the clutches of their neighbors or rivals.[78]

The disparity between the goal of sanitation – improving the nation's health – and the main means to that end – having local authorities build sanitary works – led to a widely shared view that this was to be punitive legislation. Morpeth's protest that the government was giving away vast powers otherwise

75 *Hansard's Parliamentary Debates 3rd series, 91,* 1847, 624–31, 639–40. Morpeth maintained that the 1848 bill could as well be called a bill "for consolidating, strengthening, and making more effectual the functions of local bodies in the various municipal towns of England and Wales," ibid., *98,* 1848, 738. Chadwick similarly would wish the General Board of Health had been called the "General Board of Works and Health" to designate its concern for physical causes and to help dissipate the concerns of the medical profession (Lewis, *Chadwick,* 175, 193).

76 *Hansard's Parliamentary Debates 3rd series, 91,* 1847, 623; *93,* 1847, 1101; *98,* 1848, 713–15, 797; "The Sanitary Question," *Fraser's Magazine 36* (1847): 371; Roberts, *Victorian Origins,* 68–70; Stan-ley H. Palmer, *Police and Protest in England and Ireland* (Cambridge: Cambridge University Press, 1988), 423–26; Finer, *Chadwick,* 176; Gibson, "The Public Health Agitation," 295.

77 *Hansard's Parliamentary Debates 3rd series, 93,* 1847, 729–30; *98,* 1848, 730–38.

78 Had Morpeth empowered the improvement commissions he might well have heard similar ob-jections from the municipal corporations.

obtainable only through expensive local acts was in vain. The highhanded elimination of institutions that towns had built for themselves, coupled with the gale of vilification issuing from Chadwick and the Health of Towns Association, suggested pretty plainly that towns were failures. It followed that the thrust of the legislation must be to enforce, not to facilitate. Morpeth's unwillingness to include London in the 1848 bill on the grounds that its sanitary affairs were too complicated didn't help: if sanitation were such a "boon," asked Lord George Bentinck, how could it be withheld from London? "The only reason could be that the noble Lord [Morpeth] did not believe one iota. . . ."[79]

Underlying these concerns was the accountability question. The proposed elimination or rearrangement of local government was to be in the hands of a General Board of Health, whose decisions were not subject to Parliament. It was modeled on the hated Poor Law Commission, which had recently been dissolved as a result of a scandal over accountability. Its successor, the new Poor Law Board, would be run by a minister answerable to Parliament.[80] Many opponents claimed to favor a powerful central agency that would inspect, plan, enforce environmental standards, and mandate infrastructural improvement, but only so long as those powers were vested in an accountable and/or constitutional entity: Home Office, magistracy, or common law.[81]

Historians have tended to discount such views as so much easy talk. Yet David Roberts notes that those "opposed to the growth of a bureaucratic and meddling government . . . were in no way shy about calling for an authoritarian one." For them "centralization" implied French-style technocrats; central power, so long as it was in the hands of the people's representatives, was not centralization.[82] What worried them was not a government that would act forcefully against disease but the immoderate administration of an independent Chadwick. We need also remember that "accountability" and "constitution" were animating political passions. For Cobbettian radicals, who saw a government of sinecures and patronage, accountability was the basis of their demand for democracy. Tory followers of Blackstone and Burke, on the other hand, believed that traditional institutions embodied the just balance of free-

---

79 *Hansard's Parliamentary Debates 3rd series, 93,* 1847, 1108–10; *98,* 1848, 717–20, 735, 738–39, 764, 768. Russell saw "the essential object of the Bill . . . [as] giving local bodies the power of making sanitary laws" (ibid., 799). On costs of local acts see Spencer, *Municipal Origins,* 79.

80 *Hansard's Parliamentary Debates 3rd series, 91,* 1847, 638; *93,* 1847, 1104–6, 1189–90; *98,* 1848, 764; Lewis, *Chadwick,* 167.

81 *Hansard's Parliamentary Debates 3rd series, 93,* 1847, 1095, *98,* 1848, 713–14, 722–23, 725, 727–30, 764, 798, 1175. Chadwick's preference, the Privy Council, which already served as cholera and quarantine authority, was not satisfactory because it was an extraparliamentary body (Finer, *Chadwick,* 304). Lincoln's bill seemed less problematic in this regard (Gibson, "The Public Health Agitation," 188, 202–5, 208).

82 Roberts, *Paternalism,* 40, 44, 71. Both the most enthusiastic proponents and the most vehement opponents are found among Roberts's paternalist writers (*Paternalism,* 198–200, 215, 219, 224, 232–33, 241).

dom and obligation. They saw no place for an independent Board of Health. Chadwick, by contrast, saw "accountability" as a guise for interference and obstruction. As PLC secretary he had been preoccupied with protecting scientific administration from such political "accountability."

But Parliament simply would not have an independent Chadwick with power. In meeting such criticism, Morpeth elected to protect Chadwick's independence, but at the cost of sacrificing most of his power (and a good deal of his independence too, as it turned out).[83] The resulting Public Health Act was weak, even incoherent. Lord Lincoln, Morpeth's Tory predecessor, was shocked: all that had been achieved with regard to prisons, factories, and schools; the whole tradition of "supervision by central authority, in the way of local inspection," had been bargained away.[84] Judged simply as legislation, it was not clearly an advance over the acts of 1846 and 1847. The Towns Clauses Act offered more powers to local governments; the Preliminary Inquiries Act provided for inspection and technical advising; and the Diseases Prevention Act had powers for summary action against disease-causing nuisances.[85] It is true that all of these depended on local initiative, and that this was beyond many, and maybe most, localities, but practically speaking, the same was true with the Public Health Act. As it began to be clear what would come of Morpeth's compromising, some, like Lord Lincoln, suggested that as a beginning towns simply be allowed to adopt the entire Towns Clauses Act.[86]

Why, then, was a General Board of Health so necessary? One answer is that it was necessary in order to give jobs to Chadwick and a few doctors and engineers: another Whig scheme to "feed and fatten men who were poor and lean."[87] Certainly Chadwick had a claim on Whig patronage, but other

83 Where Morpeth had proposed the endorsement of board policies through orders of council, the act utilized the provisional order mechanism, in which a great many of the board's decisions required a confirming act of Parliament (*Hansard's Parliamentary Debates 3rd series, 98,* 1848, 874–75). See also Lewis, *Chadwick,* 160–63. In trying to save the General Board of Health [GBH] in 1854 the Whigs would argue that the Home Office was the obvious place for it (*Hansard's Parliamentary Debates 3rd series, 134,* 1854, 1297–98).

84 *Hansard's Parliamentary Debates 3rd series, 99,* 1848, 689–90. The engineering press concurred: "In the actual administration of the Act, little or nothing is assigned to the Central Board. The power is almost entirely in the hands of the Local Boards. . . . And as the Local Boards are popularly selected, the power of putting the act into force ultimately belongs to the great body of inhabitants of the districts affected. There seems therefore, little reason to fear that people will be compelled to be clean, and drink wholesome water, and breathe fresh air, against their own free will and consent" ("Sanitary Laws at Home and Abroad," *Civil Engineer and Architects Journal 11* [1848]: 252–54).

85 Olien, *Morpeth,* 302, 309–10; Lewis, *Chadwick,* 138, 309.

86 *Hansard's Parliamentary Debates 3rd series, 93,* 1847, 743–46, 1103, 1108, 1189; *94,* 1847, 26–29. The 1847 bill actually included the entire Commissioners Clauses Act; see Prest, *Liberty and Locality,* 167–68. In effect, something like that happened: not only was the 1848 Act mainly permissive, its successor, the Local Government Act of 1858, let towns adopt portions of public health legislation piecemeal. Cf. MacDonagh, *Early Victorian Government,* 144.

87 *Hansard's Parliamentary Debates 3rd series, 93,* 1847, 727–28, 1100–1101, 1284; *98,* 1848, 710–11, 723, 725, 738–39, 797, 1173; Roberts, *Paternalism,* 264; Lewis, *Chadwick,* 162.

factors were at work. First, however much they had become entangled, the sanitary initiative had sprung from different roots and addressed different concerns than urban improvement. Chadwick had tackled the grand condition-of-England question, while the clauses acts simply rationalized procedure in a mundane area of administration. It is true that the switch from "labouring classes" to towns had gained Chadwick a large constituency of middle-class improvers, and equally that when linked to public health, mundane matters of rubbish removal and pothole filling suddenly became part of a glorious sanitary crusade. But if the condition-of-England problem was to be solved, and if Chadwick was to be the one to solve it, that would not happen through towns' haphazardly discovering the delights of domestic technologies.

Given the indifference to sanitary matters of Parliament and the public there was indeed danger that the sanitary fervor would dissipate and the promised public health act never appear.[88] Accordingly, there was need to magnify the vast gap between what local governments did and what public health demanded. That gap became increasingly visible in Chadwick's evolving technological vision. By 1847 the sanitary systems needed to transform society were increasingly unlike the sorts of projects local governments typically undertook on their own. In the *Sanitary Report* his emphasis had been that water and drains be available. Surface water had seemed as significant as sewer gas. Now Chadwick was pushing for "combined works." In an ideal sewer there would be no deposits and hence no deadly sewer gas. Ideal sewers were parts of coordinated water-sewage networks in which uniform flow was constantly maintained. Such a system could only work if the sewer authority controlled the water supply and if every dwelling had its water closet draining into the public sewer.[89]

The difference between typical urban improvement and true public health was the subject of a Health of Towns Association "survey" of sanitary achievements in sixty-nine towns done at the end of 1847. Ostensibly this would update the Health of Towns Commission, yet yards of sewer laid was not the main concern. Instead, towns were to be judged in terms of "correct principles" in circulation for several years (which in fact kept changing). Thus questions dealt with whether the authorities had undertaken combined works – water, house drainage, and sewerage; whether they had spontaneously rec-

---

88 On indifference see Gibson, "The Public Health Agitation," 82–83; "The Sanitary Question," *Fraser's Magazine 36* (1847): 367.

89 HOT, *Second Report*, 7. Cf. a report from William Lee, later one of Chadwick's inspectors, on Sheffield: "The sewerage, though much has been done during the last few years, is illegitimate. All these must be harmoniously worked together as parts of the same system; and we are truly convinced that this can only be done by placing them and all other sanitary arrangements under the control of one public body" (quoted by Lord Morpeth, in *Hansard's Parliamentary Debates 3rd series, 96,* 1848, 401).

ognized the need for them; and whether there were competent and trustworthy persons and institutions to undertake them.

The answers, from members or friends of the association, were overwhelmingly negative. Whatever towns were doing, it was not Chadwick-style sanitation. Several said that their towns were awaiting the guiding or coercive hand of a central authority. Most towns that had tried comprehensive sanitation (often inspired by visits of Health of Towns commissioners) foolishly found themselves deficient in power and capital. And even if they had powers and funds, like Birmingham, Leeds, and the City of London, they hadn't the skill, as was clear from the absurd and costly sewers they had built. Morpeth's bill, by contrast, would meet the needs of the powerless poor, satisfy ratepayers that their money was well spent, and ensure application of the necessary skill to sanitary works. In this view, centralization was more accountable than local democracy.[90] Morpeth quoted the survey in introducing his public health bill in February 1848. It was not a good idea. Anonymous attacks on local authorities simply confirmed the belief that this was punitive legislation.[91]

The threatened capture of the sanitary movement by urban improvement made it necessary to reiterate the principle of sanitary universality. Building fine sewers and waterworks was not enough; sanitation "proclaims a universal equality in the enjoyment of air, light, and water." Its object was "a sewer in every street of every town and village; a drain for every house; a constant and unlimited supply of good water to every family; pure air at any cost." The benevolent regimen of a disciplining network would eliminate social differences, while the costly partial works of the urban improvers only opened up one more domain in which the wealthy could distance themselves from the poor. As an opponent complained, the bill would "pass a roller over England, destroying any vestige of local preeminence, and reducing all to one dull and level monotony."[92]

In this principle of sanitary universality, Chadwick was proposing a new human right. Here, in a culture pervaded by class distinctions, a whole department of life was being withdrawn from the realm of inequality; all would henceforth sit on the same throne. While it may seem only humane, it was

90 Health of Towns Association, *Report of the Sub-Committee on the Answers Returned to Questions Addressed to the Principal Towns of England and Wales, and on the Objections from Corporate Bodies to the Public Health Bill* (London: Clowes, 1848), 3–12, 19, 22, 32–37, 40–46, 50–51, 56. Cf. Finer, *Chadwick*, 296; MacDonagh, *Early Victorian Government*, 122–26, 177. Simon, Chadwick's successor, thought Morpeth and Chadwick naive in this regard (John Simon, *English Sanitary Institutions*, 205–9, 222–23).

91 *Hansard's Parliamentary Debates 3rd series, 96*, 1848, 395; *98*, 1848, 715, 738, 788–94, 872.

92 Ibid., *98*, 1848, 713; "The Sanitary Commission, and the Health of the Metropolis," *Fraser's Magazine 36* (1847): 517. The radical Joseph Hume noted that "the object . . . was to bring such advantages within the reach of those who were not, under the present system, able to pay for them" (he included water and gas under this head): *Hansard's Parliamentary Debates 3rd series, 91*, 1847, 644–45. Cf. Prest, *Liberty and Locality*, 178, who notes that much interest in local improvement was to "insulate" the middle class.

an audacious suggestion. Make the same argument in respect to food, work, longevity, education, access to medical care, or even health in general, and it would have been rejected out of hand. Other domestic technologies – gas, electricity, telephones – did not come about as rights.[93] To all who live in dwellings with water closets and indoor water, this "toilets for all" campaign will seem an obvious step in human progress, but in its own political culture, it seemed less an appeal for minimal standards of freedom and health than an admonition about political choice: "I insist that all of you invest in toilets because I cannot trust your own prioritizing."

It can be argued that this principle of sanitary universality is implicit in the civilizing mission of the *Sanitary Report*. Perhaps it was, but we should keep well away from the view that its prominence in 1847 reflected the unfolding of sanitary destiny or even the realization of the manifesto of 1842. In Chadwick's hands sanitarianism was a paradigm, a kit of rhetorical resources applicable to many political uses, not a system of normative axioms. Sanitary universality was useful in early 1848 to highlight the need for the General Board of Health as a sort of guarantor of satisfactory sanitation, even though the legislation being considered did not embody any premise of universal sanitation.

It is worth stressing this point to emphasize that there was no sanitary teleology: the state did not have to grow as it did, the fate of the General Board of Health was not a classic tragedy. On the contrary, the history of the first decade of the "sanitary idea" is one of opportunism. For most of the period Chadwick was riding out a political storm, seeking a holdfast on which to put down roots. Sanitarianism grew and adapted. It became more detailed and technical, and the viability of various technologies of water and sewerage looked quite different in 1848 than in 1838. The nature of the sanitary problem changed as did notions of practicable solutions. In early 1838 it was stagnant ponds. In 1842 it might have been enough to make sure that people had access to water and a way of getting rid of dung heaps and dirty ditches. By 1848 "combined works" were necessary. The focus had shifted with political circumstances and with Chadwick's own career, from revolution and pleasing Peel to urban improvement and speculative capitalism in the days of the Health of Towns Commission and the Towns Improvement Company, finally to state growth as Chadwick kicked free of the sinking Poor Law Commission

93 Daniel Boorstin calls it "environmental democracy" (*The Americans: The Democratic Experience* [New York: Vintage, 1974], 307, 346–58). Cf. J. P. Goubert, *The Conquest of Water*, introduction by Emmanuel LeRoy LaDurie, trans. by Andrew Wilson (London: Polity Press, 1989). This idea that the mass market items of nineteenth-century technology should be understood as democratization appears in many disparate authors, among them E. E. Slossen, "Chemistry in Everyday Life," *Science in Literature: A Collection of Literary Scientific Essays,* ed. F. H. Law (New York: Harper, 1929), 201–3; Samuel Florman, *The Existential Pleasures of Engineering* (New York: St. Martin's Press, 1976); Rosalind Williams, "The Cultural Origins and Environmental Implications of Large Technological Systems," *Science in Context 6* (1993): 377–403.

and bullied the Whigs into putting him in charge of a new public department. Had Normanby's bills passed in 1841, or Lincoln's in 1846, or even Morpeth's in 1847; or had the Towns Improvement Company won contracts, "public health" might easily have occupied a quite different niche. Chadwick, if involved at all, might have been something like the chief inspector under the Preliminary Inquiries Act, helping towns acquire powers and plan works – what Morpeth's secretary in the Office of Woods and Forests was doing in 1847.[94] Or he might have been a great capitalist, supplying water and utilizing sewage in the great towns of Europe.

But none of these happened. So we must move now to what did, the ways in which Chadwick and his associates wielded those resources of sanitarianism in running the General Board of Health.

94 Olien, *Morpeth*, 301–3.

# 9

## Selling Sanitation: The Inspectors and the Local Authorities, 1848–1854

In the late summer of 1848, the General Board of Health began its life. After years of misery in the Poor Law Commission, Edwin Chadwick finally had authority. For the moment cholera occupied his attention, but how the board would do its main job of facilitating sanitary improvement was less clear. He was preoccupied first with colleagues. One he knew well. Lord Morpeth (seventh earl of Carlisle after October 1848), as chief commissioner of woods and forests (a minor cabinet post), was the board's president. Together they had piloted public health through Parliament and planned consolidation of the Greater London sewers commissions. Morpeth chaired and Chadwick set policy for the new Metropolitan Sewers Commission, established in November 1847. A decade earlier Morpeth had been considered a likely prime minister, but his career had stalled. In the eyes of some the "disgrace" of failing to carry public health in 1847 killed hope of significant advancement.[1]

The other member of the board was Lord Ashley, heir of the earl of Shaftesbury, "Evangelical of the Evangelicals," unsurpassed in gravity and principle. Conscience kept Ashley out of Parliament; he could no longer uphold his constituents' protectionist views. He and Chadwick had often been opponents. Ashley had pushed a ten hours' bill despite Chadwick's factory commission; in 1844 he had sponsored a select committee that highlighted the "mutton medicine" that so insidiously undermined the workhouse test.[2] Quickly they were joined by Southwood Smith, brought in first under the Diseases Prevention Act to organize the response to cholera, kept on under an 1849 act on safe burial, the fruit of Chadwick's interments report.

Morpeth exemplified political fluidity: they would sometimes disagree when it came to dealing with "Parliaments and bodies of men," he warned Chadwick. Chadwick would have to trust his judgment of what was politically

---

1 Diana Olien, *Morpeth: A Victorian Public Career* (Washington, D.C.: University Press of America, 1983), 291, 294.
2 G.F.A. Best, *Shaftesbury* (New York: Arco, 1964), 67, 110–11. Morpeth and Ashley had been close friends at Oxford, but their relationship had cooled with Ashley's snub of Morpeth's attempt to pass a compromise on the ten hours' question (Olien, *Morpeth*, 26–27, 343).

possible. Ashley, like Chadwick, exemplified rigidity. "Right" and "wrong" were as unmistakable for him as "scientific" and "inefficient" were for Chadwick. These two tactless, humorless lovers of authority and bureaucracy got on splendidly. Even before Carlisle's departure in March 1850 (to take the backwater office of chancellor of the Duchy of Lancaster), the board was not a "happy few" working tirelessly together to conquer insanitary England.[3] Chadwick, though happy enough to have him as an uncompensated servant, took umbrage at Southwood Smith's pretensions to equal status, while even from the outset, Morpeth was looking for release (even if it meant the fall of the government) from this administrative "purgatory."[4]

To appreciate the problems Chadwick faced we need to look more closely at the act the board would administer. The 1848 Public Health Act was a monster, with the head of coercive medical police and the body of local self-government. Although the General Board had some powers to act in epidemics, its main duty was to promote municipal sanitation. It did so by setting up new units of local government, called local boards of health, with powers to undertake water supply, house drainage, sewerage, and sewage treatment, and to maintain roads and regulate new construction. These local boards were to be elected, the qualification for voting varying from place to place, and they could raise a rate. Though Morpeth had insisted that local boards had "imperative" functions of mapping, watering, and sewering, nothing in the act enforced that demand.[5] Most importantly, local boards could take on the long-term (thirty year) debt needed for systemic public works, rather than being forced to build bit by bit out of annual income. Such loans required approval of the General Board of Health (GBH), to be based on a report of one of its inspectors. Local boards had to employ a clerk as legal adviser, and a surveyor, a sort of combination chief executive, public works planner, and inspector. A board could employ a medical officer to advise on necessary improvements. GBH approval was required to dismiss a surveyor. What little

3 Morpeth to Chadwick, 4 September 1848, University College London [UCL] Chadwick Papers, #1055; J. L. Hammond and Barbara Hammond, *Lord Shaftesbury*, 3d ed. (London: Constable and Co., 1925), 163–64; R. A. Lewis, *Edwin Chadwick and the Public Health Movement, 1832–1854* (London: Longmans, Green, 1952), 158, 182.

4 In 1843 Chadwick had refused to recommend Smith as a Health of Towns commissioner; in 1848 he would block his appointment to the General Board of Health and would chastise Smith for allowing himself to be celebrated as the father of sanitation. Smith to Chadwick, 29 March 1843, Chadwick to Smith, undated July, 11 August 1848, UCL Chadwick Papers #1844; Chadwick to Morpeth, 1 June, 20 August 1848, UCL Chadwick Papers #1055; Health of Towns Association, *Abstract of the Proceedings of the Public Meeting Held at Exeter Hall, December 11, 1844* (London: Charles Knight, [1845]), 31; Finer, *The Life and Times of Sir Edwin Chadwick* (London: Methuen, 1952), 339; Lewis, *Chadwick*, 35, 184. On Morpeth, see Olien, *Morpeth*, 349–66; Morpeth to Chadwick, 4 September 1848, UCL Chadwick Papers #1055.

5 *Hansard's Parliamentary Debates 3rd series, 96*, 1848, 389–91, 399; General Board of Health [GBH], "Minutes of Information Collected with Reference to Works for the Removal of Soil Water or Drainage of Dwelling Houses and for the Sewerage and Cleansing of the Sites of Towns" [to be cited as GBH, "Minutes on House Drainage"], *Parliamentary Papers [P.P.]*, 1852, 19, [1535.], 144.

bound head to body – loan sanctions and the surveyor's appointment – was resented, and might as easily inhibit sanitation as facilitate it.

Towns did not automatically have local boards of health. Where annual mortality rates exceeded 23/1000, the GBH might establish one, but it did not use that power much.[6] Much more often it responded to local initiative in the form of a petition from at least a tenth of the ratepayers. On receiving a petition the GBH would dispatch a superintending inspector to tour the district and meet with interested parties. The inspector would circulate a draft report in the locality and having received and responded to comments, write a final report. The GBH would then decide whether a local board should be established and determine its boundaries, the qualifications of electors, and its relations with existing local government. This then would be confirmed either by an order in council (for places without improvement commissions or corporations) or by a confirmatory act of Parliament.

Establishing a local board of health did give a town significant advantages with minimal obligations. True, it sacrificed the freedom to discharge its surveyor and left its public works programs hostage to the GBH's inspectors, but it gained powers for improvement hitherto available only through an expensive private act, permission to take on long-term debt and sometimes to consolidate under a single authority functions previously divided among several. The package of powers ensured more uniform services than could be counted on from the jumble of clauses an improvement commission might possess.[7] The relationship between a home improvement contractor and a customer perhaps catches best the flavor of relations between town and board. You called it in (or at least a tenth of your ratepaying neighbors did) and were told how badly you needed double-glazing or vinyl siding and how little it would cost when all benefits were added in and when the project was amortized (with proper security) over a long span. The board could not make you buy, but in setting up a local board of health it could, in effect, establish an account and make it hard for you to go elsewhere.[8] But in most respects sanitary improvement under the General Board of Health would be indistinguishable from what towns were doing under private acts.[9]

6 When it did, it was only after an appeal from the existing local government (*Hansard's Parliamentary Debates 3rd series, 135*, 1854, 234–43).
7 David Roberts, *Victorian Origins of the British Welfare State* (Hamden, Conn.: Archon Books, 1969), 111–12, 117; Edward H. Gibson, "The Public Health Agitation in England, 1838–1848: A Newspaper and Parliamentary History" (Ph.D. diss., University of North Carolina, Chapel Hill, 1955), 286. Freedom to dismiss a surveyor was often seen as an inviolable privilege of local administration and sufficient reason to oppose a local board. The requirement was quietly dropped in the 1858 Local Government Act.
8 Inasmuch as the inspectors themselves were available as private practice engineers to carry out the works they recommended, the analogy is apt. Chadwick in fact has some claim to be considered the inventor of the concept of double glazing. See Chadwick to Peel, 18 March 1845; British Library, Peel Papers, Add. Mss. 40563 f 53.
9 Hammonds, *Lord Shaftesbury*, 159–61.

Unable to mandate the new sanitation, the board had to persuade. It appealed to two sometimes competing images. One, considered later, was expertise, embodied in its inspectors. The other was accountability. The general board was the ratepayer's friend and guarantor of good government. So-called local democracies were rarely very representative either of people or of property; besides, someone, in this case central government, had to look out for the interests of absentee landowners. Both the *Sanitary Report* and the Health of Towns reports presented much evidence of waste. Through local legislation small and sometimes arbitrary groups had acquired unlimited power to tax their neighbors with no check on how that money was spent. In its 1847 survey of towns the Health of Towns Association had asked whether local units of government could be trusted to carry out so costly and complicated a task as comprehensive sanitary improvement. "Certainly not," was the response. Ratepayers were right to oppose most sanitary improvement projects, Chadwick would often assert: they would just be costly failures. In Parliament Morpeth made much of the central board's power of audit. There was much talk of "uniform procedure" and "responsible control."[10]

Outrage at public expenditure, central and local, was a long-standing hallmark of radicalism. The problem of overzealous and often corrupt improvers was real enough. Plans, estimates, budgets, accounts, audits, solicitation of bids, and supervision of contractors were foreign to many local governments. Yet hand in hand with a caution and rigor that effectively raised the burden of proof a public works project had to meet, Chadwick and his colleagues had also to encourage risk taking. They were asking towns to embark on untried schemes of unprecedented magnitude, to subscribe a significant portion of their rates for the next three decades to something that might fail utterly.[11]

I

Chadwick's salesmen were the superintending inspectors, and the warrant for a local government that was simultaneously cautious and cheap and grand and transforming was science, the only institution that combined the sharp and honest gaze of the skeptic with the true vision of the mystic. Science would take the uncertainty out of massive investment. The rest of this chapter focuses on the inspectors and their "science": first on the role of inspection, then on

---

10 Health of Towns Association, *Report of the Sub-Committee on the Answers Returned to Questions Addressed to the Principal Towns of England and Wales, and on the Objections from Corporate Bodies to the Public Health Bill* (London: Clowes, 1848), 35, 51, 57; *Hansard's Parliamentary Debates 3rd series, 96*, 1848, 736–37. On the accounting ideal in such contexts see Theodore Porter, *Trust in Numbers: The Pursuit of Objectivity in Science and Public Life* (Princeton, N. J.: Princeton University Press, 1995).

11 "The Public Health Bill: Its Letter and Its Spirit," *Fraser's Magazine 38* (1848): 444.

the approaches of individual inspectors, and finally on their handling of issues of local government, sanitary technologies, disease, and class relations.

What sanitation most required in a town were courage and confidence. While they acted in the name of science, Chadwick's inspectors were confidence men, in the most positive sense we can summon for that term. In this they had much less in common with other government inspectors – of prisons, factories, or schools – in this age of state growth than they did with those other contemporary creators of confidence, the promoters of railroads. Like the new joint stock companies described by Richard Lambert, local governments were petrified by large decisions. "How could a group of timid tradesmen . . . be persuaded to agree to . . . bold annexations, leases, purchases, or extensions?" Only by "cajolings, promises, threats, and chicanery. . . . A loud voice, a blustering manner, a little jugglery with the figures." The inspectors, no less than the George Hudsons of the day, had to be capable of "mesmerizing . . . audiences, and inducing them to swallow down wholesale the golden schemes."[12]

In most writing on the growth of the state, it is assumed that the audience for inspection is central government. Inspectors observe and document, enforce, advise, even criticize. They supply the data with which a truly scientific public administration documents problems and allocates resources.[13] But the GBH inspector had nothing to enforce. With so much power remaining local, the inspectors' reports could not be the fodder of the government behemoth, for in public health there was no such beast. Thus, their activities were not focused inward on transforming government, but outward, toward potential clients, the towns. They had to be. The General Board might well be a

12 Richard S. Lambert, *The Railway King, 1800–1871: A Study of George Hudson and the Business Morals of His Time* (London: George Allen and Unwin, 1934), 23–27. Coleridge also compared the new joint stock companies to local democracies (David Roberts, *Paternalism in Early Victorian England* [New Brunswick, N.J.: Rutgers University Press, 1979], 39).

13 This perspective characterizes those who stress Bentham's influence and even more clearly those who see government growth as an iterative process of investigation, discovery of real problems, pragmatic regulation, discovery of a need for further regulation, and so forth, the well-known "revolution in government." For a recent summary see Roy MacLeod, "Introduction," *Government and Expertise: Specialists, Administrators, and Professionals, 1860–1919,* ed. R. M. MacLeod, 1–24 (Cambridge: Cambridge University Press, 1988). The principal anti-Chadwick tract of the mid-1850s condemned a process very like that described by Oliver MacDonagh: "A report follows, piling, mountains high, the distresses to be relieved, and the remedies – of which one is the creation of a new office, moulded to the exact dimensions of our philanthropic advocate; the office is, perhaps, temporary, but an ingenious mind, with the help of annual reports, soon contrives to make it permanent. In these reports the ignorance of anyone – except the philanthropical commissioner – is set forth at great length with many piquant anecdote illustrations. . . . And so, from year to year, the profitable game of commission-ship goes on." *Engineers and Officials: An Historical Sketch of the "Health of Towns Works" (Between 1838 and 1856) in London and the Provinces, with Biographical Notes on Lord Palmerston, the Earl of Shaftesbury, Lord Ebrington, Edwin Chadwick, F. O. Ward, John Thwaites* (London: Edward Stanford, 1856), 35–36. My own views are in "Muddling in Bumbledom: Local Governments and Large Sanitary Improvements: The Cases of Four British Towns, 1855–1885," *Victorian Studies* 32 (1988): 55–83.

stableful of experts eager to sewer and water every town in the land, but they were part-timers, in work only when towns petitioned the board to adopt the act or to approve a loan request.

They had a formidable task – to persuade towns not simply to establish local boards but to take up comprehensive improvement. Though cleanliness, airiness, and roominess were widely shared ideals, people were being asked to accept a vast increase in the realm of the public. Ideally, they would internalize these new standards so well that elected local boards would enforce them as rigorously as Chadwick would have. But towns had their own public health agendas, which conformed only partly to Chadwick's. Often they were more interested in visible works, like good streets, than in works underground. The inspector then had to show that Chadwick's public health met local concerns and went even further to solve critical problems they were barely aware of. Aside from his actual visit, the inspector's main means of persuasion was his official report.[14] While the reports were addressed to the GBH, its concerns were few: boundaries and property qualifications; some indication of sufficient support for a local board to function.[15] The reports were longer (some are over 200 pages; 30 is common) than needed to convey such information, and far more widely ranging. Even statements addressed to the General Board, like William Lee's on Over Darwen – "It has rarely been my duty to bring before . . . the Board such a series of painful facts" – are clearly intended for the town.[16] They tell the GBH little, but make clear how much the town has offended the inspector.

Even the wealth of description can be seen in this light – the page after page of squalid dwellings and foul privies on one badly paved street after another. This wealth of "fact" has been key to the view that sees empirical social science as generating government growth; through the reports hitherto unrecognized conditions acquire weight and demand attention. Yet the descriptions are better seen as reflections, comparisons, and judgments, as appeals for authority rather than examples of it. The way to promulgate standards was to invite the town to see itself in a mirror constituted by the objective gaze of a cosmopolitan outsider, the inspector. One was then to declare with the outsider, "Look at this *mess!*" "How *can* you *live* like *this?*"[17] The descriptions

---

14 A microfiche edition of 399 reports in the Department of Health and Social Services Library is available as *Urban and Rural Social Conditions in Industrial Britain. Local Reports to the General Board of Health, 1848–1857* (Harvester Microfilm, 1977). The common format of the reports is "Report to the General Board of Health on a Preliminary Inquiry into the Sewerage, Drainage, and Supply of Water and Sanitary Condition of the Inhabitants of the Town of . . . in the County of . . . by. . . ." As the titles have a common format, I have simply cited them by author, town name, and year.

15 See Clark, Bristol, 1850, 5, as one of the few who explicitly addresses his report primarily to the town. After Chadwick's fall in 1854 the reports became much shorter and more narrowly focused.

16 Lee, Over Darwen, 1850, 8.

17 Cf. Mary Douglas, "Environments at Risk," *Science in Context*, eds. Barry Barnes and David Edge (Cambridge, Mass.: MIT Press, 1979), 260–75.

are less "this is so" statements than invitations – "See yourself as I see you" or "See how much worse you are than you might be" – or even exhortations: "Shame on you!" The details were important; authority to dictate the sanitary condition of a town might be contested street by street.

It is also sometimes suggested that inspection stirred sanitary action because townsfolk, officially and individually, were ignorant of local sanitary conditions until inspectors enlightened them.[18] In a strong sense the claim strains credulity. Statements like William Ranger's appeal to the Halifax aldermen "to visit the accommodations of their poorer fellow-creatures" were a part of the struggle over whether Ranger or the town's leaders knew better what its sanitary condition was.[19] Even with the growing separation of the classes, many elements of sanitary condition – water supply, drains, muck in the streets, odors, facilities for relieving oneself, complexion and stature of the people – were truly public. Even if they did not see or smell or feel what inspectors saw, smelled, or felt, townspeople knew such conditions better than inspectors ever could. What they had not done, at least at the level of collectivities, was to designate normal conditions as problems. Yet the fiction of the discovered unknown was useful to both parties. For the inspectors the new facts were products to be harvested and shipped off to the mill of responsive government; for locals the pretense of shocked revelation permitted the excuse of ignorance – how much easier to say "I didn't know" than "I know and am responsible."[20]

Description was to imply action. "Discovery" talk bypassed the vexing matter of standard setting by implying that standards already existed; it bypassed priority setting by representing action as imperative.[21] This was all the trickier for it was impossible to describe conditions fully within decent vocabulary. Thus often we get not conditions but reactions. The inspectors make their own literary limitations the basis of their appeal: "Things here are so bad that my horror transcends description." Paroxysms of revulsion, like

---

18 This view is found both in modern secondary literature and in contemporary journalists' accounts. See Roberts, *Victorian Origins*, 225–26, 233; Arthur Helps, *The Claims of Labour: An Essay on the Duties of Employers to the Employed*, 2nd ed, *to Which Is Added, An Essay on the Means of Improving the Health and Increasing the Comfort of the Labouring Classes* (London: Pickering, 1845), 196. It is noteworthy, however, that inspectors often found a long record of local groups investigating the state of the urban environment and seeking to improve it.

19 Ranger, Halifax, 1851, 23–29, 82.

20 Novelty itself helped generate a response: The "discovery" need not even be communicable; in fact, the less it could be described, the more readily it could be represented as utterly awful, and absolutely impermissible. Thus a Bristol sanitary committee wrote: "To exaggerate the state of things is literally impossible; to depict it correctly, simply hopeless; and to invite any of their fellow citizens to witness it for themselves, uninfluenced by other motives than mere curiosity, your Committee feel would be exposing their philosophy to a most unwarrantable ordeal" (Clark, Bristol, 1850, 60).

21 Roberts, *Victorian Origins*, 106–7.

shouts of "crisis," undercut caution and heightened tolerance for the Chadwickians' quick fixes.

Far from being summaries of local fact, the inspectors' reports are one-sided conversations with a local audience not unlike the self-serving dialogues of classical philosophers. The inspectors quote things said to them, but their reports are not transcripts. They describe, but also react; they praise and condemn; cajole, promise, and threaten. Finding much wrong, they highlight only some of it and often assume that what they fix will itself solve other problems.[22] Having to take seriously the desires, fears, and political complexions of the different towns they visit, they often focus on different issues and use different arguments from one report to the next. Yet their reports are also in part diaries of experiences, and efforts to explain things to themselves in a way that would allow them to make a cogent case for how public health could make things better.

## II

A great range of motives led towns to seek the act. Sometimes disease, particularly cholera, was the main concern. But often adopting the act had little to do with public health in any sense. Many towns sought relief from a tangle of jurisdictions and procedures that had grown up over the centuries and that might make widely desired changes almost impossible. In Macclesfield, a board of health was the prize in a struggle between evenly matched rivals: the corporation and the police commission.[23] Some, like well governed Halifax or Leamington, would use the act to impose order on new suburbs. The social and environmental problems of outlying regions could not be prevented from crossing borders, and the act would also expand the rate base for improvement. Fashionable suburbs of the future or watering-places-to-be, like Layton with Walbrick in Lancashire (later part of Blackpool), saw in the act a way to coerce recalcitrant landowners to accept development and new environmental standards. Railroad interests were the prime movers of "public health" in the parishes near Lancaster that would become Morecombe.[24] Finally, some towns sought a board of health to solve a particular environmental problem – usually

---

22  Roberts rightly calls their reports "essays" on "social, moral, and physical" conditions and adds, "Scarcely ever was 'moral' omitted from the formula, and scarcely ever did it include 'economic.'" Roberts, *Victorian Origins*, 211–15.

23  Smith, Macclesfield, 1850, 4–5. See also Roberts, *Victorian Origins*, 281. The resistance of improvement commissions was also an issue in Durham, Cardiff, Dover, Bristol, and Great Yarmouth. For context, see Sidney Webb and Beatrice Webb, *English Local Government from the Revolution to the Municipal Corporations Act: Statutory Authorities for Special Purposes* (London: Longmans, Green, 1922), 346.

24  Lee, Poulton, Bare, and Torrisholme, 1851, 18; Rawlinson, Poulton-cum-Seacombe, Wirral, 1851, 6. On motives for adoption see E. C. Midwinter, *Social Administration in Lancashire, 1830–1860: Poor Law, Public Health, and Police* (Manchester: Manchester University Press, 1969), 79–86.

water supply. In many places the old question of the character of the poor remained central. Whatever the problem, it was for the inspectors to show how the public health of Chadwick could be the solution.

Their reports are hardly the work of faceless bureaucrats. In some loose sense all were civil engineers, but in Victorian Britain that title was open to any who would claim it.²⁵ With the exception of Robert Rawlinson, then beginning his career, they were marginal engineers. Most were not members of the Institution of Civil Engineers, not a terribly high hurdle at the time. Henry Austin (1809–61), ex-secretary to the Health of Towns Association, was secretary to the GBH, and their first chief. James Smith of Deanston, manufacturer and drainage expert, we have seen as a Health of Towns commissioner. Edward Cresy (1798–1858) was an architectural historian, only marginally successful as an architect. Alfred Dickens (1822–66) was Charles Dickens's brother; Benjamin Herschel Babbage (1815–78) was Charles Babbage's son. As an assistant highways act surveyor in Sheffield William Lee had testified to the Health of Towns Commission about waste and ignorance in local administration. While Lee attained fame as a biographer of Defoe, George Thomas Clark (1808–98) became an antiquarian, specializing in medieval fortification. He also became a leading South Wales ironmaster. William Ranger (1800–1863) had failed as a contractor on the Great Western Railroad. He patented a new type of building stone and was professor at the short-lived Putney College of Civil Engineering, an institution patronized by Chadwick and ridiculed by most civil engineers. T. W. Rammell (1812–89) had been an enthusiast for atmospheric railroads and spent most of his post-GBH career abroad. Rawlinson and Smith of Deanston tended to be sanctimonious, Smith probably to the point of antagonizing some whose support a more tactful person might have had. Lee was fascinated by local history; Alfred Dickens shared his brother's penchant for close observation and belief in the nobility of the poor. Only Rawlinson, Ranger, Dickens, and Austin stayed after Chadwick's departure.²⁶

Recruiting this staff was no mean achievement. Those with experience in sanitary matters were deemed unqualified as being unable to unlearn bad habits. Testimonials were useless, no matter from whom. Instead, candidates were asked how they would sanitize an imaginary town. This might show how well they had read their Chadwick but not how capable they were in the field.²⁷ Since the inspectors were paid per diem they did not have the

25 On British civil engineering see R. A. Buchanan, *The Engineers: A History of the Engineering Profession in Britain, 1750–1914* (London: J. Kingsley, 1989); Charles M. Norrie, *Bridging the Years: A Short History of British Civil Engineering* (London: Edward Arnold, 1956); Gareth Watson, *The Civils: The Story of the Institution of Civil Engineers* (London: Thomas Telford, 1988).

26 In general see H. T. Smith, "Introduction," *Urban and Rural Social Conditions in Industrial Britain,* 4–7. For more positive assessments of the engineering staff see Roberts, *Victorian Origins,* 159, 166; Lewis, *Chadwick,* 187.

27 Chadwick to Morpeth, 14 September 1848, UCL Chadwick Papers #1055; General Board of

security of the civil service to look forward to. (The advantage was that they were free to build as engineers the works they approved as inspectors.) Nor was it easy to work for Chadwick. He was thoroughly convinced that he knew the business of any profession better than those trained in it – he had learned to write engineering reports in his days promoting the Towns Improvement Company; reading a book on the "philosophy of medicine" convinced him that contemporary medicine had forgotten the premonitory symptoms of cholera.[28] On the one hand he complained that the technical staff lacked initiative; on the other he followed a management philosophy that encouraged mutual spying.[29] He was particularly uneasy about Rammell, Ranger, and Lee and soon suggested to Morpeth that there be two classes of inspectors. Younger men with junior rank would do the leg work for experienced and "higher-class" men like Clark and the portly Smith of Deanston, "who looks well before a Town Council" but needed "a young and dapper man to run about him and do his biddings." Morpeth did not like the idea. (Chadwick did institute a differential pay scale, but only by promising some of the juniors, like Lee, a minimum level of annual business.)[30]

What was it like then, to be an inspector inspecting? On visiting a town the inspector was to open proceedings by taking evidence that the inquiry had been properly advertised, reading out the death rate, and then calling on any persons present to notify him of any evil.[31] In the next few days he would tour the area and hear from all who had views to present.

One often thinks of grim-faced Victorian inspectors descending Jehovah-like, swollen with middle-class wrath, forefingers pointed at transgressions of sanitary law.[32] And in some ways – in their statistics, their calculations, their catalogues of streets or of bylaws – the inspectors do exhibit audacious confidence in an orderly official world. Yet plenty of passages indicate that inspectorial authority did not go unchallenged and that they were often moved,

Health [GBH], "Report from the General Board of Health on the Administration of the Public Health Act and the Nuisances Removal and Diseases Prevention Acts from 1848 to 1854, with Appendix," *P.P.*, 1854, *35*, [1768.], 95–96. In light of Chadwick's opinions on the competence of surveyors, it is worthwhile to compare this examination with the exacting test given by the Westminster Commission of Sewers in 1844 ("Questions for Solutions by Candidates for the Situation of New Assistant Surveyor," Greater London Record Office, Archives of the Westminster Commission of Sewers [GLRO WCS], January 1844, WCS 799).

28  Chadwick to Morpeth, 20 September, 23 October 1848, UCL Chadwick Papers #1055.
29  Chadwick to Morpeth, 18 September 1848, UCL Chadwick Papers #1055: "In this entirely new and untried work, I could scarcely say that we have any that must not be regarded as unsafe hands. They will all require watching and training."
30  Chadwick to Morpeth, 7 October, 4, 7, 12 December 1848; Morpeth to Chadwick, 25 October, 5 December 1848, UCL Chadwick Papers #1055.
31  GBH, "Minutes on House Drainage," 143–44; GBH, "Report by the GBH on the Measures Adopted for the Execution of the Nuisances Removal and Diseases Prevention Act, and the Public Health Act, up to July 1849" [to be cited as GBH, "Report of 1849"], *P.P.*, 1849, *24*, [1115.], 129–35.
32  Lewis, *Chadwick*, 181.

shocked, disturbed, or simply bewildered by what they saw. This first generation of inspectors had yet to acquire the callouses of the seasoned bureaucrat. Unlike the assistant poor law commissioners, they had little need to fear
that opposition to the act would turn violent, yet it could be unpleasant, even
frightening. At Accrington in April 1849 Babbage faced protests that his very
inquiry was illegal and taunting on his tour of the town. On arrival in Merthyr
Tydvil in May 1850 Rammell was met by hundreds of angry colliers. He had
to hire a translator and organize the protesters into delegations before he could
even begin to deal with their concerns.³³

The gratuitous recountings of events like these or of casual remarks made
to them give us a much greater sense of the shock the inspectors felt than
their florid declamations of how awful the conditions were. Lee wrote of a
"joke" played on (or for) him at Reading: "A number of idle young men,
treating the repulsive condition of these . . . [privies] as a good joke, poured
several buckets full of the semi fluid nightsoil . . . over the seat and floor, in
order that I and the gentlemen who accompanied me might have ocular
evidence of the quality of its contents. There are four houses of ill fame among
these." Why, we wonder, the juxtaposition of filth and prostitution? It may
be no more than the overwhelming foreignness Lee feels: here the orienting
standards of civilization do not prevail; here people laugh at a privy with "a
hole so large . . . that a child might fall down many yards into the obscene
mass below," and doubtless all manner of other unacceptable things go on
also.³⁴

While most of the reports express outrage at the toleration of filth, it is
Rammell's on Merthyr Tydvil that exhibits the disorientation of an inspector
who finds that the prepared rhetoric simply will not do. He had been told to
expect bad conditions, found them worse than he imagined, and yet was told
the town was clean – "the west end of London, compared with what it was."³⁵
With a population of about forty-five thousand, Merthyr had neither drains
nor water supply. Attempts to apply the Nuisances Removal Act backfired:
since that act gave powers to regulate privies it put a "premium" on not
having one. The streets, covered up to eighteen inches deep in a mix of ash
and excrement, were the chief sites of waste disposal. Children voided themselves "in open chairs in the street"; men on "cinder-heaps . . . or by the sides
of walls, or backs of houses"; women waited until night and used the open
fields, resulting in debilitating constipation. Quarrels were fought with hurled
filth; it was hard to convict, admitted a magistrate, since it was hard to distinguish willfully thrown filth from the normal mode of disposal. And yet

33 Babbage, Accrington, 1850, 3, 5; Rammell, Merthyr Tydvil, 1850, 3–4. See also Raymond Grant,
 "Merthyr Tydfil in the Mid-Nineteenth Century: The Struggle for Public Health," *Welsh History
 Review, 14* (1988–89): 574–94.
34 Lee, Reading, 1850, 23.
35 Rammell, Merthyr, 1850, 24–25.

within houses all was tidy: child care seemed excellent; workmen took daily baths.[36]

Though they were there to investigate technical and legal matters, the cellars and courts, bad water and bad drains belonged to the lives of real people, and it was difficult to assess them without wondering about and reacting to the people who were their users.[37] And often it is not foul conditions but incomprehensible persons that most trouble inspectors. Conditions, after all, were in the realm of the controllable: the absence of drains accounted for muck in the streets. People were not so easily explained. How, Lee wonders, to understand an elderly salesman of religious tracts, whom he finds on a nighttime visit to a lodging house "in his natural character – a drunken, cursing, obscene wretch."[38] At Brixham, Dickens was fascinated by the sociology of immorality. Despite "roughness and noise," there were "few open prostitutes" yet "much sin before marriage" and desertion. He told of how trawler profits were divided; of the kind of youths attracted to fishing; of the need for religious training; and even of book-buying habits and reading lists. He was glad to find "a feeling of shame and disgust" despite "the practices they are publicly compelled to follow," and then jumped directly to water supply.[39] Sometimes the answer to such puzzles was only found by asking. Though rare, there is more of working-class voice in these inspectors' reports than in the *Sanitary Report*, the *Local Reports*, or the reports to the Health of Towns Commission. How do people live this way? Answers Mrs. Rignall of Ely, "The privy turns one's stomach. We never stop any longer than we can help."[40]

---

36  Ibid., 18, 24, 29–33. Even with Rammell's report Merthyr did not lose its power to stun hardened sanitarians and force them to reexamine their ideas on state responsibility. Visiting in December 1853 to review plans for the removal of a graveyard, the Manchester surgeon Philip Holland, no stranger to urban filth, found himself overwhelmed with the ubiquity of excrement: "*Everywhere*, even along roads and paths constantly frequented are visible indications of the absence of those places of accommodation generally thought indispensable." "I saw a young woman filling her pitcher from a little stream of water gushing from the surface of which was so thickly studded with alvine deposits that it was difficult to pass w/o treading in them, in some of which I saw intestinal worms, and the rain then falling was washing the feculent matter into the water which the girl was filling into her pitcher, no doubt for domestic use!" For this Manchester liberal Merthyr was "the theory of *laissez-faire* carried out to its legitimate conclusion. Nothing has been done by united action for all, everyone has been left to get his own supply of water as he could and get rid of the refuse from his own dwelling as he could." He felt that the "violent and apparently purposeless outrages that have occasionally broken out in South Wales" were now explained. So struck was Holland that he forgot to say anything in his report about the graveyard relocation (P. H. Holland to GBH, 15 December 1853, *Merthyr-GBH Correspondence*, Public Record Office [PRO] MH 13/125).

37  A few reports ignore humans, as having nothing to do with the slopes of sewers. But for the mention of a mortality rate and poor relief costs, they give no indication of being about inhabited places. See Babbage, Accrington, 1850, 27–29; Cresy, Brighton, 1849; Ranger, Croydon, 1849, 7; Ranger, Hertford, 1850; Ranger, Aldershot, 1857.

38  Lee, Ely, 1850, 31.

39  Dickens, Brixham, 1854, 7–10, 17.

40  In Lee, Ely, 1850, 22.

But tentativeness is rare. These marginal engineers took quite readily to the role of social betterment consultants. They patronized their brother professionals in the church and medicine and did not hesitate to judge their competence (measured as adherence to sanitary principles), nor to pronounce on medical and moral matters.[41] Often they dealt with medical matters in detail, demonstrating competence in statistics and familiarity with subtle theoretical distinctions.

Their reports were written at leisure, often appearing months after the inspection, allowing ample time to develop a strategy of authority. Understanding that their purpose was to effect change, the inspectors were for the most part careful to balance encouragement and chastisement. They praised individuals and criticized abstractions, like town councils of times past or bad laws. Yet when confronted with direct opposition (as from the mayor and council of Halifax), they could turn sarcastic.[42] They were less appreciative of local efforts than they might have been, a fact which surely contributed to the board's declining popularity. Especially when it was the town government itself that invited them, the inspection might provide an opportunity to show off local accomplishments as well as to identify what was still needed. Yet Cresy, writing of Brighton, could say nothing good about its sewerage; only that it cost too much, that it did not remove household wastes, and that the accounts were poorly kept.[43]

The chief manifestations of inspectorial authority in the reports are the sanitary sermons. Founded on the flimsiest of science, and without any long track record, the sanitary campaign depended on faith. The tone varies – admonitions to duty, simple moral lessons, threatenings of new plagues, or ecstatic visions of the sanitized world to come. Lee had a gift for suddenly catching his readers in a beam of contempt. He began his Ely report with a glorious review of its heritage as a cathedral town, on the grounds that while "history and antiquities" might not be "within the objects of the Report, [yet] . . . there is invariably some peculiar feature connected with the locality of every city or town which has attracted together a population . . . [and] exercises a powerful influence on the physical, moral, and social condition of the inhabitants." Unfortunately "inertia in local government" was the chief legacy of Ely's ecclesiastical past.[44]

Rawlinson appealed to decency, justice, and stability: "To allow poor people to live [in], and crowd places where the medical officer can demonstrate . . . that disease must necessarily be generated . . . [was] worse than mere negligence." There were weightier considerations than expense: "Filth, overcrowding, and neglect . . . produce vagrancy and crime. And, as civilization advances, making no adequate provision for the poor in their houses and in their education; so does crime increase. . . . There is no permanent safety for property if the condition of the poor is neglected. Relief in money is not so much required as that there shall be secured to all classes the means of health and comfort in their houses and in their person."[45]

Smith contrasted life now with life after sanitation: in "a town sewered in a perfect manner by airtight tubular sewers, and with a proper house sewerage receiving all slops in proper water-trapped orifices whereby it is instantly and completely removed from the premises, leaving no taint behind; the enjoyment of life would be much heightened, and disease and death would be greatly lessened, affording even a pecuniary saving much beyond the cost of the sewerage." A water supply would undermine "that unnatural craving for strong drink which the smells of bad sewerage create."[46] Or Smith could be the righteous sanitary socialist: "Private rights must be viewed in reference to public rights." Build as you please in the country, but not in the town: "Unless certain privileges are given up [for] . . . the general public, it would be impossible that a town could exist."[47] Quite likely such sentiments were widely shared among those investing time and effort in sanitary reform; whether Smith's hectoring bolstered their case is less clear.

As the sermons of Rawlinson and Smith remind us, sanitary reform was not just a matter of building waterworks, sewers, and street pavements. What was important were the changes these structures would generate, virtually an end to the social problems of industrialization. This had been Chadwick's promise; sewers and water were to end famine fevers, Chartist threats, drink, despair, and discontent, and to produce disciplined industrial laborers and happy proletarian families. Such concerns surfaced when an inspector showed up and started asking "how things were." By and large the inspectors encouraged this talk as part of building the will for public action. Lee continued the Playfairian argument that sanitation would end opium taking. Smith tried to figure drink expenditure in Bristol to calculate the funds available for better use when sanitary reform eliminated it. Babbage expanded on the wonders of a privy next to each house,

so placed that the most delicate female may use . . . [it] without her innate sense of modesty being shocked by the consciousness of public observation. Under such an arrangement it is hoped that a new and healthier tone of feeling will gradually spring up. Thus the sanitary Reformer, energetically sweeping away all that is detrimental to physical health, will pave

45  Rawlinson, "Further Inquiry on Macclesfield," 1851, 25; Rawlinson, Crumpsall, 1853, 16.
46  Smith, Macclesfield, 1849, 29.
47  Ibid., 1849, 48–49; cf. Lee, Reading, 1850, 52: "No man has a right to destroy and endanger the life of another, and yet there might, and most probably would be, owners of property only too glad to save their pockets, by refusing to give their tenants proper supplies of water, and thus disease might be generated."

the way for the entrance of the ray of light which will usher the Teacher and the Minister into those dark corners of our crowded towns.[48]

Still, the very process of inquiry reinforced Chadwickian reductionism. The inspectors were engineers, after all, and though they handled medical and social questions creditably, their product was public works. An undrained town needed drains, whatever their impact on disease or social relations.[49] The mode of investigation put a premium on what could be seen or smelled and counted on a brief stay. Sight, mainly of the outsides of structures, disclosed the state of a town; the epidemiologist's searching inquiries or the casual conversations that lead the ethnographer or journalist to sense the tapestry of social relations were impossible. The "public health" of the superintending inspectors was pretty much limited to plans and sermons.

## III

Local government, far more than disease, was the hook inspectors used to persuade towns to adopt the act. A local board might not build sewers, but its very existence ensured that a town had a government that could do so later. Adoption would end the squabbling of rival institutions seeking either to acquire responsibilities or to escape them. There were legions of examples of local government irrationality: of outdated rules, vast futile expenditure; overlapping, conflicting, or ambiguous jurisdictions. Leicester was classic. Its corporation had no jurisdiction over sewerage; that matter was for the parish or for surveyors to turnpike commissions.[50] At Hertford, where there were petitions and counterpetitions on the imposition of the act, Ranger added to his report the documentary record of squabbling local authorities. The Sanitary Committee of the Pavement Commission, the center of activism, found that its surveyors might remove only nuisances that obstructed traffic, not those "objectionable merely on the grounds of uncleanliness or insalubrity." Even though the governors of Christ's Hospital were willing to pay half the cost of converting an open sewer into a barrel drain, this proved impossible, as a result of disagreement about how to solve the problem and lack of authority to act. Since the drain received discharge from a prison, the committee took the problem to the home secretary, who advised them to use the Nuisances Removal Act, which allowed a sanitary authority to issue a summons on the assertion of two medical men that a structure harmed health. But no one owned the ditch so there was no one to summon. And an unannounced visit

---

48  Lee, Ely, 1850, 18–19; Smith, Bristol, 1850, 153–57; Babbage, Accrington, 1850, 37.

49  Babbage found little disease in Layton with Walbrick, but much need for sanitary technology (1850, 10). Clark judged the "sanitary condition" of Bristol on the proportion of low-rental houses, assuming that they somehow represented disease incidence (Clark, Bristol, 1850, 37).

50  Ranger, Leicester, 1849, 12–16.

from a Home Office prison inspector produced a declaration that the drain was not a nuisance.

Similar confusion followed the committee's attempt in December 1848 to require the marquis of Salisbury, as landowner, to do something about wheeled tub privies he had provided for his tenants, which it found to be "injurious to health and disgusting to the view of the inhabitants." Salisbury replied that the Town Council had endorsed the facilities and that the lessee, with whom he had "no legitimate means of interference," was responsible for keeping them clean. The lessee, with whom the committee sided but against whom it was obliged to proceed, claimed to have been forbidden by Salisbury to build proper brick cesspools. But surely, Salisbury replied, brick cesspools would put the town at risk of "infectious disease," while the tubs facilitated rapid removal of wastes and thus proper recycling – the Health of Towns Commission had made that clear. Moreover, others, including members of the Sanitary Committee, were themselves responsible for nuisances they were attributing to him.[51]

Episodes like these, documented in floods of indignant correspondence, seemed so clearly to indicate a need for reforms that would allow towns to take obvious steps to solve simple problems. How absurd for so many important folk with such mighty tools of law and capital to be unable to get the drains cleaned. Chadwick delighted in these vignettes of irrationality – so much silly English tradition that might be swept away by authoritative enactment as easily as one swept filth from the streets with a high-pressure jet.

As in Hertford, where problems persisted despite the passing of resolutions "requiring the removal of an infinite number of nuisances," the inspectors often found energetic local authorities curtailed by unworkable laws. The Accrington inspector of nuisances had probably gone beyond "strict . . . legality" in his war on piggeries, Babbage noted.[52] The advantage of blaming bad law was that it absolved individuals. Thus Clark praised Bristol's surveyor and council for their "economy and skill"; yet they could not "with their present limited powers of jurisdiction . . . work to an extended plan."[53] Or at Brixham, while there was a "Sanitary Committee," there was no responsible officer, and it could "hardly be expected that a body of gentlemen can continually act as inspectors of nuisances."[54]

In many cases a petition for a board of health reflected the hope that the GBH could settle some local conflict. Dickens found he had been invited to Brixham to settle a dispute about waterworks finance. Everyone wanted water,

51  Ranger, Hertford, 1850, 10–20.
52  Ibid.,12, 16; Babbage, Accrington, 1850, 15.
53  Clark, Bristol, 1850, 125, cf. 174–76: One could argue that the authority ought to have sought the powers it lacked. But see Rawlinson, Poulton, 1851, 8, where the problem is not the improvement act, but the failure of the commissioners to use their powers.
54  Dickens, Brixham, 1854, 23.

but there was disagreement about who should pay what for it. In such cases dictatorial central authority (provided it dictated the right things) was not objectionable. Rural Wallasey called on the inspector to bring an almost military authority to bear on the depredations of its neighbor, Birkenhead. The Leamington Improvement Commission had no power to remove a dam that impeded their drainage but was sure central government could get rid of it.[55]

Even where they could arbitrate, the inspectors often found no clear rules to guide them. Clark, investigating Leamington in October 1849, held that the local district should include the adjacent parish of Milverton on the grounds that its sanitary fate was inextricable from Leamington's. Aghast at the frontage rates Leamington charged for laying flagstones and convinced that they had solved their own sanitary problems, Milvertonians opposed the merger. Ranger, reinvestigating in November 1851, upheld them, insisting that Clark's view would result in "injustice and great inconvenience." Where Chadwick and Clark thought boundaries should reflect natural drainage, he opposed altering political boundaries. In 1856, Dickens, investigating an appeal for boundary changes, upheld Clark. He found a large part of the opposition due simply to "strong personal feeling against some of the members of the local Board of Leamington."[56] Complicating matters was a dispute about how high to set the property qualification for the new local board. Some saw it as a remedy for the existing unduly democratic local government; others as a means to greater democracy.[57] A common issue in Leamington and elsewhere was equitable rating. Suburbs sought to escape the debt burden of the older core, yet the air and water of one affected the air and water of the other; poor provisions for fire in the one heightened fire danger in the other. Here the inspectors had little power; they could only suggest a fair apportionment of debt.[58]

Perhaps the two most important provisions of the act were liberation from private bill procedure and the ability to incur long-term debt. Private bill procedure was inflexible; alterations of the sort frequently encountered in building large public works might require a return to Parliament with the

---

55 Ibid., 7–8; Clark, Leamington, 1850, 19; Rawlinson, Poulton, 1851, 7–8.

56 Clark, Leamington, "Further Inquiry," 1851, 7–8; Ranger, Leamington, 1852, 6; Dickens, "Further Inquiry with Reference to Certain Proposed Alterations to the Boundaries," 1857, 9–19; Henry Austin, "Report . . . of an Inquiry as to Certain Proposed Amendments of the Provisional Order Relating to the Parish of Leamington Priors," 1854. Dickens's advice was not taken; relations among the rival local governments were still bad a decade later, and sanitary offenses and threats were still the chief medium in which they fought out their quarrels (Hamlin, "Muddling in Bumbledom"). See also Smith, Macclesfield, 1849, 4–5, 16.

57 Clark, Leamington, 1850, 6, 28, 39; Clark, Leamington, "Further Inquiry," 1851, 6–8.

58 Dickens, "Further Inquiry," 1857, 8, 11–12, 16, 19–20; Ranger, Halifax, 1850, 7–8, 11; Smith, Macclesfield, 1850, 6, 17. Inspectors did sometimes urge that ample compensation be given to superseded improvement commissions and water companies, provided those bodies cooperated in the change. Dickens, Leamington, "Further Inquiry," 1857, 20; Clark, Bristol, 1850, 200. Cf. Lee, Reading, 1850, 50–53.

accompanying expense and risk of opposition. Much of Lee's Reading report recounted that town's fiasco with private bill procedure. In 1847 Reading had sought a local act to undertake sewerage (£60,000) and sewage recycling (£39,500) and also to improve streets, build a market, regulate housing, and purchase and enlarge waterworks (£35,000). Under the Preliminary Inquiries Act, two engineers from the Office of Woods and Forests had investigated. After twenty-five days of testimony, they quashed the scheme. The town had wasted £8000. Lee saw the problem as overreliance on oral testimony – a brief tour could have obviated hours of assertion and denial. The private act of Parliament, he insisted, was far more constraining than the GBH.[59]

While it may seem obvious that large permanent works require long mortgages, debt financing of local public works was in fact quite new. Prior to the 1830s, private bill committees had tended to see indebtedness as an inappropriate fiscal state for local governments; necessary works were to be financed by current rates and could be carried out only as fast as money came in. The active Halifax improvement commissioners accomplished a great deal, yet a debt ceiling of £3000 made it impossible even to think of systematic works. The public health act benefited from a reversal of opinion, linked no doubt to the growing faith that capital investment was the motor of progress. For Chadwick the chief rationale of inspection under the act was not to guarantee health but to assure ratepayers (and lenders) that their investments were safe from sanitary charlatans and incompetent elected officials.[60] Most towns did prosper during the Victorian period and municipal debt was slowly transformed from a sign of poor administration to one of prudent foresight. Long-term finance did ease some conflicts that impeded sanitation – such as whether occupier, lessee, or owner was to pay the capital cost of supplying a house with the new sanitation.[61]


IV

A close second to reform of government was reform of infrastructure. So often what exasperated local governments was not silly laws but inconvenient nature – water *would* run downhill; excrement insisted on accumulating. Laws to prevent nuisances were useless without drains. Sometimes it was necessary to state simple physical truths. Reading's cesspools might be safe at present, Lee wrote, but their use would ultimately saturate the subsoil, and "the inevitable

59 Lee, Reading, 1850, 7–9.
60 E.g., Rawlinson (Poulton, 1851, 8–9) worried that the Wallasey Improvement Commission, unlike a local board, could "borrow money, and spend it, without any guarantee to the ratepayers that the works are judiciously planned."
61 Clark, Bristol, 1850, 180; Ranger, Halifax, 1851, 43–44, 51; Rawlinson, Ormskirk, 1850, 23; Ranger, Leicester, 1849, 25.

result will be that the town must become uninhabitable."[62] There were ready technical solutions to an astonishing range of problems. Reading's crime rate was due to lack of public privies, a citizen noted: the police were too often absent, having "to go home or to a distance to obey the calls of nature." A public piggery outside the town would resolve conflict among Leamington's hoteliers about the stench of one another's piggeries, Clark suggested.[63]

On technical matters the inspectors were most careful to maintain a solid front. All recommended small-bore pipe sewers. There could be "but little difference . . . between persons competent to form an opinion," noted Clark.[64] On sewage recycling they tended to gush about a post-Malthusian world where every being generated the fertilizer to sustain its own existence. Smith admitted that there was no long track record of sewage farming, yet he would still make a firm commitment of the profits it would yield.[65] (In many places the public needed little convincing.)[66] In figuring the savings sanitation would generate most used a formula developed by Lyon Playfair for the Health of Towns Commission: society would save £5 funeral costs/excess death + £1/ excess illness (figured at 28 excess illnesses/death). They did cite other costs (e.g., the costs of dealing with those who would not have been drunk and disorderly had there been proper sanitation, the cost of extra soap necessitated by absence of easily cleaned pavements, property depreciation from same, pump repair costs, cesspit emptying costs, costs of labor to fetch water at 1 penny/day), but they left these out of formal calculations.[67] Finally, all recognized an obligation to try to show that all necessary works would cost less

---

62 Lee, Reading, 1850, 35, 47–48.
63 Ibid., 48; Clark, Leamington, 1850, 27.
64 Clark, Leamington, 1850, 30.
65 Cresy, Brighton, 1849, 29–31; Ranger, Enfield, 1849, 13–18; Smith, Macclesfield, 1849, 42–48. Nonetheless, in the case of coastal towns some of the inspectors saw the obvious solution as sending the sewage into the ocean (Dickens, Brixham, 1854, 45).
66 Lee, Reading, 1850, 71; Rammell, Halsted, 1852, 20; Clark, Bristol, 1850, 196–97; Ranger, Halifax, 1851, 21–22.
67 Playfair, "Report on the Sanitary Condition of Large Towns in Lancashire," Royal Commission on the State of Large Towns and Populous Districts," *Second Report,* Appendix, pt. 2, *P.P.,* 1845, *18,* [610.], 59–60. For its use and criticism see Lord Morpeth and Lord George Bentinck in *Hansard's Parliamentary Debates 3rd series 91,* 1847, 634; *93,* 1847, 1108–10. In comparison with other modes of calculation, this version of the Playfair formula would give a low estimate. In some of their calculations Smith and Clark would add lost wages, calculated at 7.5 shillings/week (considered the average adult wage) times the number of weeks of prematurity of death, and Smith would add also the cost of relief to widows and orphans (in general see Clark, Bristol, 1850, 46; Smith, Macclesfield, 1850, 13; Cresy, Brighton, 1849, 6; Clark, Wigan, 1849, 31; Ranger, Leicester, 1849, 33–34). For an early version see Thomas Ferguson, *The Dawn of Scottish Social Welfare: A Survey from Medieval Times to 1863* (Edinburgh: Thomas Nelson, 1948), 117. To portray existing conditions as irrational, inefficient, and expensive was one of the most difficult arguments for the inspectors: "There appears to be a strange and undefined dread of expense on behalf of certain persons, who do not consider that the existing condition of things is by far the most ruinously costly, directly or indirectly; directly in reducing the actual value of house property, and indirectly by generating excessive sickness and consequently causing pecuniary loss and bodily suffering" (Rawlinson, Macclesfield, 1850, 14).

than two pence per household per week, Chadwick's promised figure, though sometimes they had to admit that this sum was unrealistic.[68] In engineering design centralization was no sham. Only the GBH, advised by its inspector, could allow a local board to raise money on the security of rates to carry out public works. Deviate from Chadwickian principles and a "very serious responsibility" would be on their heads, Ranger told the Halifax council.[69]

## V

The question of disease arises in these reports less often than one might expect. Even where it did, there was little interest in determining its particular local sources. It was easy enough to find, as in Alfreton, "local causes quite sufficient to account for even a greater degree of sickness than the inhabitants have endured."[70] Diseases like consumption, which fit the Chadwickian paradigm less well, were often neglected even when these were major causes of mortality.[71]

Whatever etiological theory one subscribed to, it was possible to argue that sanitary reform was the crucial element in prevention. Medical men who rejected the claim of environmental filth as a specific cause of disease could still agree that removing such predisposing causes would improve health.[72] There was rarely a sense that contagionist and miasmatist explanations led in different directions. Those like William Budd's brother, George, who saw typhus fever as propagated "directly or indirectly from the bodies of persons already ill of it," could nonetheless argue that "a free supply of water, and the general adoption of water closets, and covered sewers will . . . tend more than any other measures to prevent the spread of fever, by giving the means of cleanliness and by carrying away from human habitations the infectious matter that is thrown off from the bodies of persons ill with fever."[73]

---

68  Cf. Roberts, *Victorian Origins,* 217, 242; Babbage, Layton with Walbrick, 1851, 40; Lee, Reading, 1850, 65.

69  Ranger, Halifax, 1851, 51–52, 83.

70  Lee, Alfreton, 1850, 9; Clark, Bristol, 1850, 51; Rawlinson, Ormskirk, 1850, 16.

71  Cresy, Brighton, 1849, 7–8.

72  Etiological explanation was flexible and vague, e.g., John Muriel of Ely: "I attribute disease in Common Muck-hill to a stagnant drain and filth of every description. . . . Such disease, although not originating in the want of sanitary arrangements, would be very much aggravated in such localities. Endemic disease has a tendency to weaken the constitution; the children in such localities have an unhealthy, cadaverous appearance. Such persons stand less chance when attacked with active disease than persons in other more healthy neighbourhoods" (quoted in Lee, Ely, 1850, 15–16; see also Ranger, Halifax, 1851, 36, 103–4; Cresy, Brighton, 1849, 10). A wide range of "filth" could be implicated, too, such as the odor of low tide (Lee, Poulton, 1851, 11). Dampness was usually a cause of disease; yet the present lack of fever in Leicester could be ascribed to wetness which dilutes "noxious matter" (Ranger, Leicester, 1849, 7).

73  George Budd to Reverend Errington, 24 January 1850. See also G. Oldham to Errington, early

As a tangible evil whose causes – invisible gases or particles – were difficult for lay opponents to contest, disease could be a means to persuade a recalcitrant corporation to acknowledge a need for sanitation.[74] At Halifax Ranger did not focus on existing disease: it, evidently, was an acceptable state of affairs, since the town had not taken steps to prevent it. But matters would get worse: the wonder was "not that the mortality is so great, but that it does not infinitely exceed its present amount." Fever was an "infallible gauge of contaminated atmosphere" and there was no doubt of the contamination. Among its constituents were the concentrated exhalations of the people of Halifax (calculated at 4212 gallons per person per day) along with their daily perspiration ("two pints of watery fluid"). The "headache, weariness, oppression, and sometimes even nausea," that townsfolk experienced were "simply caused by people breathing the poisoned air exhaled by their neighbours." Even drying clothes caused harm, by increasing humidity, which in turn prevented perspiration from evaporating and led to "re-introduction of substances for the discharge of which such careful provisions are made in nature." Natural theology was the ultimate source of authority: The townsfolk were flouting "laws founded for a benevolent purpose."[75] Ranger was pandering to class tensions here. Those who produced (and experienced) disease endangered those Ranger was addressing, who wrongly felt they ran no risk.

Thus, "disease" was a trump card. To cry that some feature of society caused disease raised the stakes, just as the cry "witch" would have amplified a complaint about an irritating neighbor in an earlier century. "Disease" could sanction almost any intervention. It was an escalation of "nuisance" (i.e., the "streets [are] infested with pigs and asses, so as to be not only a nuisance, but positively dangerous," or the cesspits were "quite [bad] enough to propagate fever of the worst description" [whether or not they actually had]).[76]

Usually talk of "disease" was couched in terms of accusations. The epidemiological question, *where the disease came from*, was less important than *whose*

December 1849; Thomas Watson to Errington, 24 December 1849 (quoted in Lee, Alfreton, 1850, 32, 35–38).

74  Thus Rawlinson threatened Wallasey with calculations of "wholesale poisoning": "If a return of the cubical volume of atmosphere affected and tainted by the nightsoil was appended to the weekly returns, some idea of the evil might be gathered from it" (Rawlinson, Poulton, 1851, 16). See also Babbage, Accrington, 1850, 17.

75  Ranger, Halifax, 1851, 31–42. Ranger is quoting a local medical man, Dr. Alexander.

76  Lee, Poulton, 1851, 11; Clark, Leamington, 1850, 10. It was also an escalation of sin: the lodging houses were "literally dens of iniquity, and the *hotbeds of disease*" (Lee, Ely, 1850, 31; cf. Lee, Reading, 1850, 57). "Disease" could solve the rhetorical problem of how to convey to readers that the filth and squalor being described were far worse than any other filth and squalor they had seen or read of, and thus in more immediate need of remedy. Thus one finds statements like the following, made by a Bristol practitioner describing a house with a bad privy: "Any one not accustomed to such scenes, would, in all probability, be seized with sudden illness, if called upon to visit it" (Clark, Bristol, 1850, 89–90). By no means is this hyperbole. The idea that the nervous system was the medium for outrage in sensibility to trigger physical illness was a respectable one in contemporary pathology. On trump cards see Douglas, "Environments at Risk," 260–75.

*fault* it was. Sometimes what seems to be theoretical conflict is better seen as the assigning and dodging of culpability. At Macclesfield, for example, the mortality rate was an unacceptable 29/1000. A committee of local practitioners tried to convince inspector Smith that the *town* was really healthy. Disease was due either to the weather or to people who came there from elsewhere, and they could be held responsible for neither. Many deaths were consumptions from "the peculiar bleakness of this locality" or from "physical degenerations . . . promoted by vitiated conditions of the atmosphere, by sudden changes of temperature, by unsuitable clothing, by crude and innutritious aliment; causes . . . always in operation in densely populated manufacturing districts."[77]

Similarly, the protesting workers told Rammell that the high mortality rate in Merthyr "was caused by the mode of life of the people, working under ground, and by want of sufficiency of food, and not by want of sanitary laws. What they wanted was more meat." Though they felt wages compensated for damage to health, employers shared this view. Rammell disagreed. Since the excess mortality was in children, labor relations could not be the cause. He offered a scenario in which structures were to blame. In Merthyr infant mortality could not so readily be ascribed to filth because even though the streets were filthy, the homes were clean and child care good. It could, however, be attributed to the poor health of breast-feeding mothers, which in turn was a result of the constipation caused by waiting until dark to defecate. Sewers and water closets would solve the problem.[78]

In Macclesfield and Merthyr the inspectors were meeting the Alisonian claim of poverty and hard work as the cause of disease. But it was being used differently – not to show the need for greater social provision but to justify resistance to public action, since, it was argued, neither work nor weather nor food was amenable to it. (Banning Irish immigration was acceptable, however, the Macclesfield medical committee decided.)[79] In response, the inspectors followed Southwood Smith: Good sanitation compensated for hard work and scanty food. Thus Clark, in his peroration to Bristol: "A powerful local government cannot, it is true, make employment plentiful, bread cheap, or spirits dear; but it is in its power to give . . . those blessings of water, air, and clean-

---

77  Smith, Macclesfield, 1849, 68–69. Cf. *Statements and Observations in Relation to the Report of William Lee C.E. to the General Board of Health on a Preliminary Enquiry into . . . the Sanitary Condition of the Inhabitants of the City of Ely* (Ely: Thomas Hicks, 1850).

78  Rammell, Merthyr, 1850, 4–5, 17, 11, 15–18, 24. Over 50 percent of deaths were of children less than five years old, a rate even more remarkable in a population skewed toward young adult immigrants. For other examples of the unwillingness to indict work see Lee, Alfreton, 1850, 12; Lee, Poulton, 1851, 15.

79  "Report of the Corporation Sanitary Committee, 3 May 1849," in Smith, Macclesfield, 1850, 61–68. By no means is this report a simple apologia; it admits insanitary conditions though it gives them a secondary role in the explanation of an excessive mortality rate.

liness which are beyond all the drugs in the Pharmacoepia."[80] In Halifax, Ranger quoted R. D. Grainger, one of Chadwick's medical inspectors, that while food, fuel, and clothing were usually seen as "the chief necessaries of life, [yet] it is less difficult for people to . . . maintain a certain degree of bodily health on scanty food, and with imperfect means of warmth, than it is for them to escape disease when immersed in a vitiated atmosphere." Unquestionably privation caused disease; all the more important that those "badly fed" should be well housed.[81] And for practical purposes "housing" meant water and drains. Housing itself was stuck so fast in the realm of market-defined commodities that the inspectors gave little attention to improving it or preventing overcrowding. You could not rebuild the bad houses in Brighton, Cresy noted, but you could fix the drains.[82]

## VI

However we judge the limits Chadwick put on acceptable intervention, he and the inspectors were sure the gifts they bestowed would make lives better and ease class conflict. Water and sewers were to be an automatic philanthropy in contrast to the haphazard effects of hospitals, schools, and religious instruction.[83] The inspectors echoed Chadwick, Morpeth, and the Health of Towns Association in insisting that it was essential that the technologies of health be available to *all*. All dwellings should be roomy, open to air and sunlight, provided with tap water and water closets, and located on drained and cleaned streets. Leamington's water was fine, Clark observed, but available only to the wealthy. The act would allow "the poor many of those domestic comforts . . . possessed by none but the rich." In Alfreton, access to water depended on the whim of the owner of a well. Though he gave water to all who needed it, Lee held this to be unacceptable dependence.[84] Here sanitation was a species of liberty; freeing the poor from the shackles of the cesspool was in its modest way a bit like freeing the slaves.

The inspectors could understand why corrupt local authorities or tightfisted shopkeepers opposed them, but not why the poor, who stood to gain so

---

80 Clark, Bristol, 1850, 180.
81 Ranger, Halifax, 1851, 37–38; cf. Ranger, Barnsley, 1852, 21; Clark, Wigan, 1849, 31; Clark, Preston, 1849, 11; Clark, Leamington, 1850, 33. At Preston the opinion remained strong that fever was less a result of insanitary conditions than of the "distressed condition of the neighbourhood, occasioned by the want of employment, and many of the common necessaries of life."
82 Cresy, Brighton, 1849, 17; Ranger, Barnsley, 1852, 38.
83 "At present, whatever may be the desire of the upper classes to raise the condition of the people, they can attempt it only by private visitings, charities, schools, and religious instruction; but their exertions are checked, at every step, by . . . the condition of the cottages" (Clark, Bristol, 1850, 176).
84 Lee, Alfreton, 1850, 19–20; Clark, Leamington, 1850, 26, 34.

much, were often ambivalent, even hostile. Cholera had recently swept the island (some of the inquiries were done during the epidemic years themselves), yet in many places public health seemed not to be particularly important.[85]

Certainly it was not apathy, if by that one means desensitization to disease and death. Ranger's observation that people in Hertford "complained of being constantly ill" suggests that they saw their health as poorer than it ought normally to be. Sometimes, as at Merthyr, health was simply a low priority. It was a boom town with no middle class. People went there not to live but to make money. Workers were willing enough to admit that they were killing themselves, but they saw immediate income as more important than environmental quality. Lee understood the failure of Ely residents to recognize the dangers of well water as ignorance of sanitary science: "The poor creatures . . . are deluded into [drinking] poison because they get it from the pump, while they acknowledge that the ditch [which recharges it] is injurious. . . . They turn with loathing from the stagnant, stinking fluid in front of their houses, but are compelled to take it, only slightly changed, from their pumps at the back."[86] Yet was this really ignorance, or a choice to use the better of two vile waters in a situation where there were no good options?

And by no means was the tone of sanitary intervention unambiguously benevolent. The theme of sanitary universality appeared more often in terms of discipline than in terms of liberty and dignity. It seemed that there was a class that was dangerous unless you kept them continually hosed down and made sure they did not fraternize under unsupervised conditions. In-house water, for example, was needed because the community pump was a site of unacceptable socialization. Queuing for water, a minor theme in the *Sanitary Report*, looms large in these reports. The morning queue in Wigan averaged 60; at Ormskirk, Rawlinson counted 117.[87] Chadwick had seen queuing mainly in terms of inefficiency, as time that could be more productively used. The inspectors emphasized immorality. In queues assignations were made; children learned bad language. At Barnsley and at Merthyr water gathering was done at night by adults. There were quarrels over turns, and, worse, "men and women rolling each other over in the grass, and behaving in the most obscene manner."[88]

Public privies were also associated with sexual license, a concern we have seen with the Health of Towns Commission. "The want of proper privy accommodation" caused "immorality," maintained an Over Darwen curate. The houses were decent, but the privies (and lack of paving and drains) led

---

85 Many reports make no mention of cholera. But see Dickens, Brixham, 1854, 30; Rammell, Merthyr, 1850, 62.
86 Lee, Ely, 1850, 24.
87 Clark, Wigan, 1849, 20–21; Rawlinson, Ormskirk, 1850, 34.
88 Ranger, Barnsley, 1852, 23; Rammell, Merthyr, 1850, 37–38. Similarly, water was needed in Enfield because for some the only source was the pub (Ranger, Enfield, 1849, 12).

to a high rate of illegitimacy; they were the "greatest . . . social and moral evil." The link was self-image; "*propriety of feelings*" was as important a goal of sanitation as "*healthy cleanliness and comfort.*"[89] Even the most innocuous sanitary undertakings might be proxies of class conflict. Was a complaint in opulent Clifton about the "dreadful stench" from a cab stand really about horse dung or "the obscene conduct of the flymen, whose conversation and conduct is quite corrupting to the morals of our children"?[90] The threat-to-health argument could be applied to any social arrangement one objected to. A Halifax man attributed the high rate of mortality to the new cheap Sunday railroad fares, which "tempted the people, who had been working in the heated atmosphere of the mills during the week, to go and expose themselves to the cold on the Sundays."[91]

The starkest statement of the political, social, and cultural costs of sanitation is the observation of the Preston reformer the Reverend William Clay that rate of mortality in Preston jail was only one seventeenth that in the town, because of "cleanliness, proper food, good air, regular hours, exercise, sobriety, and medical attention." "The great mass of the people" might do as well "if they would only strive to do for themselves what discipline and order do for the prisoners." Statistically, the comparison is ludicrous: the jail population fluctuated; the age structure was very different from that of a town population. But no irony is intended: only a view that "health" is the opposite of ordinary inclinations and actions.[92]

All the same, these engineers were not ideological dupes. If they tended to reduce problems to structures that is hardly surprising: they were engineers. Yet engineering was no mere building profession for at least some of them; it embodied a vision of equilibrium and equitable distribution. Rawlinson, whose stature would have allowed him to move in many directions, remained an inspector, preoccupied with what is best called justice: sanitation was one of the few compensations available to those disenfranchised in so many other ways. Clark, too, thought sanitary legislation must "protect the lives of the poor." Where the high walls of the rich blocked life-giving air, the sanitarian might bring them down.[93]

89 Ranger, Hertford, 1850, 11–12; Lee, Over Darwen, 1853, 16, 25. See also Rammell, Halsted, 1852, 16; Ranger, Halifax, 1851, 17; Babbage, Accrington, 1850, 37.
90 Clark, Bristol, 1850, 94.
91 Ranger, Halifax, 1851, 28–29.
92 Clark, Preston, 1849, 6.
93 Clark, Bristol, 1850, 89. In his Ormskirk report Rawlinson included a statement to the working poor on "the Advantages of Local Government." He argued that their opposition to sanitary reform could be understood only in terms of ideological deception and false class consciousness. Bad conditions that were simply costly and unpleasant for the rich were for the poor "productive of poverty, degradation, extreme misery, sickness, and premature death. It is most suicidal, therefore, in the poor to blindly resist works of improvement; they should rather aid . . . in the work. The honest, hard-working resident looks around and contemplates the vast accumulation of neglected filth which has taken place; he has also most probably suffered by sickness, either in

## VII

Yet things had changed. By the early 1850s an insanitary environment was less a culpable offense than a publicly remediable condition that victimized the innocent poor. There is little of the anger and horror of the poor so clear in Kay's 1832 pamphlet. It was "unfair to tax the poor with being dirty," if they had no "means of removing the reproach," argued Ranger. It was even unfair to tax them with opium taking, added Lee, for "where there is much dampness and a depressed sanitary condition . . . the poor inhabitants . . . become low-spirited, lose all energy, feel their misery without the power to control external circumstances, and endeavor to forget it in the temporary excitement of these noxious drugs."[94] If there was less need to rant about the subhuman poor, it was because the most important social issues had been resolved. Revolution no longer seemed imminent. The ten hours' bill had passed in 1847; no Spitalfields weavers still petitioned for the ancient Statutes of Labourers. The great poor law issues of how to create character and enforce work had faded.[95] When a Halifax medical officer noted of overcrowding that "it is difficult to suggest a remedy for the evil, because it is generally the result of poverty and not of inclination on the part of the recipients," he was appealing to a notion of poverty as natural and neutral, the product neither of unsound policy nor of wanton laziness.[96] He could not have said that a decade earlier.

The new focus was on the physical and political problems of people in groups: in short, the problem of effective local government. In Merthyr and elsewhere, topography caused "ill-feeling between neighbours, and . . . frequent quarrels." Whatever was discarded from higher houses washed down on houses below. Only proper drainage could create harmony.[97] Asking "Who is to blame?" for filth in Bristol, Clark answered both, "Everybody, except the occupant" and "no one": landlords bore responsibility, as did leading citizens and those who were too greedy or insufficiently educated, but the "grand defect" was "powerless and irresponsible government." At times the vision is explicitly socialist: in matters of health "the futility of private

his own person or in his family; but his reply to any argument for improvement is probably evaded by throwing all the blame upon 'The Irish,' or upon 'the landlords.' . . . I would seriously appeal to the working man who resists it, and ask if he can justify such conduct to himself" (Rawlinson, Ormskirk, 1850, 23).

94 Ranger, Halifax, 1851, 18; Lee, Ely, 1850, 18; cf. Watson in Clark, Leamington, 1850, 8; Clark, Bristol, 1850, 173; J. L. White in Rammell, Merthyr, 1850, 18.

95 Those who raise poor law issues usually do so in connection with lowering costs through sanitary measures. Cresy, Brighton, 1849, 8–9; Rawlinson, Crumpsall, 1853, 18.

96 In Ranger, Halifax, 1851, 17–18.

97 Rammell, Merthyr, 1850, 29, 31. See also Rammell, Halsted, 1852, 18; Lee, Over Darwen, 1853, 23; Smith, Macclesfield, 1850, 27.

exertion, and the mutual dependence of the inhabitants on each other," became clear.[98]

Did all this preaching have an effect? Probably not. The local boards that were established were overwhelmed with local matters. What they did depended not only on what they conceived public health to be, but on accidents of personality, the tact and competence of those they hired (chiefly their advisory and executive officers, the clerk and surveyor), and all manner of unforeseen contingencies: lawsuits by disgruntled riparian landowners, economic cycles, even international events like the American Civil War, which spurred infrastructure projects in the cotton North as a way to offset the unemployment caused by the Union blockade. In many towns, the most important feature of the act was to establish a coherent local government with responsibility for the urban environment. Remarkably, a number of towns – Leicester, Merthyr, Croydon, Macclesfield, Ely – accepted the obligation of full sanitation and moved quickly to do precisely what Chadwick expected of them, though with mixed results. What stuck in most places was some sense of public health as the most noble of causes. Whatever a "board of health" did – the filling of the most trivial pothole – became an act of charity, a fulfilling of God's laws, a part of the march of progress. In Macclesfield the friends of "public health" fought "filth, misery, vice, and crime." Both clergy and medical men found that "the *same* causes operate to render their services necessary in the *same* localities," wrote Lee.[99]

98 Clark, Bristol, 1850, 168–69, 174–76; Lee, Ely, 1850, 30; cf Dickens, Leamington, "Further Inquiry," 1857, 18. See also Oliver MacDonagh, *Early Victorian Government, 1830–1870* (London: Weidenfeld and Nicolson, 1977), 151; Gerry Kearns, "Private Property and Public Health Reform in England, 1830–1870," *Social Science and Medicine 26* (1988): 187–99.

99 Rawlinson, Macclesfield, 1849, 3; Lee, Reading, 1850, 37.

# 10

## Lost in the Pipes

In 1844, Arthur Helps, one of the new career bureaucrats, friend of Slaney and Morpeth, wrote that "it is evident that the health of towns requires to be watched by scientific men, and improvements constantly urged on by persons who take an especial interest in the subject. If I were a despot, I would soon have a band of Arnotts, Chadwicks, Southwood Smiths, Smiths of Deanston, Jones, and the like."[1] As we have seen, sanitation was to be a democratizing technology; a new human right that would be the new basis of citizenship. But as Helps saw, the democratizing technology had no room for democracy itself: notwithstanding the inspectors' sermons, many towns were unenthusiastic about Chadwick's combined works. But science might do what friendly persuasion could not. The despotism of nature – the laws of physics, economy, health – embodied in self-scouring pipe sewers might drive sanitary rationality into every British hamlet.

Yet where Chadwick had power to rationalize sanitation, as in London from late 1847 to late 1849 and in towns seeking loans under the Public Health Act from 1848 to 1854, he found that unruly democracy prevailed in the world of engineering too, sometimes in the form of uncooperative nature, or of negligent people, or of unforeseen events. There was no simple formula of sanitation, but instead a vast number of inescapable decisions – about standards, responsibilities, priorities, authority – and people made them not as Chadwick would have them do, by applying his system, but on the basis of trust, tradition, convenience, gain, fear, and so forth. As some remarked at

---

1 Arthur Helps, *The Claims of Labour: An Essay on the Duties of Employers to the Employed, the 2nd ed, to Which Is Added, an Essay on the Means of Improving the Health and Increasing the Comfort of the Labouring Classes* (London: Pickering, 1845), 135–36. The Jones may be R. L. Jones, who would become a member of the Metropolitan Sanitary Commission. On Helps see David Roberts, *Paternalism in Early Victorian England* (New Brunswick, N.J.: Rutgers University Press, 1979), 25, 36. Themes in this chapter are also developed in Christopher Hamlin, "Edwin Chadwick and the Engineers, 1842–1854: Systems and Anti-Systems in the Pipe-and-Brick Sewers War," *Technology and Culture 33* (1992): 680–709.

the time of Chadwick's fall in 1854, cleanliness was all very well, but if people had to be cleansed by Chadwick, many would as soon stay dirty.[2]

Chadwick's reign did end in the summer of 1854. When the Board of Health came up for renewal a broad consensus of members of Parliament decided that the price of its continuance was Chadwick's exit. These included philosophical radicals like Joseph Hume and William Molesworth, metropolitan radicals like Benjamin Hall, and some of the country Tories who had opposed the 1848 bill, like Joseph Henley. Even the active support of Lord Palmerston, the home secretary, and the government's offer to put the board in the Home Office, which would have satisfied those opponents in 1848, was not enough. Henceforth a single member of Parliament would supervise the few inspectors necessary to continue the mundane business of the act. While there was talk of another post, Chadwick never returned to public service.[3]

Technological controversy, in its strong sense of legitimate debate about the characteristics of good technologies, has not figured much in accounts of Chadwick's fall. Instead, historians have tended to treat Chadwick's policies as Chadwick saw them: as obviously the right ones. Thus Finer writes that had Chadwick prevailed in imposing pipe sewerage, "it would have provided, from the standpoint of to-day, the greatest single justification for the sanitary despotism of the Board." In their view the tragedy is one of good ideas in the hands of one too bold.[4] After Carlisle's departure in March 1850 there was no one to massage egos and suggest compromises and Chadwick was quickly in trouble, antagonizing the professions and mismanaging campaigns to bring London safe water, good sewers, and state cemeteries.[5] Those he had ignored or ridiculed or swept aside – the parliamentary agents and ignorant

---

2 *Hansard's Parliamentary Debates 3rd series, 135,* 1854, 997.

3 Ibid., *134,* 1854, 1297–98, 1301; *135,* 1854, 973–74, 990, 1138–39, 1223–24; J. L. Hammond and Barbara Hammond, *Lord Shaftesbury,* 3d ed. (London: Constable and Co., 1925), 166–68.

4 S. E. Finer, *The Life and Times of Sir Edwin Chadwick* (London: Methuen, 1952), 451, 501; cf. R. A. Lewis, *Edwin Chadwick and the Public Health Movement, 1832–1854* (London: Longmans, Green, 1952), 181, 328–29; Oliver MacDonagh, *Early Victorian Government, 1830–1870* (London: Weidenfeld and Nicolson, 1977), 141, 150. Finer, 483, for example, calls the main anti-Chadwick polemic, the anonymous *Engineers and Officials,* "a scurrilous pamphlet. . . . A travesty, written with every violence of expression and with an evident dishonesty of purpose." This is a book of more than two hundred pages, well researched, and by no means uniformly critical of Chadwick *(Engineers and Officials: An Historical Sketch of the "Health of Towns Works" (Between 1838 and 1856) in London and the Provinces, with Biographical Notes on Lord Palmerston, the Earl of Shaftesbury, Lord Ebrington, Edwin Chadwick, F. O. Ward, John Thwaites* [London: Edward Stanford, 1856]). Chadwick's successor, John Simon, did not agree with Finer and Lewis; he saw Chadwick's General Board of Health as "far too unconditional and dogmatic." It failed to "distinguish between opinions and knowledge, and was imperatively pressing large rules of practice, and seeking from Parliament new powers of coercion, in cases where lessons of experience were still wanting" *(English Sanitary Institutions, Reviewed in Their Course of Development, and in Some of Their Political and Social Relations* [London: Cassell and Co., 1890], 225, 228–29).

5 On these questions see Finer, *Chadwick,* 390–411; Lewis, *Chadwick,* 261–74.

engineers, and the dogs of vestrydom – were no longer nipping at his heels but biting deep and drawing blood.

There were many glad to see Chadwick go. Botched initiatives didn't help. But they, and the anticentralization tirades of country squires, would not alone have toppled the board. Its fate was tied to its technologies. The question was not simply whether these worked, but what it meant to say that they worked, and who had the power to decide.[6] In short, Chadwick's approach depended on acceptance of his philosophy of technology, which was more than a philosophy of state growth.

To the degree there was such a thing, the guardians of technological possibility were the civil engineers. They and Chadwick should have gotten on famously. Engineering is, after all, the most utilitarian of the professions, "greatest good at least cost" its central precept. Underlying sanitary reform was the idea of "the city as a natural system," as Davison puts it, and this too was an engineering concept: the city was a machine that performed more or less well.[7] Beyond that, they stood to profit more directly than anyone else. The engineer's fee was 5 percent of the cost of works; surely they would have been enthusiastic about getting works built. Indeed, in the summer of 1844, as engineers roamed the country to harvest the projects stimulated by the Health of Towns Commission, the water engineer Thomas Hawksley wrote to Chadwick, "Pray keep the pace up."[8]

But on several technical issues Chadwick found himself in deep disagreement with the civil engineers: on the practicality of constant high-pressure water and sewage recycling and most importantly on the relative merits of large-diameter brick sewers versus small-diameter earthenware pipe sewers, the "pipe-and-brick sewer war" of the early 1850s. With the exception of sewage recycling, historians have tended to see these questions as illegitimately contested. They have suggested that engineers were resistant to innovation, jealous of an outsider who knew their business better than they, embarrassed that their solutions cost more and worked less well than Chadwick's; further, that the engineers and the venal politicians who fed on their authority were guilty of magnifying small failures in hopes of returning to their old practices and pelf, which included building vast underground sewer-gas generators – sewers of "vicious construction," Chadwick called them.[9] Thus Finer writes that their criticism of Chadwickian technology "came as manna to the lead-

---

6 *Hansard's Parliamentary Debates 3rd series, 134,* 1854, 1300, 1309; *135,* 1854, 978, 983–84, 1347–48.

7 G. Davison, "The City as a Natural System: Theories of Urban Society in Early Nineteenth-Century Britain," *The Pursuit of Urban History,* eds. D. Fraser and A. Sutcliffe, 349–70 (London: E Arnold, 1983).

8 Hawksley to Chadwick, undated, c. early October 1844, UCL Chadwick Papers #960.

9 General Board of Health, "Minutes of Information Collected with Reference to Works for the Removal of Soil Water or Drainage of Dwelling Houses and for the Sewerage and Cleansing of the Sites of Towns," *P.P.,* 1852, *19,* [1535.], 29 [to be cited as GBH, "Minutes on House Drainage"].

erless, discontented cottage ratepayers and slum-owners . . . [who] could emerge from their odium to claim that they were . . . not the 'dirty party' but 'the efficiency party.' "[10] Following this line, the most charitable view of the engineers is as semiliterate technicians, barely competent to carry out Chadwick's reforms, and then only after much coercion and persuasion, and grumbling all the while.

But many of those who opposed Chadwick were neither pretenders, rogues, nor fools – people like Thomas Hawksley, who built waterworks in more than one hundred British towns, and Joseph Bazalgette, builder of greater London's main drainage and long-time chief engineer of the Metropolitan Board of Works.[11] Their record in sanitary public works far outstrips that of any of Chadwick's loyalists. Chadwick's controversy with the engineers is more fruitfully seen as one of conflicting technological styles. Engineers shared Chadwick's goal of well drained towns but had different ideas about design, expertise, and the social role of the engineer. Their response was not one of opposition to efficiency, cheapness, or the state, but only to Chadwick's dogmatic advocacy of ideal and finely tuned sanitary systems. Their argument may be summarized in three statements: first, there was no point in worrying about perfect sanitary systems because one would never be in the position of building one. Second, one should think not of principles and dogmas, but of adapting of tools to situations. Third, the "right" solution was right for the client; there was no single right answer.[12] None of this made sense to Chadwick's master-planner mind – it all seemed equivocation. Unable to communicate effectively with them, he became suspicious, hostile, and

10 Finer, *Chadwick*, 440, 451–52; see Lewis, *Chadwick*, 90. Cf. Henry Austin, "Further Report from the Consulting Engineer to the General Board of Health on the Croydon Drainage," *P.P.*, 1852, *96*, (1009.), 5–6 [to be cited as "Further Report on Croydon"].

11 Lewis, *Chadwick*, 352–53. On Hawksley see G. M. Binnie, *Early Victorian Water Engineers* (London: Thomas Telford, 1981), 14–30; "Memoir of Thomas Hawksley," *Minutes of Proceedings, Institution of Civil Engineers 117* (1893): 364–76. On Bazalgette see G. C. Clifton, "The Staff of the Metropolitan Board of Works: 1855–1889: The Development of a Professional Local Government Bureaucracy," (Ph.D. diss., London School of Economics, 1986).

12 Early Victorian engineers are sometimes presented as hostile to state growth. Finer, for example, finds them "intensely individualistic even for an individualistic age" and adds that "in their ruthless eruptive animal energy, the engineers showed a swashbuckling disdain for the social evils around them" (Finer, *Chadwick*, 439–40). They did tend to think in terms of the demands of clients rather than abstract notions of public good. Their purported opposition to state regulation was, at least in some cases, a concern about the qualifications of the regulators more than the idea of regulation. Robert Stephenson's remarks on railroad regulation are not dissimilar to Chadwick's on sanitary works: "The extraordinary feature of the Parliamentary legislation and practice consists in the anomalies, incongruities, irreconcilabilities, and absurdities." Such "inexperienced tribunals" should give way to "a commission . . . of practical men of acknowledged . . . ability. . . . What we ask is knowledge. 'Give us,' we say, 'a tribunal competent to form a sound opinion. Let it . . . judge of the desirability of all initiatory measures . . . delegate to it the power of enforcing such regulations . . . devolve on it the duty of consolidating . . . [the] laws, and of making such amendments therein, as the public interest . . . may require . . . all we ask, is that it shall be a tribunal that is impartial, and that is thoroughly informed.' " Stephenson, "President's Address," *Minutes of Proceedings, Institution of Civil Engineers 15* (1855–56): 136.

ever more doctrinaire. That is the reason to call this a tragedy, for it need not have turned out that way.


I

The Westminster engineers with whom Chadwick battled in the early 1850s were an elite. Their home was the Institution of Civil Engineers, founded in 1818 by four student engineers, kept alive by Thomas Telford's willingness to accept the presidency. It was located in Great George Street, Westminster, across from Parliament because the bulk of an engineer's work came from schemes requiring private bills. Even in their early days the civils had seen themselves as sanitary engineers. The "removing [of] noxious accumulations as by the drainage of towns and districts to prevent the formation of malaria, and secure the public health," was one of the missions in their 1827 charter.[13] By the 1850s several had experience in water supply, somewhat fewer in large-scale town sewering.[14]

They were a touchy bunch. Many came from humble backgrounds and were self-educated. Early Victorian engineering held enormous possibilities for social mobility. George Stephenson, illiterate collier, died a landed gent. They scorned higher mathematics, formal training, and professional certification, all characteristics of French civil engineering, which they despised (and Chadwick revered). Rule-of-thumb algorithms were preferred to physical theory; what you built mattered; whether you were a calculus whiz was moot.[15] While the works they built were reason enough for pride, their mode of work encouraged arrogance: they made their livings selling confidence to investors and parliamentary committees.

Early on Chadwick had been uncharacteristically respectful of engineers. In the *Sanitary Report* he had ridiculed illiterate and poorly trained parish and sewers commission surveyors, but to the truly scientific engineer he offered a vast field of profitable activity. There was to be a whole new civil service of

---

13  C. M. Norrie, *Bridging the Years: A Short History of British Civil Engineering* (London: Arnold, 1956), 50. On the structure of the British engineering profession see Gareth Watson, *The Civils: The Story of the Institution of Civil Engineers* (London: Thomas Telford, 1988); F. R. Conder, *The Men Who Built the Railways; a Reprint of F. R. Conder's Personal Recollections of English Engineers*, ed. Jack Simmons (London: Thomas Telford, 1983); *The Education and Status of Civil Engineers, in the U.K. and in Foreign Countries, Compiled from Documents Supplied to the Council of the Institution of Civil Engineers* (London: Institution of Civil Engineers, 1870); R. A. Buchanan, "Engineers and Government in Nineteenth Century Britain," *Government and Expertise: Specialists, Administrators, and Professionals, 1860–1919*, ed. Roy M. MacLeod, 41–58 (Cambridge: Cambridge University Press, 1988).

14  The elder Rennie had prepared sewerage plans for Liverpool and for Westminster in 1807–9. In most respects his design principles were the same as Chadwick's: good gradients and rapid flow. Greater London Record Office, Archives of the Westminster Commission of Sewers, WCS 873 [to be cited as GLRO, WCS], reports 1807–8 by John Rennie.

15  Hawksley to Chadwick, undated 1845, UCL Chadwick Papers #960.

regional engineers who would improve health, augment prosperity, and settle squabbles about drainage works. They, not the doctors, would have the central place in sanitation. "The great preventives," he wrote in the *Sanitary Report*, "are operations for which aid must be sought from the science of the civil engineer, not from the physician."[16]

That harmony persisted through the Health of Towns Commission despite the unpleasantness with Robert Stephenson over the viability of constant-service water. As promoter of the Towns Improvement Company during those years, Chadwick was trying to raise capital for a massive campaign of public works. If it worked, he would become the clearinghouse for engineering employment on a vast scale. Some engineers looked to Chadwick as a patron, a role he was quite happy to play. In mid-1844, he mentioned to Thomas Hawksley that he was urging Glasgow to consult Hawksley on its water. He wrote to Hawksley's competitor, J. F. Bateman, that he was urging Manchester to consult Bateman, though he could do so more enthusiastically were Bateman to bone up on sanitation. Both were asked to experiment with flow through pipes, though Chadwick could not promise to pay for the experiments.[17] There was something here for all: for Chadwick success as a company promoter, for young engineers international reputations as pioneers in a new field. If there was less enthusiasm than one might think, this was because many were already employed on railroads and others were Chadwick's competitors. But there was no sense of conflict between the profession's interests and Chadwick's sanitation.

But by mid-1845 strains had developed. Chadwick's patronage had turned out to be unimportant – he could not deliver work to those he favored; they found they could get commissions without him. He also failed to realize that engineers served clients; they did not command them.

All this is manifest in Chadwick's worsening relations with the young Nottingham water engineer Thomas Hawksley.[18] Hawksley was living proof of the feasibility of constant-service water. The system he had built in Nottingham was cheap and worked well. In the summer of 1844 Chadwick had invited Hawksley to associate himself with the new Towns Improvement Company he was launching. It would build combined sanitary works (mainly, it seemed at first, in Continental towns). For Chadwick the rationale for combined works was as much economic advantage as adequate sanitation.

---

16 Edwin Chadwick, *Report on the Sanitary Condition of the Labouring Population of Great Britain*, ed. M. W. Flinn (Edinburgh: Edinburgh University Press, 1965) [to be cited as Chadwick, *Sanitary Report*], 393, 396.

17 William Lindley to Chadwick, October 1842–February 1844; UCL Chadwick Papers #1235; Chadwick to Thomas Hawksley, 5, 9 July 1844, UCL Chadwick Papers #2181/5; Chadwick to J. F. Bateman, 16 September 1844, UCL Chadwick Papers #2181/4.

18 Anthony Brundage, *England's "Prussian Minister": Edwin Chadwick and the Politics of Government Growth, 1832–1854* (University Park: Penn State University Press, 1987), 101–12; Lewis, *Chadwick*, 120–21; Binnie, *Early Victorian Water Engineers*, 14–30.

With one company supplying all services, one could pave roads with the waste tar from gas manufacture, and so forth.[19] Hawksley was willing, and together they joined the other circumambulating engineers seeking customers. Having failed at Paris and Lyons, they looked to midsized English towns: Leicester, Lancaster, Bristol, Exeter, and Derby. They had no charter, no capital, only promises and a list of directors. Chadwick himself was paying most of the expenses.[20]

A year and a half with no contracts convinced Hawksley that combined works did not appeal. The profitability of sewage irrigation was unproved and there was little enthusiasm for constant-service water.[21] Despite Chadwick's protests that he was as ruthless as any of them, canny northern men of business saw the company as do-gooders playing at capitalism, and they were right. The technologies Chadwick was selling were to be profitable but something else – order, control, harmony, even health – underlay them. The reasons they wanted water and drains, like protecting Liverpool warehouses from fire and making sure that the streets to them were passable, weren't good enough for Chadwick. And however much Chadwick claimed Hawksley's reputation would soar through a connection with the Health of Towns Commission, Hawksley did not need him or it.[22]

In autumn 1845, as the deadline approached for towns to lodge private bills for public works projects, their diverging ideas of the engineer's role led to a clash and then a split. To be taken seriously they needed money for surveys, Hawksley told Chadwick, but there was none.[23] A few weeks later, when Hawksley accepted a retainer from a Preston water company, Chadwick challenged him to stand firm for sanitary truth. The Preston plan (waterworks without drainage) was another of those projects for "carrying out singly and separately" works that promised "immediate profit" regardless of "future convenience." To accept such a project would be hypocrisy; their enemies would rejoice. A month later he commanded Hawksley to sever the connection on the grounds of his obligation to the Towns Improvement Company.[24]

But what was hypocrisy to Chadwick was to Hawksley work "of a profitable and reputable character." He was a water engineer, these people wanted water, and he would work within the limitations the client outlined. In the

19  Chadwick to Thomas Hawksley, 11 August, 19 September, 16 November 1844, UCL Chadwick Papers #2181/4, 5.
20  Chadwick to Thomas Hawksley, 27 February, 5 July 1845, UCL Chadwick Papers #2181/7, 11; Chadwick to John Easthope, 31 October 1844, UCL Chadwick Papers #2181/8; Lewis, *Edwin Chadwick*, 117–20.
21  Chadwick to Thomas Hawksley, 25 May 1845, UCL Chadwick Papers #2181/9.
22  Chadwick to Hawksley, 10, 12 July 1845, UCL Chadwick Papers #2181/11; Hawksley to Chadwick, 11 July 1845, UCL Chadwick Papers #960.
23  Hawksley to Chadwick, 5 August 1845, UCL Chadwick Papers #960.
24  Chadwick to Thomas Hawksley, 31 August, 26 September 1845, UCL Chadwick Papers #2181/ 11, 13.

next few months Hawksley took command of the relationship. He had better connections and more sensitivity to local politics than Chadwick. There were places that did want water and sewerage and might accept sewage irrigation too. But the Manchester water promoters, "keen sensible and active minded," must "see their way clearly before they embark in a speculation; I therefore recommend to you not to complicate the water supply in *this instance* with sewage." Likewise with Leicester: Chadwick's estimates of irrigation profits were too bold; better to drop that for now. And Chadwick must make sure to offer plenty of local control.[25]

Chadwick did not heed the advice and in January Leicester engaged Hawksley privately to supply water. Chadwick saw this as "treachery," personally and intellectually. He was deeply hurt, was a great hater, and never reconciled with Hawksley. He began to see engineering as a trade of merchants in evidence who would support any project if the fee were right. Hawksley, who appreciated that civil engineering was a world of shifting coalitions, was willing to go on if Chadwick would accept that larger towns, perhaps for reasons of politics and patronage, were unlikely to want combined works and that an engineer's duty to a client was higher than that to a company or an ideal. But he would not commit his career to promoting an unpopular and possibly unrealistic technological dream. Given that, he would happily speak on Chadwick's behalf "to the many capitalists with whom I am connected."[26]

It was indeed a dispute about integrity, but whose? Chadwick's was an integrity of principle. You adopted right principles, stuck to them, moved heaven and earth and sewage to make the world conform. Hawksley's was an integrity based in trust: someone trusted you to look after his interests. To trade those interests for a vague vision of a better tomorrow was a betrayal. Still, bad relations with Hawksley did not mean bad relations with engineers generally. Well into 1848 most engineers were favorable to sanitary reform. The engineering press praised Roe's egg-shaped sewers and was happy to see passage of the Public Health Act.[27]

The break began in autumn 1847. The Poor Law Commission collapsed

25 Hawksley to Chadwick, 29 September, 5, 16, 17, 23, 26 October 1845; 14 January 1846, UCL Chadwick Papers #960.
26 Chadwick to Robert Slaney, 6 September 1845, UCL Chadwick Papers #2181/11; to P. H. Holland, 26 January 1846, UCL Chadwick Papers #2181/14; Hawksley to P. H. Holland, 8 February 1846, UCL Chadwick Papers #960. For Chadwick's reflections see General Board of Health, "Report from the General Board of Health on the Administration of the Public Health Act and the Nuisances Removal and Diseases Prevention Acts from 1848 to 1854, with Appendix," *P.P.*, 1854, *35*, [1768.], 25 [to be cited as GBH, "Report of 1854"].
27 Braithwaite, Wicksteed, and Walker in discussion of James Green, "The Sewerage of Bristol," *Minutes of Proceedings, Institution of Civil Engineers* 7 (1848): 101–7; "Sanitary Laws at Home and Abroad," *Civil Engineer and Architects Journal* 11 (1848): 252–54; Playfair, "Report on the Sanitary Condition of Large Towns in Lancashire," Royal Commission on the Health of Towns and Populous Districts, *Second Report, P.P.*, 1845, *18*, [610.], Appendix, pt. 2, 8. The chief anti-Chadwick polemic, *Engineers and Officials*, 44–47, also saw a consensus until 1847.

just as the new sanitary institutions were blossoming. Within the year Chadwick had three new bases of power. Besides the General Board of Health, from which he could steer adopting towns to follow his proposals, he was effectively in charge of the sanitation of London. Both Lincoln and Morpeth had omitted London from their public health bills, ostensibly on the grounds that a law for midsized market towns would not work for a vast city, but in fact to avoid opposition from the powerful City of London Corporation. They had been much criticized for this cowardice (or prudence) and the 1848 bill passed only with promises that London would soon be dealt with. To begin the process, the government appointed a five-member Metropolitan Sanitary Commission, whose not so secret mission was to manufacture the authority needed to disband the older sewers commissions. Its three most active members were Chadwick, Southwood Smith, and the former Health of Towns commissioner Richard Owen. As well as this investigatory body, it also established an executive authority, the twenty-two-member consolidated Metropolitan Sewers Commission, chaired by Morpeth and dominated by Chadwick and his experts. His two sewerage theorists, John Roe and now John Phillips, became its chief surveyors, while the engineer Henry Austin, former secretary to the Health of Towns Association (and future secretary to the General Board of Health), served as consulting engineer in a loose supervisory capacity. Though the Sanitary Commission finished its work in late 1848, and Chadwick lost control of the Metropolitan Sewers Commission in October 1849 (as a result of lack of progress and factional strife, the commissioners, including Chadwick, were recalled and replaced with a new body unlinked to the factions), these institutions, with the Board of Health, constituted a nucleus of authority that rivaled the Institution of Civil Engineers.[28]

The Sanitary Commission's main strategy was the old one of denouncing the sewers commissions, particularly their inability to deal with the coming cholera.[29] But Chadwick painted with a broad brush. The true laws of sanitation were so well known and widely disseminated that "well-informed minds earnestly directed toward the attainment of the object" would not fail to follow them. Sewers built in defiance of them harmed health and wasted money. He insinuated that engineers, paid on commission, systematically overbuilt. Citing Joseph Gwilt's claim that a cabbage stalk could decompose in a large sewer without harming health, he would claim that engineers were unconcerned with health. Finally, sewer building was to be seen as an arcane

---

28  Finer, *Chadwick*, 356–78; Lewis, *Chadwick*, 216–237; [Metropolitan Sanitary Commission], *Register of Papers, Health of Towns Commission*, undated, Public Record Office [PRO], HO 45/416.

29  Behind the scenes Chadwick was reassuring the clerks and surveyors of the old commissions that work could be found for them if they were willing to adopt the new technical and administrative practices. "All they want is emancipation and security to induce them to work well with us." Chadwick to Morpeth, 3, 4, 5 August 1847, UCL Chadwick Papers #1055. He would later conclude that he had been overly sanguine.

specialty. It was beyond the competence "of ordinary professional engineering and architectural practice," and also that of "popular administrative bodies."[30]

Meanwhile, at the Metropolitan Sewers Commission a team of surveyors was having a field day uncovering the absurdities of past sewerage. They found plenty to horrify the press, lines of sewer of "of all shapes and sizes, from squares nearly to circles, and . . . various modifications and combinations of these forms, differing greatly in very short distances, that of the outfall being frequently one of the smallest parts, – they are generally without artificial bottoms, – the sides, in parts, are built upon or supported by piles, which project to a great extent." Gradients were often "from, instead of to, the outfall." In them were "pits or cesspools" filled with "dead dogs and cats, offal from slaughter houses, vegetable refuse, stable dung, privy soil, ashes, tin kettles and pans, broken stone-ware, as jars, pitchers, etc.; bricks, pieces of wood, etc.," in deposits up to three feet deep.[31] Surely someone must be responsible for such a state of things, and it was easy enough to see that someone as private practice engineers. A president of the Institution of Civil Engineers had endorsed flat-bottomed sewers, Chadwick had already triumphantly announced.[32]

At the General Board of Health a year later, Chadwick confronted the same resistance to comprehensive change that he had met in promoting the Towns Improvement Company. People felt safer with little bits of sanitation and more trusting of traditional engineers who did not assault them with sanitary sermons. On the one hand Chadwick met such concerns by making clear that what was needed was novel and outside the scope of customary practice: "an entirely new system of sewerage . . . combined with a new system of house drainage, with a new system of water supply, and with a new system of removing and applying the refuse of towns to agricultural production." On the other, he reassured ratepayers that caution was no longer necessary. Their resistance to sanitary works was understandable: they had so often been the victims of old style engineers. But under the GBH there would be no cost overruns. Chadwick was in a stronger position than in 1845. Loan requests from adopting towns crossed his desk; his inspectors were loyal to combined

30 Metropolitan Sanitary Commission, *First Report, P.P.*, 1847, *32*, [888.], 2, 24–25, 39–42, 49, 51; "Report by the General Board of Health on the Measures Adopted for the Execution of the Nuisances Removal and Diseases Prevention Act, and the Public Health Act up to July 1849," *P.P.*, 1849, *24*, [1115.], 63 [to be cited as GBH, "Report of 1849"]; GBH, "Minutes on House Drainage," 36.

31 T. Lovick and J. L. Hale, "Report on the State of Sewers in the Surrey and Kent District, near Borough," *Times,* 7 August 1848, 8f.

32 "Metropolitan Commission of Sewers," *Times,* 14 January 1848, 3; 28 January 1848, 3; 3 February 1848, 4. The president was Telford's successor, James Walker (Metropolitan Sanitary Commission, *First Report*, Evidence, 36, 41); for Walker's response see discussion of James Green, "The Sewerage of Bristol," *Minutes of Proceedings, Institution of Civil Engineers 7* (1848), 105. By contrast, Roe credited Walker with having recognized the desirability of curved-sided sewers (*Sanitary Report*, Appendix 1, 373).

works and eligible to undertake as private engineers the projects they approved as inspectors. The frugal ratepayer would see the economy of employing the inspector who had already done the preliminary work.[33]

In its first annual report the board warned Great George Street what to expect from the inspectors. In the case of a town that already had plans for sanitary works, the inspector was to ignore them until he had determined "the applicability of established [Chadwickian] principles." The inspector would be accountable for any "delay and expense in the examination of plans which *prima facie* are erroneous in principle."[34] As late as 1854 he was still defending private practice for inspectors: no one else was competent.[35]

The tactics worked. By a mix of inspectorial vetoes and promises that they had a cheaper and better product than orthodox engineers, the inspectors won a significant amount of business. Chadwick was surely delighted when Hawksley complained that "able professional men are wrongfully injured . . . for the gain of Government Inspectors."[36]

## II

The basis of Chadwick's campaign was to be a new science of hydraulics that would open up unrecognized possibilities in economical sewerage design. "The new systems . . . are as distinct from the old works, as old roads on the best engineering construction, differ from railways," he wrote in 1854.[37] To understand the sewerage doctrines Chadwick was espousing is no easy matter. "Correct principles" kept changing, nor was there unanimity among Chadwick and his associates at any given time. Only in 1854 was there clearly an "arterial–venous" system of town drainage, with a steam engine as a heart, veins distributing sewage to the countryside, and arteries returning water to the town.[38] There were also disagreements about priority in design, one of

33  GBH, "Report of 1849," 54–56, 64–65.
34  "Instructions of the General Board of Health to the Superintending Inspectors," in GBH, "Report of 1849," 132–34.
35  On the inspectors see GBH, "Report of 1854," 45–46. Austin disagreed ("Further Report on Croydon," 10–11).
36  Thomas Hawksley, *Letter to the Most Hon. Marquis of Chandros, M.P., in Relation to the Exercise of Some of the Most Extraordinary Powers Assumed by the General Board of Health and the Superintending Inspectors to the Great Grimsby Improvement Bill* ([London]: 1854), 7; idem, in discussion of James Leslie, "Observations on the Flow of Water through Pipes, Conduits, and Orifices," *Minutes of Proceedings, Institution of Civil Engineers 14* (1854): 295. This was an important issue in Parliament's consideration of the board in 1854 (*Hansard's Parliamentary Debates 3rd series, 134,* 1854, 1299–1300; *135,* 1854, 991–93).
37  GBH, "Report of 1854," 45.
38  The clearest version is from F. O. Ward, a surgeon, publicist, and politician, presented to a Sanitary Congress in Brussels in September 1856. Ward drew explicitly on Harvey, speaking of the analogues of the heart (a steam engine) and of blood (water, "our *liquid* food"). See "Circulation or Stagnation" in *Circulation or Stagnation, Being a Translation of a Paper by F. O. Ward Read at the Sanitary Congress Held at Brussels in 1856 On the Arterial and Venous System for the Sanitation of Towns,*

the main reasons for the fall of the Chadwick-dominated consolidated Sewers Commission in 1849. Some argued that if sewage recycling were to be taken seriously it was essential to decide how it was to be done before one could determine where the sewers were to go. Chadwick would start with house drains and street sewers, mainly because it was the easiest place to start. Others argued that designing a *system* of sewers required knowing how much water could be relied upon to flow through them. Their priority was to control the water supply.[39]

But before any sanitary works could begin, even before plans could be approved, a town had to be surveyed on a large scale (i.e., five to ten feet to the mile). If in retrospect this seems an obvious thing to do, it was not so obvious for a local authority possessing minimal borrowing powers and building sewers bit by bit: at most one needed levels for the street being sewered.[40] Only when one began to think of *systems* of works did surveys become vital; without one there was no way to coordinate sewers, to make branches join mains at proper angles and levels.[41] Surveys were unpopular in towns adopting the Public Health Act: full of enthusiasm for sanitation, the new boards were being asked to devote their money, and worse, their time, to an intangible. The Barnard Castle Local Board, one of the first, complained until it convinced the inspector, William Ranger (who was also its engineer), to persuade the General Board to waive the requirement of a survey (on the grounds that a refusal would lead to the election of a board uninterested in sanitation).[42]

Ideally, a system of sanitary works required public control of the water supply and some means of recycling the sewage, preferably by irrigation. In practice both were optional, the former because the water companies had been able in 1848 to block proposals to make water a fully public service, the latter because there was no well tried and widely applicable means of sewage

with a Statement of the Progress Made for Its Completion Since Then by Sir Edwin Chadwick, Formerly Chief Executive Officer of the First General Board of Health (London: Cassell and Co., 1889), 11–17. For an earlier instance (April 1853) see C. Fowler in discussion of John Thornehill Harrison, "On the Drainage of the District, South of the Thames," *Minutes of Proceedings, Institution of Civil Engineers 13* (1853): 107: "Thus the water being pumped into the town, and becoming charged with organic matter, would be pumped back into the country, to fulfill its proper purpose of reproduction." "In both instances [city and body] Nature would work by a principle of circulation to support and sustain life, in perpetual succession."

39 *Times*, 21 July 1849, 6b; 24 July 1849, 8d; 27 July 1849, 6f; 30 July 1849, 3b; 31 July 1849, 7c; 4 August 1849, 4e; 24 September 1849, 3f; 28 September 1849, 5b; 4 October 1849, 6c; 20 October 1849, 4e. Cf. Metropolitan Sanitary Commission, *First Report,* 25, 39–40, 49, Evidence, 61.

40 Metropolitan Sanitary Commission, *First Report*, 44.

41 As John Phillips put it, without a survey "it is impossible to put sewers in such positions so that they may join together hereafter as part of a complete system. . . . Without such a plan . . . the arrangement of the sewers must be guesswork" and "an absolute waste of money." Phillips, Metropolitan Sanitary Commission, *First Report*, Evidence, 61–62.

42 Barnard Castle Local Board to General Board of Health [GBH], 31 August, 6 November, and undated 1850; Ranger to GBH, 22 February 1851, *Barnard Castle-GBH Correspondence*, PRO MH 13/15.

recycling. Otherwise, the most conspicuous and controversial part of Chadwickian doctrine was "tubular drainage." This, "the second revolution" in sewerage, had come along only in the beginning of 1848 (hence the disingenuousness of "correct principles" long known).[43] But by 1849 Chadwick was assuring the inspectors that "it may be taken as demonstrated that such removal [of waste water from houses] may be best effected by means of impermeable tubular drains, which will allow of no escape of noxious gases; and from the comparative smoothness, and the better adaptation of forms and concentration of the stream, will allow of the best scour and consequently the least deposit."[44]

The "first revolution" had been that of John Roe, who had been Chadwick's exemplary sewerage engineer from 1842 to 1847. Roe had been appointed surveyor to the Holborn and Finsbury Commission of Sewers in 1838, having served for seven years as clerk of works. He was grammar school–educated, self-taught in engineering. He favored egg-shaped brick sewers. They were strong and unlikely to clog since the increased velocity produced by pinching the sides would keep sediment suspended. He held that sewer junctions should be made on a tangent since right-angled junctions caused turbulence and, consequently, deposition. Most importantly, he had developed a simple means for the hydraulic flushing of sewers. An operator would accumulate a head of water behind a board dam; when released, this water would rush down, scouring the sewer. Costly manual cleaning would no longer be needed.[45]

By late 1847, John Phillips, a former bricklayer who had been elected surveyor to the Westminster Commission in 1846 by one vote, had superseded Roe. The two were very different. Roe was modest, practical, uncomfortable with doctrine, and he got on well with orthodox engineers. Phillips was an arrogant, mercurial theorist. Like Chadwick he made enemies easily and could not conceive any legitimate disagreement with his views. His complaints about the Westminster Commission echo Chadwick's frustrations with the PLC. "Power to do things properly . . . is taken from me, or rather has never been given to me. One is obliged to act by rules . . . highly unscientific and prejudicial" – all to swell the profits of builders.[46]

Phillips offered two new ideas: first, that one could substitute significantly smaller earthenware pipes for Roe's small oval brick sewers; second, that Roe's flushing gates could be done away with, since a proper system of sewers would

43 General Board of Health, *Report on the Supply of Water to the Metropolis,* Appendix II, *Engineering Reports and Evidence,* P.P., 1850, 22, [1282.], 113–15.

44 "Instructions of the General Board of Health to the Superintending Inspectors," 130.

45 Royal Commission on the Health of Towns and Populous Districts, *First Report,* P.P., 1844, 17, [572.] [to be cited as HOT, *First Report*], Evidence, qq 108–72, 369–95, 807, 1075–1113, 1748–1940, 2094–2130, 4480–4528, 5345, 5423–46, 5827–46. On Roe, see *Minutes of Proceedings, Institution of Civil Engineers 39* (1874–75): 297–98.

46 John Phillips, Metropolitan Sanitary Commission, *First Report,* Evidence, 42–45, 73.

flush itself continually; sediment would never accumulate. Chadwick had long been intrigued with pipes; they could cut drainage costs by more than half. At his suggestion Roe had experimented with them in 1842. By 1847 they were being used in Manchester, and even in London by some of the unregenerate surveyors of the old sewers commissions.[47] But no one was looking to pipes as *the* answer. Pipes might clog; it would be imprudent to dispense with flushing entirely, Roe felt. Moreover, most agreed that at somewhere around a foot in diameter, brick became cheaper than pipe, especially when quality and durability were considered.[48]

At issue then was not the use of pipes but the conviction that one could engineer cheap and elegant *systems* of pipe sewerage. Phillips's dream was a network of converging and diverging small-bore sewers. Having flushed a high-level sewer, water would flow into a lateral collector which would distribute it to the next level of local sewers, to be collected again and perhaps flush several small sewers before reaching the outfall. This constant flow at constant velocity would end all accumulation.[49]

What Chadwick took from Phillips was not the complicated convergings and divergings but the idea of a cheap self-cleaning system. The reason for rejecting pipes had been that they were impossible to clean, since they were too small for someone to crawl into. Self-cleaning eliminated that problem. And small meant cheap: the other great objection to existing sewerage practice was that sewers were "so very expensive, as to offer very formidable obstructions to the extensive voluntary adoption of works of sanitary improvement." Chadwick downplayed Phillips's warning that without control of the water supply, it was imperative to build sewers big enough for human entry.[50]

Since they would be self-cleaning, pipe sewers could be small. But how small? In part this was a question of use. Should sewers accommodate surface drainage and rainfall or just sanitary sewage? If the former, should one plan for two inches of rain per hour or per day? In general, Chadwick would suggest that surface drainage must be accommodated by other means, perhaps by old sewers. But as we shall see, he also tried to demonstrate a much greater discharge from small-bore sewers than anyone had suspected.[51]

Phillips also believed that pipe sewerage would solve the sewer ventilation problem. As early as 1834 Parliament had addressed the question of what could be done about the offensive, if not deadly, eructations that rose from seething

47 GBH, "Minutes on House Drainage," 37; Beriah Drew, Joseph Gwilt, E. D'Ianson, J. Newman, John Roe, J. Billing, Metropolitan Sanitary Commission, *First Report*, Evidence, 88–89, 102, 106, 115, 155–56, 186–88.
48 J. Roe, J. Gwilt, J. Newman, Metropolitan Sanitary Commission, *First Report*, Evidence, 82–84, 99, 116; Edward Gotto, John Grant in GBH, *Report on the Supply of Water to the Metropolis*, Appendix II, *Engineering Reports and Evidence*, 135–36, 156.
49 John Phillips, Metropolitan Sanitary Commission, *First Report*, Evidence, 45, 49–52.
50 Ibid., 49–51; GBH, "Minutes on House Drainage," 62.
51 GBH, "Minutes on House Drainage," 14, 62.

vats of sewage into houses and streets.[52] Phillips's answer was downward ventilation. The continuous rush of sewage would draw off the bad gases – ideally,
of course, there would be no gas since the sewage would be at the outfall
before it could decompose.[53] No longer would sleepers inhale "disease and
death" in the "foul air from the sewers, drains, and cesspools." Cholera would
vanish.

A final element of Chadwick's sewerage doctrine was "combined back
drainage": collecting the drainage of several dwellings in a pipe that ran between the backs of houses on adjoining parallel streets. It was a substitute for
running a drain beneath each house to a main sewer in the street. It was
cheaper than orthodox house drainage and probably safer, in eliminating the
potential for sewer gas seeping into one's living quarters.[54] The objection was
that it required neighborly cooperation. Those at the head of the drain would
suffer from any blocks caused by downstream neighbors. Chadwick insisted
the sewers would not clog – theory and experiment said so. But even if they
did and had to be replaced yearly, that would be better than suffering the
effects of "large drains, detaining and spreading deposits, and facilitating decomposition within the walls and beneath the floors of . . . dwellings."[55]

What was most controversial in the early 1850s was not the proposals themselves so much as the knowledge that warranted their use. Should one look
to science or practical experience to solve sewerage problems? In 1847, with
his new power bases, the sanitary and sewers commissions, Chadwick sought
to finish the job of establishing the technical details of sanitation. A great deal
of the Sanitary Commission's first report dealt with the applicability of hydraulic theory to sewer design. Despite pages bristling with equations, the
commission decided that it was not applicable. According to Austin, the use
of formulae in town drainage led "almost invariably" to error. There were
problems of scaling up, and little understanding of the effects of friction, or
turbulence, or additional inputs. What was needed was a massive research
program on flow through pipes.[56]

Austin thought the Royal Engineers or the new College of Engineering at

52 "Select Committee on Metropolis Sewers," *P.P.*, 1834, 15, (584.); Beriah Drew, Metropolitan
Sanitary Commission, *First Report*, Evidence, 88–89.
53 Phillips, Metropolitan Sanitary Commission, *First Report*, Evidence, 45, 69; Rawlinson, "The
Drainage of Towns," *Minutes of Proceedings, Institution of Civil Engineers* 12 (1852): 39.
54 GBH, "Minutes on House Drainage," 42–43, 126–27, 136.
55 Ibid., 36.
56 See its highly technical charge: Metropolitan Sanitary Commission, *First Report*, iii, 1. Also Henry
Austin, John Phillips, ibid., Evidence, 127–28, 53. The Health of Towns Commission had been
more sanguine about the use of theory. Asked whether these "theoretical deductions" were "confirmed by practice," Butler Williams of the Putney College of Civil Engineering replied, "These
direct and necessary conclusions of the application of theoretical investigation . . . [were] fully
confirmed by experience." HOT, *First Report*, Evidence, qq 5827–5935; see also qq 369–95, 807–
48, 1071–1116, 2090–2130.

Putney might do this, but Chadwick arranged for it to be done by a Trial Works Committee of the Metropolitan Sewers Commission. Roe designed a series of experiments to determine discharge in tubes of various diameters laid at various gradients and with variously arranged inputs. This was not random empiricism; two hypotheses for increasing flow rate had emerged from the Sanitary Commission's theoretical explorations. First, both Roe and Phillips stressed that velocity increased with depth so sewage would flow faster in a narrow channel than in a broad one. The second, from the Reverend Morgan Cowie, principal of the Putney College of Engineering, was that sewage as a falling body must accelerate. A sewer initially full would soon be only half full and thus able to receive more sewage. Further, the force of sewage entering from branches would accelerate the flow in the main sewer even more; it was well known that the cross-sectional area of two merging streams was much less than the sum of their separate areas. In principle, then, there was no need for an increase in diameter along a line of sewer, for velocity would increase to compensate for increasing volume. One had only to ensure that the outfall could withstand the issuing jet of sewage.[57]

What a seductive idea – in theory one could deliver any amount of sewage through a tube of any size. One need not worry about clogging since any obstacle would generate the pressure to effect its own removal. But as even the pipe sewerage "fanatic" Austin admitted, all these hypotheses left out "friction, that most important and ever varying item, [about which] we indeed know little or nothing."[58] The Trial Works Committee would find the limits of acceleration.

The trials were done in spring and summer 1849. For almost the whole time Roe was too ill to supervise. Carried out mainly in the sewers themselves by poorly trained assistants, the trials produced widely ranging and often bizarre results. In some trials discharge fell as gradient increased. In one case doubling steepness increased discharge time by a third; in another a pipe at a gradient of 1:160 took 39 minutes to discharge, 51 minutes at 1:120, and 55 minutes at 1:60.[59] Yet sheet after sheet of such data was transferred to beautifully colored graphs. The fiasco became clear only in October as the Trial Works Committee was summarizing its work. Enough data could be salvaged

---

57  The Reverend Morgan Cowie and Edward Cresy in Metropolitan Sanitary Commission, *First Report*, Evidence, 133–55, 158–59.
58  GBH, "Minutes on House Drainage," 33–34; Austin in Metropolitan Sanitary Commission, *First Report*, Evidence, 128; Finer, *Chadwick*, 443.
59  J. Medworth, "[Reports on Discharge with Junctioned Four Inch Pipes at Various Inclinations]," *Trial Works Committee Papers*, September 1849, Greater London Records Office, Archives of the Metropolitan Commission of Sewers [to be cited as GLRO MCS], 193. Thus at 1:480, a 4 inch sewer, 30 feet long, 1/4 full at its head, took 17.5 minutes to discharge 20 cubic feet of water; at 1:240, it took 23 minutes. But this relation was not constant: Usually 1:240 took less time than 1: 480; see also *Trial Works Committee Minutes*, 1849, GLRO MCS 192.

to give reasonable curves, but the committee disowned the bulk of the experiments.[60]

Chadwick was livid. Having long championed scientific over amateur administration he found that his own amateurs had ruined his only chance to compile the mass of data needed to sweep the field of the vexing engineers. He fumed at Joseph Medworth, one of the supervisors: could it be so hard to time the transit of a certain amount of water from one end of a pipe to the other? His job was to experiment, not explain, replied Medworth; maybe the results weren't sufficient for a new hydraulic theory and were "nothing approaching to mathematical accuracy," but they were surely good enough "for practical purposes."[61] Chadwick sent the data on to the now retired Roe, asking him to derive tables showing what size of pipe to use to drain a certain number of houses though a sewer of a certain gradient. Roe too could get little from them, and the warrant for the tables he eventually produced was his twenty years' experience of sewerage engineering. They indicated sewers not significantly smaller than Hawksley's.[62]

A massive research program with no results! Though there were rumors of botched experiments, the raw data were unavailable. Hawksley and his friends were limited to snide remarks, which could be dismissed as professional jealousy.[63] Still, one could cultivate the aura of empiricism. Roe's tables became the centerpiece of a campaign to depict orthodox engineers as bound to obsolete theories or unconfirmed rules of thumb. "Rules are laid down," and "tables are blindly put forward . . . without . . . instruction or explanation,"

60 "We are sorry that we are unable to recommend to the court to place confidence in the comparative results deduced from the experiments in the Fleet Sewer, as they do not seem to have been conducted with sufficient care when Mr. Roe was not personally superintending, and are thus contradictory when compared with each other. We the more regret this, as the opportunity was a very good one for obtaining valuable results, and we had hoped that proper care would have been taken by the Officers in charge, to secure accuracy" ("Report of the Trial Works Committee," *Trial Works Committee Papers*, December 1849, GLRO MCS 193, 6). As of July there was still full confidence ("[Metropolitan Sewers Commission]," *Times*, 24 July 1849, 8). In a September 1849 defense of the experiments it was argued that they showed some claims were wrong: The work was of a "cautionary or of a prohibitory or negative character" ("[Metropolitan Sewers Commission]," *Times*, 21 September 1849, 5).

61 Medworth in GBH, *Report on the Supply of Water to the Metropolis*, Appendix II, *Engineering Reports and Evidence*, 186–87, 190–93. It was rare for Chadwick to criticize a friendly witness: Before Chadwick's dressing down, Medworth was claiming great significance for the results. Medworth was correct that general trends were clear in some cases. On steep sewers, it was found that acceleration was significant, but once a sewer was full, additional inputs did not appear to increase its discharge ("Report of the Trial Works Committee," *Trial Works Committee Papers*, December 1849, GLRO MCS 193, 21–27).

62 Roe to Cowie, 19 February 1849, GLRO MCS 192; Roe to Austin, 9 February, 19 June 1852, UCL Chadwick Papers #206; Chadwick to Roe, 19 December 1851, 30 March 1852; Roe to Chadwick, 2, 9 March 1852, UCL Chadwick Papers #1704. Given that Hawksley's sewers were to accommodate much more rainfall than Roe's, their views of sewer capacity were actually even closer.

63 J. W. Bazalgette and Hawksley in discussion of Leslie, "Observations on the Flow of Water through Pipes," 49–53. Cf. Lewis, *Chadwick*, 223–24; Finer, *Chadwick*, 443.

complained Austin. The local boards could hardly question these "hypothetical dogmas founded upon a display of algebraic signs and quantities," yet their use led to "serious constructive error."[64] (Chadwick's engineers did not invariably use Roe's tables, however. When Robert Rawlinson drained 550 acres at Hitchin through a twenty-inch sewer, Roe protested that his tables called for a sixty-inch sewer. The same discharge with a twenty-inch pipe would require a flow of four miles per minute.[65])

## III

Deserted by theory and by experiment, Chadwick was left only with the engineer's classic appeal. He represented experience, he claimed, against their dogma. But the engineers, who saw themselves bound by "honest facts" not "unproved theoretical schemes," would have none of it, and they had cultivated the image of empiricism far longer than he. The good engineer, explained Robert Stephenson, had immeasurable, irreducible experience. On joining the Metropolitan Sewers Commission (after Chadwick's departure) he had recognized the "bewildering local circumstances and domestic difficulties." He "envied the self-confidence . . . [and] daring . . . of non-professional men who had not hesitated to lay down definite rules, to meet all cases of this most indefinite branch of . . . practice." James Rendel, the institution's president, noted the "great difference between mere theoretical speculations, and actual practical experience." In matters of sewers "engineers must deal with towns as they found them, and not according to pre-conceived opinions," he added.[66] The engineers' appeal to authority was no less self-serving than Chadwick's: the principle that each case required the unique prescription of an ethical practitioner was what kept "professionals" in business.

Despite Chadwick's denials, his board was doctrinaire, and it was the appropriateness of being doctrinaire more than the doctrine itself that engineers objected to. They had been slow to see Chadwick as a threat; a few had

---

64 Austin, Metropolitan Sanitary Commission, *First Report*, 128; GBH, "Minutes on House Drainage," 66–68. See also their use by William Lee, "Report in Communication from the General Board of Health and Reports from the Superintending Inspectors of the Board, Made to the Secretary of State in Relation to the Reports of the Metropolitan Sewers Commission in Respect to the Operation of Pipe Sewers," *P.P.*, 1854, 45, [1891.], 18–20 [to be cited as GBH, "Reports of the Superintending Inspectors"].

65 Rawlinson, "Drainage of Towns," 41; Roe to Chadwick, 1, 8 December 1852, UCL Chadwick Papers #1704; Roe, Haywood, in discussion of Rawlinson, "Drainage of Towns," 96–99, 52. Rawlinson and Austin developed their own rules of thumb, which did not depend on hydraulic formulae (Rawlinson in discussion of J. W. Bazalgette, "The Drainage of London," *Minutes of Proceedings, Institution of Civil Engineers 24* [1864]: 317; Austin in *Trial Works Committee Minutes*, GLRO MCS 192, 47–52).

66 Stephenson in discussion of Rawlinson, "Drainage of Towns," 85; Rendel in discussion of George Donaldson, "An Account of the Drainage of the Town of Richmond," *Minutes of Proceedings, Institution of Civil Engineers 11* (1851): 421; see also *Engineers and Inspectors*, 10.

complained in 1848 about the tone of the Sanitary Commission's reports but active opposition did not develop until 1852.[67] By then a good deal of pipe sewerage had already been laid, most of it in London. Some towns that had adopted the Public Health Act were beginning to plan sanitary works, and engineers were finding their schemes rejected and their competence questioned.

The "pipe-and-brick sewers war" of 1852–55 occurred on two levels. On one level it was a personal dispute between Chadwick and Hawksley, fueled by mutual dislike and charges of unethical practice. Hawksley claimed that under the guise of inspecting them, one of the inspectors had copied his plans and used them elsewhere, and that another had hired away a staff member to learn his professional secrets. This war was fought in nasty letters, pamphlets, and contemptuous remarks in public meetings.[68] But on a broader level the conflict was about technology assessment. Chadwick's most developed treatment is the board's "Minutes on House Drainage" of autumn 1852, which included Roe's tables. The engineers' views appear in a series of discussions on pipe and brick sewers at the institution.

There was a good argument for large brick sewers, which Chadwick had ignored. They could accommodate heavy rainfall, and also soil moisture, if top and sides were left unmortared. To be sure, pipes might be self-scouring if water ran through them constantly, but that was rarely the case. And hydraulic science was not the only factor to consider. What about congealed grease, for example, or indurated road mud? If they clogged, they would have to be excavated, cleaned out, and relaid. One might have to expose a long section to locate a block. A pipe that clogged once was likely to clog again at the same spot because of the difficulty of realigning pipe sections. Rigid pipes did not stand up well to distorting forces, like heavy carts passing overhead. Defects in workmanship, like thin walls or poor firing, were harder to detect in pipes, and it was hard to connect pipe sections: mortar tended to ooze inside and block flow. Adding a drain to a pipe sewer was clearly a larger job than with a brick sewer. While pipes were certainly cheap, one had to think of the commerce disrupted in replacing them. That made them unsuitable for busy streets. It was also dangerous to put pipes in very deep excavations because of the costs and risks of stabilizing adjacent buildings should repair be needed.[69] The consensus (one that included some of Chad-

67  In discussion of Green, "The Sewerage of Bristol," 95, 101, 104.

68  Chadwick to Charles May, 30 June, 20 July, May to Chadwick, 22 June, 7 July 1852, UCL Chadwick Papers #1375; *GBH–Durham Correspondence*, 1850, PRO MH 13/66; Hawksley, *Letter to the Marquis of Chandros,* 8–9; Lewis, *Chadwick*, 299.

69  In discussion of Green, "The Sewerage of Bristol," 101, 107; Rawlinson, "Drainage of Towns," 41, 43, 66; Donaldson, "Richmond," 410, 416; Rammell and Ranger in "Reports of the Superintending Inspectors," 75, 77; Thomas Wicksteed, "Copy of a Report by Thomas Wicksteed, C.E. on the State of the Works of Drainage and Sewerage in the Town of Croydon," *P.P.*, 1854, 61, [450.], 5.

wick's own engineers) was that pipe sewers, significantly larger than those Chadwick proposed, were good for short, steep runs of sewer; larger brick sewers were better for long, flat runs. That ran directly counter to Chadwick's claim that because velocity increased with depth, it was in flatter places that smaller pipes were most needed. And while theory might warrant two-, three-, four-inch pipes, experience preferred six- and nine-inch pipes.[70]

The only significant effort at mediation was Robert Rawlinson's November 1852 address to the institute, "Drainage of Towns." Rawlinson, who would later become chief inspector for the successor agencies of the General Board of Health, was known throughout his long career for his diplomacy. He needed it. He was the only one in the Chadwick camp who could have managed the mission; the others were far too feisty.

Rawlinson quickly made clear that he would espouse no dogma. He would unequivocally defend neither pipes nor any guidelines on size. There were always trade-offs; practical engineers would eventually arrive at optimal designs: "Discussion rarely makes converts, but facts are stubborn things." His defense of Chadwick was downright apologetic: the engineer "anxious after truth will not denounce a system, because some men push it to extremes" – and three inches was surely too small for any drain. In his conclusion he reiterated that his purpose was simply to begin a discussion; "positions unduly assumed" would surely "be overthrown."[71]

The deference was strategy, not capitulation. Ex cathedra pronouncements à la Chadwick would only irritate, but it might be possible to shift the focus to historical, political, and social aspects of sewerage. Rawlinson held that "the progress, if not the permanence of civilization," depended on finding "the best system of town sewerage and house drainage" and appealed to the old Chadwickian equation, "Misery, pauperism, vice and crime find a forcing-bed in the unsewered parts of towns, and amidst the foul air of undrained houses." Bad sewerage caused the degeneration of the race; those who grew up in foul environments were "left . . . shattered, feeble, febrile, and disorganized." With so much at stake there must be a right answer – a five-by-three-foot brick sewer or a fifteen-inch pipe could not both be right, he insisted. Cost mattered: "If that man is a benefactor . . . who makes two blades of wheat grow, where one only grew before, he is likewise so . . . who con-

---

70 On sewer sizes see GBH, *Report on the Supply of Water to the Metropolis*, Appendix II, *Engineering Reports and Evidence*, 108–11, 135–36, 156; Rawlinson and Haywood in discussion of Rawlinson, "Drainage of Towns," 35, 51.

71 Rawlinson, "Drainage of Towns," 35–36, 40–41, 100. Haywood, the surveyor of the City of London, alluded sarcastically to Rawlinson's independence: The "reports emanating from the Board of Health" had "left on his mind, an impression, that the empirical rules therein laid down, were required to be implicitly followed." The only position Rawlinson assumed was that sewer systems should be built for house drainage rather than rainfall. Heavy rain would not get into the sewers, anyway, and there were other means, such as street layout and pavement design, to facilitate surface drainage (Rawlinson, Haywood, Hawksley, Bazalgette in ibid., 29–33, 45–47, 58, 67).

structs two lineal yards of effective sewer, for the price that has before been expended upon one yard."

With this style of argument the engineers were utterly at sea, indeed they could see no argument here at all. That cheaper was better was a truism, as was the proposition that there was a best answer so long as there was agreement on the criteria of assessment. Rawlinson's only specific claim was that it was inhumane to design sewers that required manual cleaning. He appealed to the analogy of chimney sweeps. When it learned of their work and lives, the public had decided that the employment of climbing boys was intolerable. If it was wrong for boys to climb chimneys, it was wrong for men to go into sewers, Rawlinson proclaimed, and even more important: "More lives have been destroyed in foul sewers, than ever were lost in crooked chimneys."[72] The engineers rejected the analogy. Making sewers accessible was not the same as designing them to require manual cleaning. The workers in question were free adults, who were generally healthy and well paid and worked relatively short hours.[73]

It was on the heels of Rawlinson's paper that the Metropolitan Sewers Commission directed its newly appointed chief engineer, Joseph Bazalgette, to investigate pipe sewerage. In its earlier incarnation under the Chadwickians, the commission had built pipe drains and sewers in several desperately unsanitary London neighborhoods. There were also newly sewered towns under the GBH: Rugby, Sandgate, Croydon, Tottenham, St. Thomas Exeter, Ottery St. Mary, Barnard Castle. And several independent engineers had used pipes elsewhere. Bazalgette visited them all. In Richmond and in London he had pipe sewers opened for inspection. Of 122 London pipe sewers (nine to fifteen inches in diameter), he found 66 with deposits more than two and one half inches deep (another 47 had smaller deposits) and 23 cracked or broken. At

---

72 Rawlinson, "Drainage of Towns," 25–28. Rawlinson's was a milder version of Chadwick's condemnation: "There are some descriptions of labour which it is improper for human beings to perform, and which ought to be forbidden as being false in principle, and belonging to a low state of art, and as being ignorant or interested excuses for the avoidance of the trouble and expense of practicable and efficient substitutes. Putting men to crawl or creep through channels filled with foul ordure, and to breathe noxious gases . . . is one example of such labour. Putting children to crawl through channels, filled with soot, to cleanse them, is another." "Those whose lot it is to perform offensive and filthy labour have their perceptions blunted; their work, rendering them filthy in their persons, excludes them from the society of more cleanly and respectable astrains [*sic* artisans]; their occupation is supposed to necessitate and justify the constant use of ardent spirits, and they become degraded in condition, and a separate caste. The prevention of such degradation . . . is of itself a matter of social and civic gain. As is usual, however, in the operation of really correct principles, it will be found to be attended also with pecuniary saving." Minimum sewer sizes for human passage were two feet, six inches, by two feet for crawling; three feet, six inches, for crouching; four feet for stooping (GBH, "Minutes on House Drainage," 20–30).

73 Haywood, Bazalgette, Stephenson, in discussion of Rawlinson, "Drainage of Towns," 46–47, 68, 85. The claims appear true. E. D. I'Ianson and J. Newman in Metropolitan Sanitary Commission, *First Report*, Evidence, 105, 116. They worked from eight to four o'clock, earned almost twenty-five shillings/week.

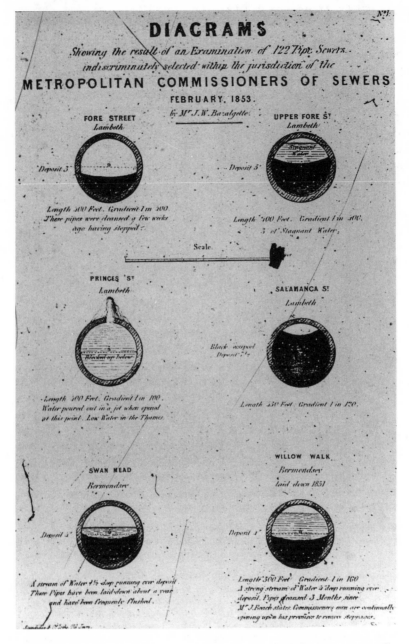

Illustrated in the most graphic way, Joseph Bazalgette's claim that many metropolitan pipe sewers were clogged would be contested in the next two years by Chadwickian engineers; the main issues of dispute were the appropriate criteria for judging the performance of public works (from "Copy of the Reports of Mr Bazalgette to the Metropolitan Commission of Sewers Relating to the Application, State, and Examination of Tubular Pipe Drains and Sewers," *P.P.*, 1852–53, 95, [668.]).

Richmond he found five cracked or broken pipes in eleven examined. Rugby reported twenty stoppages; at Sandgate there were many stoppages and broken pipes. In Manchester and Salford, on the other hand, large, thick-walled pipe sewers appeared to work well.[74]

By no means was Bazalgette uniformly negative; his reports were certainly not the smear campaign Chadwick's associates made them out to be. In the main he confirmed Phillips and Roe: pipe sewers required an ample flow of water, "more water . . . than the houses supply, and . . . frequent flushings." Once deposits started to form, they would harden and resist hydraulic scour. To prevent breaks more attention had to be given to ensuring a level and firm foundation. Accordingly, the Metropolitan Sewers Commission decided that pipe sewers must be at least nine inches in diameter, at a gradient of at least 1:200, a standard that pretty much reflected local practice. Stronger restrictions might have been imposed; the pipe sewers Bazalgette was replacing in St. Giles were two to four times steeper and nevertheless had clogged. In Chadwick's view, of course, all this was wrong headed. A smaller pipe would increase velocity and prevent deposition.[75]

Just as Bazalgette was completing his work the Croydon scandal erupted. Among the first towns to adopt the Public Health Act, the south London suburb of Croydon had completed the "combined works" of water, tubular drainage, even sewage recycling by early summer 1852. In August a fever epidemic began, striking eighteen hundred in a population of sixteen thousand in the next six months, causing seventy deaths.[76] At roughly the same time, breakages and blockages – from flannel, hay, shavings, paper, hair, sticks, kittens, a night cap, a cat, pigs' entrails, a bullock's heart – began to be discovered in the pipe sewers, about one hundred cases in all. Several inches of raw sewage covered some cellar floors; sewage saturated the ground.[77] Compounding

74 "Copy of the Reports of Mr Bazalgette to the Metropolitan Commission of Sewers, Relating to the Application, State, and Examination of Tubular Pipe Drains and Sewers," *P.P.*, 1852, *96*, (668.), 3–12 [to be cited as Bazalgette, "Report to the Metropolitan Commission of Sewers"]; T. W. Rammell, in GBH, "Reports of the Superintending Inspectors," 57, 63–67.

75 Bazalgette, "Report to the Metropolitan Commission of Sewers," 4–7, 12; Austin, "Further Report on Croydon," 21–22. The commission's decision came in January, before Bazalgette's random openings of metropolitan pipe sewers.

76 Thomas Page, "Report upon the Proceedings, the Plan for Sewerage, Its Engineering Features" [to be cited as Page, "Engineering Report"], in *Reports by Neil Arnott, M.D. and Thomas Page, C.E. on an Inquiry Ordered by the Secretary of State Relative to the Prevalence of Disease at Croydon and to the Plan of Sewerage,* *P.P.*, 1852, *96*, [1648.], 26, 30 [to be cited as Arnott and Page, *Croydon Reports*]. Cf. Neil Arnott, "Medical Report," in ibid., 5; Lewis, *Chadwick*, 315–17; Simon, *English Sanitary Institutions,* 225. The board's investigator, R. D. Grainger, claimed only fifteen hundred cases and forty-one deaths ("Medical Report," in *Statement of the Preliminary Inquiry by T. Southwood Smith, Esq., M.D., and John Sutherland, Esq, M.D. on the Epidemic at Croydon; Together with Reports by R. D. Grainger, Esq. and Henry Austin Esq. to the General Board of Health on the Circumstances Connected with the Epidemic Fever at Croydon, P.P.,* 1852, *96*, [1683.], 12) [to be cited as GBH, *Croydon Reports*]).

77 Croydon Board of Health to Home Office, 23 December 1853, PRO HO 45/5105.

the problem for the GBH was that the engineer in charge was William Ranger, one of its inspectors. Indeed, inspector Ranger had approved plans engineer Ranger had adapted from preliminary plans by the Croydon surveyor Thomas Cox and George Donaldson, a Chadwick appointee to the Metropolitan Sewers Commission staff. On the grounds that their design was too costly, Ranger had reduced sewer sizes throughout the system, replacing six-inch with four-inch sewers, and so on.[78]

In early January 1853, with the fever worsening, the GBH investigated. Bazalgette had already visited the Croydon works in November, at the beginning of his tour, and what a hostile Metropolitan Commission of Sewers might make of his report did not bear thinking.[79] Thus it was an illustrious delegation that went to Croydon: Henry Austin, chief of the engineering inspectors, and three medical men – Southwood Smith himself; R. D. Grainger, an eminent anatomist and cholera observer for the board; and the Liverpool sanitarian John Sutherland.

Smith and Sutherland reported quickly, blaming the fever on a mix of general constitution of the atmosphere (fever had been widespread that autumn), contagious transmission (the epidemic had been imported from a nearby village), and, as local causes, the "excessive and long continued prevalence of rainy weather." Given that he had been claiming for almost three decades that bad fever meant bad sewerage, Smith's appeal to everything except miasms of filth may seem tendentious. So it was. But as we have seen, all these elements – atmosphere, contagion, and dampness – were legitimate parts of an explanation of a disease outbreak. As with destitution years earlier, it was what was missing from the explanation that was significant.[80]

Grainger took the same general strategy. He represented Croydon as intrinsically unhealthy. There were miasms: they arose in cleaning old sewers, emptying cesspools, and spreading night soil, all in contravention of GBH instructions. And with such overcrowdedness (seven people in two hundred square feet in some dwellings), it was no wonder that there was fever.[81] Focusing on the breakages and blockages, Austin too blamed the town. The chief problem was bad connections between house drains and public sewers, and these were the responsibility of Croydon's surveyor, Cox. Also, things had been put into the pipe sewers that should not have been. But ever so

78 Ranger to GBH, 6 June 1850, *GBH–Croydon Correspondence*, PRO MH 13/59. Ranger denied the systematic reduction (Ranger to GBH, 11 August, 19 September 1853, *GBH–Croydon Correspondence*, PRO MH 13/59).
79 Bazalgette's report was not in fact particularly hostile (Bazalgette, "Report to the Metropolitan Commission of Sewers," 1).
80 Thomas Southwood Smith and John Sutherland, "Statement of the Preliminary Inquiry," in GBH, *Croydon Reports*, 4; idem, "Draft Report on Fever at Croydon," 19 January 1853, *GBH–Croydon Correspondence*, PRO MH 13/59. On the relations of Sutherland and Grainger to the GBH see Lewis, *Chadwick*, 196.
81 Grainger, "Medical Report," in GBH, *Croydon Reports*, 6–35.

grudgingly, he admitted that Ranger's downsizing had been unwarranted. Worse, it had slipped past the Board's scrutiny, a fact that Austin's excuse – "It would not be supposed that you [the GBH] would direct an examination of every minute portion of the many plans for which your sanction is demanded" – could not disguise.[82]

But for this tiny admission the reports acquitted the General Board of Health entirely. There the matter might well have ended had not Chadwick decided to squeeze a bit more credit from the affair by obtaining an "independent" confirmation. In early February, the board invited the home secretary, Lord Palmerston, to commission Neil Arnott, one of the authors of the 1838 reports, and Thomas Page, an engineer in the Board of Works, to investigate the Croydon case as independent experts.[83]

But Arnott and Page did not confirm the findings. Arnott found evidence that the promised downward ventilation was not occurring; instead, the new sewers seemed a network for distributing deadly poison throughout the town. Gas was rising through the network and out through drains. There was no effective surface drainage. Groundwater was seeping into the pipe sewers (intended only for household drainage), overtaxing the filtering plant, and contaminating the nearby River Wandle. Page found a correlation between fever and the new sewers, a matter on which the board's doctors had been silent. Ranger, he felt, had been arbitrary in his downsizing. His other economies, like eliminating provisions for surface drainage and opting for minimal sewage treatment, were responsible for many of the residents' complaints. He agreed that Cox had not supervised house connections carefully and had accepted poor-quality pipe.[84]

But Page also took up broader issues of the board's philosophy of technology.[85] He recognized that one could only judge success or responsibility within a framework of assessment. Ranger's design was acceptable in terms of GBH doctrine, though the actual work was not; nor was the Board's oversight.[86] From the perspective of the state of the art in pipe sewerage,

82 Austin, "Engineering Report," in GBH, *Croydon Reports,* 38–43.

83 Molesworth to Palmerston, 8, 11, 14 February 1853, PRO HO 45/5104L; Arnott, "Medical Report," in Arnott and Page, *Croydon Reports,* 5; Smith to Chadwick, 9 February 1853, UCL Chadwick Papers #1844.

84 Arnott, "Medical Report," in Arnott and Page, *Croydon Reports,* 6–8, 12; Page, "Engineering Report," in ibid., 26–33.

85 We need not see Page as disinterested: It was plain that the civil engineers of Great George Street and the Bazalgettians in the Metropolitan Sewers Commission were rejecting Chadwick and pipe sewerage. An ambitious engineer might see these institutions, not Chadwick's board, as the loci of power (Arnott and Page to Home Office, 9 April 1853, PRO HO 45/5104L; Walter Lewis, "Report on Health in Croydon," *GBH–Croydon Correspondence,* 1854, PRO MH 13/59, 38).

86 Board policy required approval of the plans, of the works before they had been covered, and of the works in action and a guarantee that the contractor maintain them in good order for five years (GBH, "Report of 1849," 63). This appears not to have been followed, and such scrutiny never did become typical.

Ranger's sewers were too small, long, and thin. But judged in terms of health and cleanliness, the entire project was wanting. Repair and inspection were difficult and there was no adequate provision either for surface drainage or for prevention of river pollution. The main blame fell on neither Cox nor Ranger, but on the "author or promoter of the mischievous system," who was "sitting in self-gratulation far away from the scene of strife."[87]

Politically, Croydon was simply an embarrassment. That Chadwick's friend Arnott had been so critical was particularly telling.[88] Left with its cracking sewers, bewildered as to whom to trust to fix them, Croydon appealed to Thomas Wicksteed, an old-school water engineer.[89] Following long traditions of professional ethics, he and Ranger agreed that Wicksteed would focus on what still needed doing, like surface drainage and sewage disposal. There had been recrimination enough. The local board was anxious to dodge the accusation that it had misplaced its trust. Cox was its chosen scapegoat.[90]

More importantly, Croydon revealed unresolved ambiguities about the role of the GBH. First, it was hard to square Ranger's performance with the board's claim to embody science. Ranger seemed to have followed no particular design rule. As Page had recognized, the board was loud on principle, weak on detail. Second, exactly what did the inspector's job entail? Leaving aside the dubious practice of letting an inspector inspect his own works, was inspection simply a matter of an official gentleman's stating that he saw nothing wrong, or did it imply an acceptance of responsibility? Moreover, how much should it focus on plans, how much on execution? Finally there was the propriety of network thinking. As Austin was reluctantly admitting, half networks – pipe sewers without constant water – might be worse than none. If the GBH had anything to offer over the private bill route, it was its claim to embody a systematic, scientific approach that would produce health, order, and comfort in the most economical way. That claim was in jeopardy in the summer of 1853.

Croydon and Bazalgette put the board on the defensive. Chadwick did not understand that Bazalgette wished to learn, not win, and responded with characteristic aggression. In August Austin officially replied to Page.[91] In Oc-

87 Page, "Engineering Report," 32, 46–48, 52.
88 Both the board and Henry Drummond, M.P., one of its most vehement opponents in 1848, asked for the complete evidence on which Arnott and Page had based their report (Arnott to Chadwick, 27 April 1853, UCL Chadwick Papers #193; Page to Home Office, 22 July 1853, PRO HO 45/5104L).
89 Cox to GBH, *GBH–Croydon Correspondence*, 3 September 1853, PRO MH 13/59. The Home Office also obtained a further report from Goldsworthy Gurney, PRO HO 45/5104L.
90 "Ranger–Wicksteed Meeting," 23 July 1853; GBH to Croydon, 3 March, undated March 1854; Walter Lewis, "Report on Health in Croydon," 1854; Croydon Local Board to GBH, 28 October 1853, in *GBH–Croydon Correspondence*, PRO MH 13/59.
91 The board also implied bias, suggesting that Arnott and Page had suppressed some of the evidence

tober, Palmerston himself surveyed towns with pipe sewerage works and found them satisfied, despite some blockages and bad work by contractors. He forwarded the responses to the Cabinet and to the Metropolitan Sewers Commission "to show the cheapness and efficiency of the tubular system."[92] The next spring, complaining that Bazalgette's reports were being circulated to discredit it, the board asked its inspectors to review Bazalgette's findings.[93] Chadwick published a vindication of the board's work, though it was much milder than the one he would have written had not Shaftesbury, Rawlinson, and Austin insisted on moderation.[94] Finally, a new Metropolitan Sewers Commission more sympathetic to pipe sewerage polled Bazalgette's assistants. Like Bazalgette himself, many had been hired during Chadwick's reign. Some, like George Donaldson, had tried and rejected pipe sewerage; others, like John Grant and Thomas Lovick, remained enthusiasts. In the main they did not contest Bazalgette's facts: there were records enough of blockages and break-ages in pipe sewers.[95]

## IV

Accordingly, the controversy was one of what those facts meant to the good engineer. Austin set the tone in responding to Page. Pipe sewerage must be seen as a system of interacting components. That it worked well in some places proved that failures were not "inherent" but due to causes that could be "entirely avoided." The Tottenham and Rugby respondents had noted that their pipe sewers worked because they controlled the water and kept the sewers well flushed. The very "progress of sanitary improvement" depended on pipes; without them universal drainage, and consequently universal health, was unaffordable. Thus the only "true course" for engineers was to "assist in

they had heard in Croydon. GBH to Palmerston 13, 27 July 1853; Page to Palmerston, 21 July, 2 August 1853, PRO HO 45/5104L.

92 Rugby Local Board to Home Office, 25 October 1853; Sandgate Local Board to Home Office, 26 October 1853; Tottenham Local Board to Home Office, 1 November 1853; R. Dymond and Sons to Home Office, 31 October 1853; Barnard Castle Local Board to Home Office, 16 November 1853, PRO HO 45/5105.

93 Tom Taylor, "Introductory Letter," in GBH, "Reports from the Superintending Inspectors," 4.

94 Lee to Chadwick, 9 November 1852, UCL Chadwick Papers #1201; Rawlinson to Chadwick, 26 January 1854, UCL Chadwick Papers #1645; "Croydon Case Materials," UCL Chadwick Papers #60.

95 Bazalgette, "Report to the Metropolitan Commission of Sewers," 12–13; *Engineers and Inspectors*, 76–77; Donaldson, "Richmond," 407–13; Lee in "Reports of the Superintending Inspectors," 15–17; "Copies of Reports to the Metropolitan Commission of Sewers on the Working of Pipe Sewers, of the District Engineers, Messrs. Lovick, Grant, Cooper, Donaldson, and Roe," *P.P.*, 1854–55, *53*, (281.), 3–6, 29–33, 36–40, 42. Bazalgette pointed that while he found 66/122 pipes with deposits greater than 2.5 inches, Donaldson, Cooper, and George Roe found 42/119 with greater than 2 inches, and even Grant's own survey found 20 percent of over two hundred sewers with blockages. There had been questions about the circumstances of Bazalgette's unannounced inspections – the pipes had been opened at night by a contractor with an animus to pipe sewerage.

remedying its defects, and determining . . . the conditions and limitations of its use."[96] Here Austin was appealing to the scientist's concept of replication: one did not reject an important discovery because some, presumably with poor technique or faulty equipment, could not replicate it. That some could was enough.

Conventional engineers rejected this analogy for various reasons. Page argued, in effect, that technology differed from science: It was all very well that pipe sewerage worked under controlled conditions but it was to be used where many conditions – like the cooperation of the populace in not drowning kittens in the water closet, or the perverse tendency of the roads to produce a sticky grit – were uncontrollable. Indeed, the number of things that could cause failures indicated a very narrow domain of successful application. Even with "inquisitorial inspection" there was no way to keep all "improper substances" out of the drains, noted Haywood of the City. Whether or not they needed to be capacious enough for human cleaning, sewers had to be repairable and inspectable; the good engineer planned for things going wrong rather than relying on them not to. Croydon had only five manholes in seventeen miles of sewer.[97]

For the most part, this argument simply didn't register with Chadwick and the inspectors. We told you, Lee complained, that ample water was required: "Similar omission of precautions clearly needed, and against express instructions for the prevention of the admission of road detritus into pipe sewers without sufficient water, are made the foundation of an hypothesis, that smooth channels or pipes are unsuited." The same principle applied with uncooperative people. The failures in St. Giles were not to count against the system, explained Lee, because they occurred among the wretched Irish.[98] Perhaps Lee meant that in an old market town where folk knew how to behave the system would work better, but the argument came close to repudiating the key rationale for an automatically working sanitary system: to civilize. Austin suggested the St. Giles Irish simply needed to be better educated in the use of sanitary appliances, but all along the argument had been that sanitation was the precondition for education. Page's view, by contrast, was that "as the population cannot be hastily fitted for the sewerage, the sewerage must be fitted . . . for the population."[99]

---

96 Austin, "Further Report on Croydon," 6–7, 13; Tottenham Local Board to Home Office, 1 November 1853; Rugby Local Board to Home Office, 25 October 1853; GBH to Home Office, 17 October 1853, PRO HO 45/5105.

97 Page, "Engineering Report," 49; Haywood in discussion of Harrison, "Drainage . . . South of the Thames," 91. Even Austin acknowledged the need for better inspection ("Further Report on Croydon," 26). On road grit see Donaldson in "Reports of the District Engineers," 24–28; cf. Finer, *Chadwick*, 449. Finer accuses Bazalgette of having "little conception of scientific method" in thinking that a few failures "discredited the system."

98 Lee in GBH, "Reports from the Superintending Inspectors," 8–14, 17.

99 Austin, "Further Report on Croydon," 23; Page, "Engineering Report," 48.

A second issue was what "failure" meant. It should not refer to "local and temporary accident," argued the Chadwickian John Grant. Instead one should measure breakages and blockages against the amount of pipe sewerage in place, or the costs of repair, not in some false absolute sense. As Grant calculated it, that meant one problem per three miles of pipe sewers and per 125 house drains in four years: a reasonable rate. But Bazalgette argued that he was not interested in comparisons, because he was not claiming that "a system" had failed, or that one "system" was better than another; what was at issue was the use of a particular tool: if "pipe sewers required more perfect workmanship and greater care than is ordinarily obtainable . . . these facts might become sound reasons *for a more limited application* of pipe sewers."[100]

Indeed, Bazalgettian engineers downplayed any notion of system beyond the set of works one coordinated to a particular set of circumstances. "The experienced engineer would adapt the means to the requirements in each individual case," rejecting the "blind and exclusive advocacy of one system for every variety of circumstances," declared Bazalgette. "Practical authorities" knew, observed Stephenson, "that mere abstract principles did not hold good, in questions of the sewerage of towns, where so many local circumstances and domestic occurrences, interfered with the perfect working of even the best-designed plan." Wicksteed complained of the "great evil" of promising "panaceas, when the very nature of the work . . . required variations in levels, sizes of sewers, and materials, not only varying with different localities, but also in each locality."[101]

"Local circumstances" went well beyond topography and soil structure: they included that which most troubled Chadwick, a view that each town must be free to shape its future. In outlining Croydon's choices Wicksteed made clear that it was not for him to dictate a solution. Sewer size was "a ratepayers' question, not an engineering one." Towns able to afford "a permanent work" would probably prefer a large brick sewer. Smaller places might "postpone the larger work until they could better afford it" and use cheaper pipe sewers.[102] There was no single technical answer.

Because they assumed a "system," which one must either support or oppose, was at stake, GBH inspectors had a hard time recognizing that conventional engineers did favor the use of pipes. Lee claimed, falsely, that Robert Stephenson opposed all use of pipes. Austin claimed it was the engineers, not the board, who were doctrinaire – brick sewers were used in half the systems it approved. To them the phenomenon of engineers using pipes made sense only in terms of hypocrisy.[103] For Chadwick and for William Lee, the most

100 Grant and Bazalgette in "Reports of the District Engineers," 29–33, 35–37 (italics mine).
101 Bazalgette and Stephenson in discussion of Rawlinson, "Drainage of Towns," 67, 84–85; Bazalgette in discussion of Donaldson, "Richmond," 415; Wicksteed, "Croydon Report," 5.
102 Wicksteed, "Croydon Report," 5.
103 Lee in GBH, "Reports from the Superintending Inspectors," 49. Cf. Stephenson's statements,

dogmatic of the inspectors, the main tactic was to reiterate old maxims: anything other than pipes would generate disease; manual sewer cleaning was unthinkably inhumane; ventilation was unnecessary; conventional engineers were unqualified, hypocritical, and usually corrupt. The widespread "misrepresentation" and "suppression of facts" were the work of an "organized opposition" trying to escape accountability to continue its huge profits.[104]

Austin, Rammell, Ranger, and Rawlinson were more pragmatic, however, willing to modify doctrine in light of experience. Rammell and Ranger compensated for fragility by laying pipes in concrete jackets or on puddled clay. Rammell admitted that hydraulic pressure did not clear clogs. If not a necessity, regular flushing was certainly a wise precaution. Austin admitted that it was unwise to try back drainage in older built up areas: "In many instances . . . back drainage has been pushed too far, and has thus been made the means of dispute and dissatisfaction, particularly when stoppages have subsequently occurred . . . but this only proves that back drainage is no more suited to all occasions than pipe sewers are fitted to all occasions" – Bazalgette or Hawksley might have said the same.[105] Equally, there were some striking successes to learn from. Very long flat pipe sewers, nearly a mile in length at gradients on the order of 1:1000, were working well at Exeter, Tottenham, and soon at Ely. By mid-1854, 284 places had petitioned for the act; local boards were at work in 170.[106]

Still, pragmatism meant real trade-offs. After more than a year trying to get a decent set of plans, sections, and estimates for a modest sewerage project in Leicester, Austin gave in: effectively what Harris, the surveyor, was proposing was to get a few thousand pounds to start building an unnecessarily large brick sewer and see how far he got with it – all quite acceptable to Wicksteed and Stephenson. Reluctantly approving the request, Austin thought he might still convince Harris to use pipe.[107] After his ouster from the Metropolitan Sewers Commission in October 1849 Chadwick was horrified to learn that his successors would not require houses to be connected to the new sewers they

which Lee is citing, in discussion of Rawlinson, "Drainage of Towns," 84–86; Austin, "Further Report on Croydon," 4–5; Finer, *Chadwick*, 450.

104 Lee in "Reports from the Superintending Inspectors," 24, 46–48, 51; GBH, "Report of 1854," 31–35, 45, 49.

105 Rammell and Ranger in "Reports from the Superintending Inspectors," 57, 74–75, 77–78; Austin, "Further Report on Croydon," 19; Henry Austin, "On a Few Points in Relation to the Drainage of Towns," *Transactions, National Association for the Promotion of Social Science 1* (1857): 422–29; cf. Page, "Engineering Report," 32.

106 Lee in "Reports from the Superintending Inspectors," 22–24; R. Dymond and Sons to Home Office, 31 October 1853, PRO HO 45/5105; "Ely Sanitary Works," *The Builder 14* (1856): 134; Finer, *Chadwick*, 437.

107 Wicksteed to GBH, 3 October 1851; S. Stone to GBH, 18 September, 2 October, 13 November 1851; 11 June, 31 August 1852; GBH to Leicester, 15 September 1851; Austin, "Further Reports on Leicester Drainage," 9 October 1852, 4 January, 18 April 1853, *Leicester–GBH Correspondence*, PRO MH 13/111.

were building. But many engineers, even those deeply and genuinely concerned with health, like Liverpool's James Newlands, did not endorse this democratizing despotism. It seemed unnecessary and impractical to antagonize owners or occupiers by making them buy domestic technologies.[108] One should not dwell on the incompleteness of the works, but take the opportunity to build what one could.

A good place to stop, with these engineers fretting about the minutiae of their trade: socket joints, butt joints, or half sockets; nine- or fifteen-inch pipes; full brick or half; grit-catching gratings and grit-reducing pavements. They show us "public health" changing from idea to institution. It was not in all respects the sort of institution Chadwick favored. The urban improvers had turned out to be the most powerful constituency in favor of public health. In the next half century they would be active in building sanitary works, not as rapidly or systematically as Chadwick would have liked, but on the whole successfully. In its six years Chadwick's General Board of Health sanctioned roughly a half million pounds of loans for water and sewerage; by 1905 local authority debt in England and Wales for those purposes was nearly one hundred million pounds.[109]

The role of the state in all this was quite different from what Chadwick would have preferred. Page had recognized a great flaw in the board's constitution. It was one thing to advise; to insist that things be done in a particular way was effectively to accept responsibility. Where works were being carried out by elected local boards and their surveyors and contractors, overseen only occasionally by an inspector, this was an impossible role for the state, however excellent its technologies. Robert Rawlinson, who stayed on to become chief engineering inspector for the Local Government Act Office (1858–71) and then the Local Government Board, developed a quite different philosophy of inspection. He had made a vow, Rawlinson told the Royal Sanitary Commission in 1869, "that nothing should force me to attempt to compel a community to do what was even for their own benefit. . . . If persons are unwilling to receive you, you must shake the dust from your boots and go somewhere else where they will. My whole life's experience goes to this, that you cannot compel unwilling men." Even where a local authority wholeheartedly embraced sanitary improvement, many things could go wrong: cost overruns, buildings damaged in the laying of sewers. Where the sanitary authority was hostile, maintaining the works would prove impossible. The inspector's job was simply a loose benevolent oversight to make sure that "the plans and estimates . . . [were] not outrageously bad."[110]

108 Chadwick to Morpeth, 1 November 1849; Morpeth to Chadwick, 2 November 1849, UCL Chadwick Papers #1055; GBH, "Report of 1854," 29; Lewis, *Chadwick*, 334; C. Hamlin, "James Newlands and the Bounds of Public Health," *Transactions of the Historic Society of Lancashire and Cheshire 143* (1994): 117–39.

109 *Thirty-fifth Annual Report of the Local Government Board, P.P.*, 1905–6, *35*, [cd. 3105], cciii.

110 Royal Sanitary Commission, *First Report, P.P.*, 1868–69, *32*, [4128.], Evidence, qq 217–20, 522–

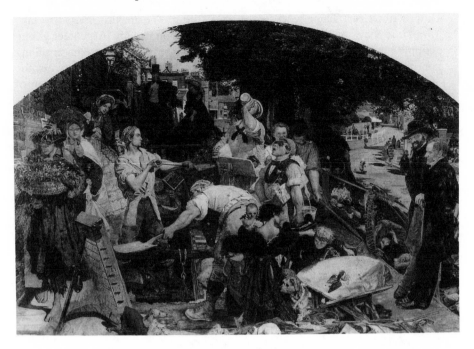

H. Ford Madox Brown, *Work* (with permission of Manchester City Galleries).

Good changes, these? Arguably the most famous painting of a broken up street, H. Ford Madox Brown's, *Work*, completed in 1863, celebrated the act of public health rather than the idea. The ruddy, white clad navvies at the center of the picture are building sanitary works – whether a water or a sewer

23, 575, 614–17, 688, 690–91. Even with his more militant conceptions of central government intervention, John Simon, the nation's chief medical officer from 1858 to 1871, was not prepared to deal with these problems. For Simon the solution was simply to ignore the reality of the engineering problems and to require local authorities to solve them in whatever way they chose. The technical aspects of sanitary engineering ought to be no part of the business of central government, he insisted: "It is the end, not the means, government is interested in. . . . If the result can be got by earth closets, if it can be got by carts, if it can be got by porters carrying refuse on their shoulders, it is no affair of Government, so long as the result is obtained. It is only, I think, on results that Government is entitled to insist: namely that there shall be freedom from nuisance" (ibid., q 2004). The political scientist Christine Bellamy calls this a "political–diplomatic" administration characterized by "general guidelines which are not so much task objectives as parameters for the long-term exploitation of influence and for the conduct of negotiations. . . . Agents seek movement rather than achievement, an acceptable outcome rather than the technically correct solution. Their aim is to minimize error and avoid the breakdown of relations, rather than maximize performance . . . characterized by flexibility, discretion, and influence" (*Administering Central-Local Relations, 1871–1919: The LGB in Its Fiscal and Cultural Context* [Manchester: Manchester University Press, 1988], 115–17). Cf. C. Hamlin, "Muddling in Bumbledom: Local Governments and Large Sanitary Improvements: The Cases of Four British Towns, 1855–1885," *Victorian Studies 32* (1988): 55–83.

line is not clear. Their work is real and lasting. We are not invited to take the same view of the darker figures who surround them: A genteel young couple – wealth with nothing useful to do; a ragged girl, with younger sibling on hip, selling flowers – grinding and hopeless poverty; and two thinkers, the Christian socialist F. D. Maurice and Thomas Carlyle, "whose condition of England question" was here being solved in the full shovels of dirt."[111]

111 Gerard Curtis, "Ford Madox Brown's *Work*: An Iconographic Analysis," *Art Bulletin* 74 (1992): 623–36.

# CONCLUSION

This book has reexamined a foundational period in the history of modern public health, an institution usually portrayed as jointly the product of two integrated events: the rise of science (here, epidemiology and bacteriology in particular) and the rise of states which are both democratic and bureaucratic, like that which took shape in nineteenth century Britain. Each reinforces the other. The rationale for the state is that it is scientific, rational. Science gains credibility from its link to administration; its proof is its practicality.

That perspective is exemplified in Oliver MacDonagh's *Early Victorian Government, 1830–1870*. There the combination of conditions – the "irreducible brute matter of the new and unprecedented social problems" – and knowledge of them – "exposure of the actual state of things" – drive society toward "collectivism." Once it was "demonstrated that ventilation mechanisms saved miners' lives or that water sanitation drastically reduced the death rate, it was practically speaking impossible to resist the state interference implied in insisting upon these precautions, the state being the only agency which could insist and enforce effectively." In technical matters like sanitation (one of MacDonagh's exemplars), the only other criterion for action was a problem-solving science. Fortunately this was available, for the pre-Chadwick period was one of maturation in engineering and medicine: "the rejection of a priori assumptions, empirical investigation, the building up of a corps of trained, examined and tried men." Thus, "when arterial drainage was called for, the newly invented glazed and earthenware pipes could be produced and transported cheaply and in great numbers almost overnight. . . . When novel ventilation or sanitary appliances were called for, there were men with some measure of exact knowledge who could and would eagerly take up the challenge." Without the rise of these new professions "measures of state interference would have been unthinkable"; the presence of these new "bodies of professionals who were beginning to apply the correct method of investigation" meant that "in every technical difficulty the administration had men to turn to; for every technical measure of regulation and control they had men to call on to enforce it."[1]

MacDonagh's determinism is driven by both the realities of the past – those "bare facts" – and the need to reach a particular present: "Resolved . . . [those problems] had to be."[2] It privileges the concrete (indeed, one might say that it privileges "concrete" itself). "Facts" are real – yards of sewer either exist or do not; persons either die or recover from cholera. These facts are either known or unknown, and science is mainly the business of collecting and organizing them. Just as inquiry is straightforward, so too action: public actions either work or don't. When they don't, the persistence of the problems sooner or later imposes true solutions; these both constitute and justify this "rational" government.[3]

All this I have tried to problematize; in the place of facts, observations of them, and obvious actions, I offer conflict, ideology, and rhetoric. Does this mean saying there is no dung in the dooryard, only dung discourse? Or that there are no yards of sewer needing to be built or cholera cases awaiting prevention? Not at all. In a broad sense and in the long term, the MacDonagh model describes changes that occurred, real problems that were gradually solved. It also reflects (and affirms) the perspectives of many of those who devoted their careers to solving such problems. But in its breadth, it misses much of the confusion and complexity of the particular. More importantly, it fails to acknowledge that conditions do not *explain* changes in social thought or in institutions.[4] The historical record, after all – and equally the record to which policymakers responded in Commons committee rooms or municipal halls – is a record of accounts, not of tons of excrement. Those accounts were parts of political struggles in which many things were at stake. They were not snapshots, but strategies of representation, and what is omitted from them is as weighty as what was included. In one sense we know this already in knowing that different political units have responded differently to industrialization

1 Oliver MacDonagh, *Early Victorian Government, 1830–1870* (London: Weidenfeld and Nicolson, 1977), 3–4, 6, 20.

2 Even, one might add, at significant cost to other social values. Note MacDonagh's appraisal of Chadwick: "We must not allow ourselves to be over-prejudiced by . . . [Chadwick's] unscrupulous behaviour as a royal commissioner, by his immediate desire to crush working class resistance to the factory system and his own despotic poor law legislation or by his failure to see or care for the dangers to liberty involved in his ultimate plan for a preventive forestalling and inquisitorial police. . . . His leading concepts of centralization, professionalism, expert training and a powerful inspectorate, which form the hard core of all his social planning, were the right ones to secure the sort of government demanded by the new, vast, complex, urbanized, and mobile society" (ibid., 5, 20, 175).

3 Ibid., 8.

4 Cf. E. P. Thompson's construal of the kind of process MacDonagh describes: "We forget how long abuses can continue 'unknown' until they are articulated: how people can look at misery and not notice until misery itself rebels" (*The Making of the English Working Class* [Harmondsworth, U.K.: Penguin, 1968], 377).

and urbanization of the sort that took place in early-nineteenth-century Britain and still do.[5]

If we deny that conditions explain, the role of science must shift too. Scientific truths do not precede and dictate action; science is a resource parties appeal to (or make up as they go along) for use wherever authority is needed: to authorize themselves to act, to compete for the public's interest and money, to neutralize real or potential critics.[6] Here again, to admit the contingency and constructedness of science does not require waiving our right to assess alternative approaches to public health problems. It does require us to acknowledge that in making judgments we are privileging certain criteria; and, equally, helps us appreciate the complexity of public health interventions which, because they transform the conditions of their application, have more the character of a leap of faith toward a new world than of the application of well proven solutions to well-defined problems. Here too we can be misled by the representation of science, much as we are by the claim that conditions are inherently problematic and their discovery is the only criterion for their remediation. How much easier to say that the solution to the condition-of-England problem is derivable from hydraulic theorems than to say there is no solution – but only a darkling plain of struggling and ignorant armies (essentially what Peel and Sir James Graham thought privately in spring 1842). That sort of use of science began to be common in early Victorian government, where blue-bound tomes with tens of thousands of items of "evidence" underwrote every new experiment for transforming public life (and equally every resistance of the establishment), and it has become commonplace in Western societies.[7] What we call the application of science is often the manufacture of the authority needed to fool ourselves that we know what we are doing in cases in which we have lost other means of making ourselves act.

Finally, to reject the determinism of "conditions" also requires us to think differently about the Victorian sanitary achievement: that monumental infrastructure is even more remarkable as an achievement of public persuasion than one of bricks and mortar. Its presence really tells us little about the problems those works were undertaken to solve, which, as we have seen, were various.

5  The case of nineteenth-century France offers the most striking contrast. See Ann La Berge, *Mission and Method: The Early-Nineteenth-Century French Public Health Movement* (Cambridge: Cambridge University Press, 1992).
6  David Collingridge and Colin Reeve, *Science Speaks to Power: The Role of Experts in Policy-Making* (New York: St. Martin's Press, 1986); Michel Foucault, *Power/Knowledge: Selected Interviews and Other Writings, 1972–1977* (New York: Pantheon, 1980).
7  Of the many purposes of the blue books, Thompson writes, "reform comes low on the list." They were undertaken as "a means of 'handling and channelling' discontent, procrastinating . . . or purely from an excess of utilitarian officiousness." "The hand-loom weavers and framework knitters were duly inquired into as they starved," he adds. Curiously, the only area where he would not regard the blue-book-writing bureaucrats as architects of repression was sanitation (*Making of the English Working Class*, 375–81). Cf. MacDonagh, *Early Victorian Government*, 6.

But it tells us a great deal about the people who undertook to solve them. How, one wonders, did they persuade themselves to do that?

Why take this new perspective? One reason is that the presumption of under- rather than overdetermination gives us a better sense of history in the making. By embracing an historical positivism; by substituting power, the empirical entity manifest both in change and in inertia, for a post hoc rationality, we descend to the level playing field of 1838. We can visit the camps, see the world from the protagonists' viewpoints, and watch a conflict unfold over what public health is to be. By extirpating destiny we recover possibility. Determinist histories deny real options. Intentionally or not, they are winners' histories; those who lost are disenfranchised for eternity as those who were bound to lose. The Alisonians thus become the Luddites of public health.[8]

But, one may argue, the Alisonians deserved to lose. Sure, there were options, but the choices Chadwick made were shrewd, practical, and beneficial: in short, rational. Complex traditional medicine was a reservoir for obfuscation; it offered no clear direction for disease prevention. Despite their noble philanthropy, hand-wringing humanitarian doctors had no coherent response to the demographic and industrial realities of England and Scotland in the 1830s. The complaints of Wakley and the *Times?* – so much grandstanding. And can Hamlin really want a world in which filth rules – no water, no sewers?

To the last point first. Chadwick has been so dominant a figure in the history of public health, and the changes for which he fought have seemed so central and necessary, that it may well seem revisionist petulance to criticize him, another of those mean jokes from which the dead cannot defend themselves. As we have seen, Chadwick insisted that his public health – derived from the law of gravity – was beyond criticism. All parts of it were of a piece: the diseases that counted were those caused by filth; in a counterfactual scenario where there was no filth they would not exist (and all would be well besides); filth removal via the optimal technologies that only a powerful and independent unit of government could build and administer was the only politically and practically viable way to prevent them.

For many of us the most important part of Chadwick's achievement will be this program of public sanitary structures. Yet water and sewers do not imply Chadwick himself, his institutions, his representations of class relations, any more than punctual railways require the person and culture of Mussolini. Technologies do have political implications, but they also, as Richard Sclove

8 That was Thompson's great project: Free artisans did not have to become dull proletarians; laissez faire was not the obvious economic philosophy in a country with a long heritage of legislation regulating commerce, manufacture, and labor. Thompson too took on the determinism of the revolution-in-government historians though his larger concern was with wresting the industrial revolution from some "standard of living" historians who would sanctify the past as an embodiment of economic theory.

points out, have multiple and shifting meanings in a particular set of social and cultural circumstances.[9] Chadwick knew that. His attempt to manage those meanings was the source of both his success and his undoing. On the one hand, his ability to tie sanitation to political stability was far more important to home secretaries in the mid-1840s than any epidemiological data he might have offered. Yet to represent it as a tool of government control was equally to cast it as a weapon to be used against those it was meant to help. However pleasant, this proposed new right to environmental quality was part of a campaign of eliminating rights championed by the Cobbettians – a right, sometimes manifest in food, to the produce of the nation, and a right to local and individual freedom.

By no means must an institution of public health that builds sanitary public works and is concerned with filth-borne diseases be one that denies the importance of food, work, and chronic disease: Almost all medical men in the 1830s and early 1840s would have agreed that water and sewers as well as sufficient food and healthy work were necessary for health. Nonetheless, in 1842 a decision to pursue one form of public health, sanitation, was a decision not to pursue another. Similarly, in 1848, the decision to establish the General Board of Health was equally a decision about the competency of certain persons and institutions. Individuals, municipal governments, companies of investors, existing professions could not be trusted with comprehensive sanitation; only a powerful and independent institution of state could.

As for other options, it is quite true, as I pointed out in chapter 1 and elsewhere, that there were no well-developed institutional alternatives to the public health Chadwick chose to offer. Nor can we say that a public health institution dominated by Alison, or by Rumsey and the poor law medical officers, or by the Institution of Civil Engineers, would necessarily have been more satisfactory – by whatever standards one chooses – than the one Chadwick tried to invent. The question is counterfactual and unanswerable. It presupposes not only a definition of what the mission of public health should be, but also knowledge of what alternative factors might have combined to cause whatever illnesses one chooses to focus on, and an appraisal of the political viability of alternative policies.[10]

9  Richard S. Sclove, *Democracy and Technology* (New York: Guilford Press, 1995), 20–21. On the politics of technologies see Bruno Latour, "Where Are the Missing Masses? The Sociology of a Few Mundane Artifacts," *Shaping Technology/Building Society: Studies in Sociotechnical Change,* eds. Wiebe E. Bijker and John Law, 225–58 (Cambridge, Mass.: MIT Press, 1992).

10  In trying to understand the causes of improvements in mortality rate, historians and demographers writing in response to the suggestions of Thomas Mckeown have raised such questions, though they do not usually ask about alternative health policies. That literature is large; for statements of the rival cases see Simon Szreter, "The Importance of Social Intervention in Britain's Mortality Decline, c. 1850–1914: A Reinterpretation of the Role of Public Health," *Social History of Medicine* 1 (1988): 1–37; Sumit Guha, "The Importance of Social Intervention in England's Mortality Decline: The Evidence Reviewed," *Social History of Medicine* 7 (1994): 89–113; Simon Szreter, "Mor-

But in the main, I take this approach less to criticize the choices taken – though I do a good deal of that – than to insist that choices were being made and that they involved profound and permanent questions that continue to need to be recognized. For what is most important about the debate of the 1830s–1850s is its scope. Partly because there were no well entrenched institutions – even Chadwick's Board of Health was the residuum of legislative compromise – debate involved grand questions of rights and obligations, of human dignity and freedom. What Alison and the others were doing, with varying success, was to keep alive a set of questions that Chadwick would suppress as matters of empirical inquiry, or rational action, or technical fine-tuning.

I see that kind of debate as necessary – then, now, always. Public health belongs to social justice quite as much as to civil engineering or epidemiology. It is inescapably, not incidentally, a matter of political philosophy in the grandest and broadest sense. Actions to deal with disease must deal with notions of what obligations people owe to each other or to governments or governments to people. These in turn involve culture: ideas not only of what disease is, and when and why it exists, but also of what persons should be like and how they become that way, of what standards can command public assent as preconditions of human dignity or alternatively of public safety. Ultimately, one may argue that where there is knowledge of disease prevention and of the factors that sustain life and health, the map of the availability of those factors is the map of the rights that exist in the society.[11]

To see the rise of modern public health as a choice rather than as an adaptation of institutions to conditions is also to change the way we think about the public health of the present. More than in other institutions, driven by the whims of markets or polities, professions rely for their senses of identity and mission on history. These thorny issues were surely settled definitively at some time in the past, professionals assure themselves; we are thankful we need not undergo the exhausting process of reinventing or rejustifying ourselves. Yet professions do not always adapt to changing circumstances; they may well (and public health has) find themselves bewildered by new challenges or changing institutions, which cannot be negotiated with the old maps.[12] To

---

tality in England in the Eighteenth and the Nineteenth Centuries: A Reply to Sumit Guha," *Social History of Medicine* 7 (1994): 269–82.

11 Such a perspective is evident in Stephen Kunitz, *Disease and Social Diversity: The European Impact on the Health of Non-Europeans* (New York: Oxford University Press, 1994); Jan-Olof Drangert, *Who Cares About Water? Household Water Development in Sukumaland, Tanzania* (Linköping: Linköping University Studies in Arts and Sciences, 1993).

12 Magali Sarfatti Larson, *The Rise of Professionalism* (Berkeley: University of California Press, 1977); Randall Collins, "Market Closure and Conflict Theory of the Professions," *Professions in Theory and History*, eds. Michael Burrage and Rolf Torstendahl, 24–43 (London: Sage, 1990). On public health in particular see the several papers in *A History of Education in Public Health: Health That Mocks the Doctors' Rules*, eds. Roy Acheson and Elizabeth Fee (Oxford: Oxford University Press,

go back to the beginning, to recover possibility in the past, is one very important way to open our eyes to the possibilities we confront in the present. But to unlock long closed institutions requires a particular sort of historical key, the sort I have tried to provide here, one that stresses contingency. To acknowledge what began in the 1830s as profoundly contingent gives us permission to recognize that public health is everywhere and always contingent in similar ways, but it is also to give us some hope of being able to manage those contingencies with some success.[13]

1991), and Jane Lewis, *What Price Community Medicine? The Philosophy, Practice, and Politics of Public Health Since 1919* (Brighton: Wheatsheaf Books, 1986).

13 For such a use of history see Daniel Fox, *Power and Illness: The Failure and Future of American Health Policy* (Berkeley: University of California Press, 1993), 16–18.

# SELECT BIBLIOGRAPHY

## MANUSCRIPT SOURCES

British Library, Peel Papers
Greater London Records Office, Archives of the Metropolitan Commission of Sewers, the Westminster Commission of Sewers
National Library of Wales, Harpton Court Mss (G. C. Lewis)
Public Record Office, Kew, Archives of Poor Law Commission, Home Office, General Board of Health
Royal College of Physicians of Edinburgh, Alison Papers
Shrewsbury Records Centre, Slaney Diaries
University College London, Chadwick Papers

## SECONDARY SOURCES

Acheson, Roy and Fee, Elizabeth, eds. *A History of Education in Public Health: Health That Mocks the Doctors' Rules.* Oxford: Oxford University Press, 1991.
Ackerknecht, E. H. "Anticontagionism Between 1821 and 1867." *Bulletin of the History of Medicine, 22* (1948): 562–93.
Anderson, Warwick. "Excremental Colonialism: Public Health and the Poetics of Pollution." *Critical Inquiry, 21* (1995): 640–69.
Ashton, T. S. *Economic and Social Investigations in Manchester, 1833–1933: A Centenary History of the Manchester Statistical Society.* 1934; reprint, Fairfield, Conn.: Augustus M. Kelley, 1977.
Ashworth, William. *The Genesis of Modern British Town Planning: A Study in Economic and Social History of the Nineteenth and Twentieth Centuries.* London: Routledge and Kegan Paul, 1954.
Bahmueller, Charles. *The National Charity Company: Jeremy Bentham's Silent Revolution.* Berkeley: University of California Press, 1981.
Bellamy, Christine. *Administering Central–Local Relations, 1871–1919: The Local Government Board in Its Fiscal and Cultural Context.* Manchester: Manchester University Press, 1988.
Berridge, Virginia. "Health and Medicine." *The Cambridge Social History of Britain, 1750–1950,* vol. 3, *Social Agencies and Institutions,* ed. F. M. L. Thompson, 171–242. Cambridge: Cambridge University Press, 1990.
Best, G.F.A. *Shaftesbury.* New York: Arco, 1964.

Binnie, G. M. *Early Victorian Water Engineers*. London: Thomas Telford, 1981.

Bonar, James. *Malthus and His Work*. 1924; reprint, New York: Augustus M. Kelley, 1966.

Boorstin, Daniel. *The Americans: The Democratic Experience*. New York: Vintage, 1974.

Briggs, Asa. *Victorian Cities*. Harmondsworth, U.K.: Penguin, 1968.

Brotherston, J. H. F. *Observations on the Early Public Health Movement in Scotland*. London: H. K. Lewis, 1952.

[Bruce, Henry Austin]. *Letters of the Rt. Hon. Henry Austin Bruce, G.C.B., Lord Aberdare of Duffryn*. Oxford: printed for private circulation, 1902.

Brundage, Anthony. *England's "Prussian Minister": Edwin Chadwick and the Politics of Government Growth, 1832–1854*. University Park: Pennsylvania State University Press, 1988.

Brundage, Anthony. *The Making of the New Poor Law: The Politics of Inquiry, Enactment, and Implementation, 1832–1839*. New Brunswick, N.J.: Rutgers University Press, 1978.

Buer, M. C. *Health, Wealth, and Population in the Early Days of the Industrial Revolution*. London: Routledge, 1926.

Bynum, W. F. "Cullen and the Study of Fevers in Britain." *Theories of Fever from Antiquity to the Enlightenment*. eds. W. F. Bynum and V. Nutton, 135–47. Medical History, Supplement 1. London: Wellcome Institute for the History of Medicine, 1981.

Bynum, W. F. "Hospital, Disease, and Community: the London Fever Hospital, 1801–1850." *Healing and History: Essays for George Rosen*, ed. Charles Rosenberg, 97–115. New York: Science History, 1979.

Bynum, W. F. "Ideology and Health Care in Britain: Chadwick to Beveridge." *History and Philosophy of Life Sciences, 10* (supplement) (1988): 75–87.

Bynum, W. F. *Science and the Practice of Medicine in the Nineteenth Century*. Cambridge: Cambridge University Press, 1994.

Cage, R. A. *The Scottish Poor Law, 1745–1845*. Edinburgh: Scottish Academic Press, 1981.

Childers, Joseph. "Mr. Chadwick Writes the Poor." *Victorian Studies, 37* (1994): 405–32.

Chitnis, Anand. *The Scottish and Early Victorian English Society*. London: Croom Helm, 1986.

Clark, G. Kitson. *Churchmen and the Condition of England, 1832–1885: A Study in the Development of Social Ideas and Practice from the Old Regime to the Modern State*. London: Methuen, 1973.

Clark, G. Kitson. "Hunger and Politics in 1842." *Journal of Modern History, 25* (1953): 355–74.

Coleman, William. *Death Is a Social Disease: Public Health and Political Economy in Early Industrial France*. Madison: University of Wisconsin Press, 1982.

Coleman, William. "Health and Hygiene in the *Encyclopedie*: A Medical Doctrine for the Bourgeoisie." *Journal of the History of Medicine, 29* (1974): 399–421.

Coleman, William. *Yellow Fever in the North: The Methods of Early Epidemiology*. Madison: University of Wisconsin Press, 1987.

Coles, Nicholas. "Sinners in the Hands of an Angry Utilitarian: J. P. Kay (-Shuttleworth), *The Moral and Physical Condition of the Working Classes in Manchester (1832)*." *Bulletin of Research in the Humanities, 86* (1985): 453–88.

Cooter, Roger. "Anticontagionism and History's Medical Record." *The Problem of Medical Knowledge: Examining the Social Construction of Medicine*, eds. P. Wright and A. Treacher, 87–108. Edinburgh: Edinburgh University Press, 1982.

Cowherd, Raymond. *Political Economists and the English Poor Laws: A Historical Study of the Influence of Classical Economics on the Formation of Social Welfare Policy*. Athens: Ohio University Press, 1977.

Crowther, M. A. *The Workhouse System, 1834–1929, the History of an English Social Institution.* Athens: University of Georgia Press, 1982.

Cullen, M. J. *The Statistical Movement in Early Victorian Britain: The Foundations of Empirical Social Research.* New York: Barnes & Noble/Harvester, 1975.

Cunningham, Andrew. "Medicine to Calm the Mind: Boerhaave's Medical System, and Why It Was Adopted in Edinburgh." *The Medical Enlightenment of the Eighteenth Century*, eds. Andrew Cunningham and Roger French, 40–66. Cambridge: Cambridge University Press, 1990.

Davison, Graeme. "The City as a Natural System: Theories of Urban Society in Early-Nineteenth-Century Britain." *The Pursuit of Urban History*, eds. D. Fraser and A. Sutcliffe, 349–70. London: Edward Arnold, 1983.

Dean, Mitchell. *The Constitution of Poverty: Toward a Genealogy of Liberal Governance.* London: Routledge, 1991.

DeLacy, Margaret. "The Conceptualization of Influenza in Eighteenth-Century Britain." *Bulletin of the History of Medicine*, 67 (1993): 74–118.

DeLacy, Margaret. "Influenza Research and the Medical Profession in Eighteenth-Century Britain." *Albion*, 25 (1993): 37–63.

DeLacy, Margaret. *Prison Reform in Lancashire, 1700–1850: A Study in Local Administration.* Stanford, Calif.: Stanford University Press, 1986.

Delaporte, François. *Disease and Civilisation, the Cholera in Paris, 1832*, trans. A. Goldhammer. Cambridge, Mass.: MIT Press, 1986.

Digby, Anne. *Making a Medical Living: Doctors and Patients in the English Market for Medicine, 1720–1911.* Cambridge: Cambridge University Press, 1994.

Donajgrodzki, A. P. " 'Social Police' and the Bureaucratic Elite: A Vision of Order in the Age of Reform." *Social Control in Nineteenth Century Britain*, ed. A. P. Donajgrodzki, 51–76. London: Croom Helm, 1977.

Douglas, Mary. "Environments at Risk." *Science in Context*, eds. Barry Barnes and David Edge, 260–75. Cambridge, Mass.: MIT Press, 1982.

Douglas, Mary. *Purity and Danger: An Analysis of the Concepts of Pollution and Taboo.* London: Routledge and Kegan Paul, 1966.

Durey, Michael. *The Return of the Plague: British Society and Cholera, 1831–2.* Dublin: Gill and MacMillan, 1979.

Eastwood, David. *Governing Rural England: Tradition and Transformation in Local Government, 1780–1840.* Oxford: Clarendon Press, 1994.

Edsall, Nicholas C. *The Anti-Poor Law Movement, 1833–44.* Manchester: Manchester University Press, 1971.

Engelhardt, Dietrich von. "Causality and Conditionality in Medicine around 1900." *Science, Technology, and the Art of Medicine: European–American Dialogues*, eds. Corinna Delkeskamp-Hayes and Mary Ann Gardell Cutter, 75–104. *Philosophy and Medicine*, 44. Dordrecht: Kluwer Academic Publishers, 1993.

Evans, Robin. *The Fabrication of Virtue: English Prison Architecture, 1750–1840.* Cambridge: Cambridge University Press, 1982.

Eyler, John M. *Victorian Social Medicine: The Ideas and Methods of William Farr.* Baltimore: Johns Hopkins University Press, 1979.

Fee, Elizabeth. "Public Health, Past and Present: A Shared Social Vision." Introduction in George Rosen, *A History of Public Health*, ix–lxvii. Baltimore: Johns Hopkins University Press, 1993.

Ferguson, Thomas. *The Dawn of Scottish Social Welfare: A Survey from Medieval Times to 1863.* Edinburgh: Thomas Nelson, 1948.

Finer, Herman. *English Local Government.* London: Methuen, 1933.

Finer, S. E. *The Life and Times of Sir Edwin Chadwick.* London: Methuen, 1952.

Finer, S. E. "The Transmission of Benthamite Ideas, 1820–1850." *Studies in the Growth of Nineteenth Century Government,* ed. Gillian Sutherland, 11–32. Totowa, N.J.: Rowman and Littlefield, 1972.

Fissell, Mary. "The Disappearance of the Patient's Narrative and the Invention of Hospital Practice." *British Medicine in an Age of Reform,* eds. Roger French and Andrew Wear, 92–109. London: Routledge, 1991.

Fissell, Mary. *Patients, Power, and the Poor in Eighteenth-Century Bristol.* Cambridge: Cambridge University Press, 1991.

Flinn, M. W. "Medical Services under the New Poor Law." *The New Poor Law in the Nineteenth Century,* ed. Derek Fraser, 45–66. London: Macmillan, 1976.

Foucault, Michel. *Discipline and Punish: The Birth of the Prison,* trans. Alan Sheridan. New York: Vintage, 1979.

Frank, Johnann Peter. *A System of Complete Medical Police; Selections from Johann Peter Frank,* ed. Erna Lesky. Baltimore: Johns Hopkins University Press, 1976.

Fraser, Derek. *Power and Authority in the Victorian City.* Oxford: Blackwell, 1979.

Fraser, Derek. *Urban Politics in Victorian England.* London: Macmillan, 1976.

Frazer, W. M. *Duncan of Liverpool.* London: Hamish Hamilton, 1947.

Frazer, W. M. *A History of English Public Health.* London: Balliere, Tindall, and Cox, 1950.

Gallagher, Catherine. "The Body Versus the Social Body in the Works of Thomas Malthus and Henry Mayhew." *The Making of the Modern Body: Sexuality and Society in the Nineteenth Century,* eds. Catherine Gallagher and Thomas Laqueur, 83–106. Berkeley: University of California Press, 1987.

George, M. Dorothy. *London Life in the Eighteenth Century.* New York: Harper Torchbooks, 1965.

Gibson, Edward H. "The Public Health Agitation in England, 1838–1848: A Newspaper and Parliamentary History." Ph.D. diss., University of North Carolina, Chapel Hill, 1955.

Goubert, J. P. *The Conquest of Water,* intr. Emanuel LeRoy LaDurie, trans. Andrew Wilson. London: Polity Press, 1989.

Grant, Raymond. "Merthyr Tydfil in the Mid-Nineteenth Century: The Struggle for Public Health." *Welsh History Review, 14* (1988–89): 574–94.

Gray, Robert. "Medical Men, Industrial Labour and the State in Britain, 1830–1850." *Social History, 16* (1991): 19–43.

Griffith, G. Talbot. *Population Problems in the Age of Malthus,* 2d ed. New York: Augustus M. Kelley, 1967.

Griffiths, A. R. G. *The Irish Board of Works, 1831–1878.* New York: Garland, 1987.

Guha, Sumit. "The Importance of Social Intervention in England's Mortality Decline: The Evidence Reviewed." *Social History of Medicine, 7* (1994): 89–113.

Hamlin, Christopher. "Could You Starve to Death in England in 1839? The Chadwick–Farr Controversy and the Loss of the 'Social' in Public Health." *American Journal of Public Health, 85* (1995): 856–66.

Hamlin, Christopher. "Edwin Chadwick and the Engineers, 1842–1854: Systems and Anti-Systems in the Pipe-and-Brick Sewers War." *Technology and Culture, 33* (1992): 680–709.

Hamlin, Christopher. "Edwin Chadwick, 'Mutton Medicine,' and the Fever Question." *Bulletin of the History of Medicine, 70* (1996): 233–65.

Hamlin, Christopher. "Environmental Sensibility in Edinburgh, 1839–1840: The 'Fetid Irrigation' Controversy." *Journal of Urban History, 20* (1994): 311–39.

Hamlin, Christopher. "James Newlands and the Bounds of Public Health." *Transactions of the Historic Society of Lancashire and Cheshire, 143* (1994): 117–39.

Hamlin, Christopher. "Muddling in Bumbledom: Local Governments and Large Sanitary Improvements: The Cases of Four British Towns, 1855–1885." *Victorian Studies, 32* (1988): 55–83.

Hamlin, Christopher. "Predisposing Causes and Public Health in the Early Nineteenth Century Public Health Movement." *Social History of Medicine, 5* (1992): 43–70.

Hamlin, Christopher. *A Science of Impurity: Water Analysis in Nineteenth Century Britain.* Bristol and Berkeley: Adam Hilger/University of California Press, 1990.

Hammond, J. L. and Hammond, Barbara. *Lord Shaftesbury,* 3d ed. London: Constable and Co., 1925.

Harrison, Brian. *Drink and the Victorians: The Temperance Question in England 1815–1872.* Pittsburgh: University of Pittsburgh Press, 1971.

Hart, Jenifer. "Nineteenth-Century Social Reform: A Tory Interpretation of History." *Past and Present, 32* (1962): 39–61.

Haskell, Thomas. "Capitalism and the Origins of the Humanitarian Sensibility." *American Historical Review, 90* (1985): 339–61, 547–66.

Hennock, E. P. "Central/Local Government Relations in England, an Outline." *Urban History Yearbook* (1982): 38–47.

Hennock, E. P. "Urban Sanitary Reform a Generation before Chadwick?" *Economic History Review,* 2d ser. *10* (1957): 113–20.

Henriques, Ursula R. Q. *Before the Welfare State: Social Administration in Early Industrial Britain.* London: Longman, 1979.

Hilton, Boyd. *The Age of Atonement: The Influence of Evangelicalism on Social and Economic Thought, 1785–1865.* Oxford: Clarendon Press, 1988.

Himmelfarb, Gertrude. *The Idea of Poverty: England in the Early Industrial Age.* New York: Random House, 1985.

Hodgkinson, Ruth G. *The Origins of the National Health Service: The Medical Services of the New Poor Law, 1834–1871.* London: Wellcome Historical Medical Library, 1967.

Ignatieff, Michael. *A Just Measure of Pain: The Penitentiary in the Industrial Revolution, 1750–1850.* New York: Pantheon, 1978.

Inkster, Ian. "Marginal Men: Aspects of the Social Role of the Medical Community in Sheffield, 1790–1850." *Health Care and Popular Medicine in Nineteenth Century England: Essays in the Social History of Medicine,* eds. John Woodward and David Richards, 128–63. London: Croom Helm, 1977.

Jewson, N. D. "The Disappearance of the Sick-Man from Medical Cosmology, 1770–1870." *Sociology, 10* (1976): 225–44.

John, Angela. *By the Sweat of Their Brow: Women Workers at Victorian Coal Mines.* London: Routledge, 1984.

Jones, E. D. and Falkus, M. E.. "Urban Improvement and the English Economy in the 17th and 18th Centuries." *Research in Economic History, 4* (1979): 193–233.

Jones, Gareth Stedman. "Rethinking Chartism." *Languages of Class: Studies in English Work-*

*ing Class History, 1832–1982,* ed. Gareth Stedman Jones, 90–178. Cambridge: Cambridge University Press, 1983.

Jones, I. G. "Merthyr Tydfil: The Politics of Survival." *Llafur: Journal of Welsh Labour History,* 2 (1976): 18–31.

Kearns, Gerald P. "Aspects of Cholera, Society, and Space in Nineteenth Century England and Wales." Ph.D. diss., Cambridge University, 1985.

Kearns, Gerry. "Cholera, Nuisances, and Environmental Management in Islington, 1830–1855." *Living and Dying in London,* eds. W. F. Bynum and Roy Porter, 94–125. *Medical History,* Supplement, 11. London: Wellcome Institute for the History of Medicine, 1991.

Kearns, Gerry. "Private Property and Public Health Reform in England, 1830–1870." *Social Science and Medicine,* 26 (1988): 187–99.

Keith-Lucas, Brian. "Some Influences Affecting the Development of Sanitary Legislation in England." *Economic History Review,* 2d ser. 6 (1953): 290–96.

Keith-Lucas, Brian. *The Unreformed Local Government System.* London: Croom Helm, 1980.

Kilpatrick, Robert. " 'Living in the Light': Dispensaries, Philanthropy and Medical Reform in Late Eighteenth Century London." *The Medical Enlightenment of the Eighteenth Century,* eds. Andrew Cunningham and Roger French, 254–80. Cambridge: Cambridge University Press, 1990.

King, Lester. *The Philosophy of Medicine: The Early Eighteenth Century.* Cambridge, Mass.: Harvard University Press, 1978.

King, Lester. "Some Problems of Causality in Eighteenth-Century Medicine." *Bulletin of the History of Medicine,* 37 (1963): 15–24.

Knott, John. *Popular Opposition to the 1834 New Poor Law.* New York: St. Martin's Press, 1986.

Kunitz, Stephen. *Disease and Social Diversity: The European Impact on the Health of Non-Europeans.* New York: Oxford University Press, 1994.

La Berge, Ann. *Mission and Method: The Early-Nineteenth-Century French Public Health Movement.* Cambridge: Cambridge University Press, 1992.

Lambert, Richard S. *The Railway King, 1800–1871: A Study of George Hudson and the Business Morals of His Time.* London: George Allen and Unwin, 1934.

Lambert, Royston. *Sir John Simon and English Social Administration.* London: McGibbon and Kee, 1965.

Latour, Bruno. *Science in Action.* Cambridge, Mass.: Harvard University Press, 1987.

Lawrence, Christopher. "The Nervous System and Society in the Scottish Enlightenment." *Natural Order: Historical Studies of Scientific Culture,* eds. Barry Barnes and Steven Shapin, 19–40. Beverly Hills: Sage, 1979.

Leavitt, Ian and Smout, Christopher. *The State of the Scottish Working-Class in 1843: A Statistical and Spatial Inquiry Based on the Data from the Poor Law Commission Report of 1844.* Edinburgh: Scottish Academic Press, 1979.

Lewis, Jane. *What Price Community Medicine? The Philosophy, Practice, and Politics of Public Health since 1919.* Brighton: Wheatsheaf Books, 1986.

Lewis, R. A. *Edwin Chadwick and the Public Health Movement, 1832–1854.* London: Longmans, Green, 1952.

Lobo, Francis. "John Haygarth, Smallpox, and Religious Dissent in Eighteenth Century England." *The Medical Englightenment of the Eighteenth Century,* eds. Andrew

Cunningham and Roger French, 217–53. Cambridge: Cambridge University Press, 1990.

Loudon, I. S. L. "The Origins and Growth of the Dispensary Movement in England." *Bulletin of the History of Medicine,* 55 (1981): 322–42.

Loudon, Irvine. *Medical Care and the General Practitioner.* Oxford: Clarendon Press, 1986.

Lubenow, William C. *The Politics of Government Growth: Early Victorian Attitudes toward State Intervention, 1833–1848.* Newton Abbott: David and Charles, 1971.

MacDonagh, Oliver. *Early Victorian Government, 1830–1870.* London: Weidenfeld and Nicolson, 1977.

MacDonagh, Oliver. "The Nineteenth Century Revolution in Government: A Reappraisal." *Historical Journal, 1* (1958): 52–67.

MacLeod, Roy M. "Introduction." *Government and Expertise: Specialists, Administrators, and Professionals, 1860–1919,* ed. Roy M. MacLeod, 1–24. Cambridge: Cambridge University Press, 1988.

Mandler, Peter. "The Making of the New Poor Law *Redivivus.*" *Past and Present, 117* (1987): 131–57.

Mantoux, Paul. *The Industrial Revolution in the Eighteenth Century: An Outline of the Beginnings of the Modern Factory System in England.* Chicago: University of Chicago Press, 1983.

Marston, Maurice. *Sir Edwin Chadwick (1800–1890).* London: Leonard Parsons, 1925.

Mather, F. C. *Public Order in the Age of the Chartists.* Manchester: Manchester University Press, 1959.

McCord, Norman. *The Anti–Corn Law League, 1838–1846.* London: George Allen and Unwin, 1958.

Midwinter, E. C. *Social Administration in Lancashire, 1830–1860: Poor Law, Public Health and Police.* Manchester: Manchester University Press, 1969.

Mort, Frank. *Dangerous Sexualities: Medico–Moral Politics in England since 1830.* London: Routledge and Kegan Paul, 1987.

Novak, Steven J. "Professionalism and Bureaucracy: English Doctors and the Victorian Public Health Administration." *Journal of Social History,* 6 (1973): 440–62.

Olien, Diana. *Morpeth: A Victorian Public Career.* Washington, D.C.: University Press of America, 1983.

Palmer, Stanley H. *Police and Protest in England and Ireland.* Cambridge: Cambridge University Press, 1988.

Pelling, Margaret. *Cholera, Fever, and English Medicine, 1825–1865.* Oxford: Oxford University Press, 1978.

Peset, José Luis. "On the History of Medical Causality." *Science, Technology, and the Art of Medicine: European-American Dialogues,* eds. Corinna Delkeskamp-Hayes and Mary Ann Gardell Cutter, 57–74. *Philosophy and Medicine,* 44. Dordrecht: Kluwer Academic Publishers, 1993.

Peterson, Audrey. "The Poor Law in Nineteenth Century Scotland." *The New Poor Law in the Nineteenth Century,* ed. Derek Fraser, 171–93. London: Macmillan, 1976.

Pickstone, John V. "Dearth, Dirt, and Fever Epidemics: Rewriting the History of British 'Public Health', 1780–1850." *Epidemics and Ideas: Essays on the Historical Perception of Pestilence,* eds. Terence Ranger and Paul Slack, 125–148. Cambridge: Cambridge University Press, 1992.

Pickstone, John V. "Ferriar's Fever to Kay's Cholera: Disease and Social Structure in Cottonopolis." *History of Science, 22* (1984): 401–19.

Pickstone, John. *Medicine and Industrial Society: A History of Hospital Development in Manchester and Its Region, 1752–1946.* Manchester: Manchester University Press, 1985.

Poovey, Mary. *Making a Social Body: British Cultural Formation 1830–1864.* Chicago: University of Chicago Press, 1995.

Porter, Dorothy. "Introduction." *The History of Public Health and the Modern State,* ed. Dorothy Porter, 1–44. Amsterdam: Rudolpi, 1994.

Porter, Dorothy and Porter, Roy. *Patient's Progress: Doctors and Doctoring in Eighteenth-Century England.* Stanford, Calif.: Stanford University Press, 1989.

Porter, Dorothy and Porter, Roy. "The Politics of Prevention: Anti-Vaccinationism and Public Health in Nineteenth Century England." *Medical History, 32* (1988): 231–52.

Porter, Roy. "Cleaning up the Great Wen: Public Health in Eighteenth-Century London." *Living and Dying in London,* eds. W. F. Bynum and Roy Porter, 61–75. *Medical History,* Supplement, 11. London: Wellcome Institute for the History of Medicine, 1991.

Poynter, J. R. *Society and Pauperism: English Ideas on Poor Relief, 1795–1834.* London: Routledge and Kegan Paul, 1969.

Prest, John. *Liberty and Locality: Parliament, Permissive Legislation, and Ratepayers' Democracies in the Nineteenth Century.* Oxford: Clarendon Press, 1990.

Redlich, Josef and Hirst, Francis, *The History of Local Government in England, Being a Reissue of Book I of Local Government in England.* 2d ed. Intr. and epilogue Bryan Keith-Lucas. New York: Augustus M. Kelley, 1970.

Reid, Donald. *Paris Sewers and Sewermen: Realities and Representations.* Cambridge, Mass.: Harvard University Press, 1991.

Richards, Paul. "R.A. Slaney, the Industrial Town, and Early Victorian Social Policy." *Social History, 4* (1979): 85–101.

Richards, Paul. "The State and Early Industrial Capitalism: The Case of the Handloom Weavers." *Past and Present, 83* (1979): 91–115.

Richards, Paul. "State Formation and Class Struggle." *Capitalism, State Formation, and Marxist Theory,* ed. Philip Corrigan, 49–78. London: Quartet, 1980.

Richardson, Ruth. *Death, Dissection, and the Destitute.* London: Penguin, 1988.

Riley, James C. *The Eighteenth Century Campaign to Avoid Disease.* London: Macmillan, 1987.

Roberts, David. *Paternalism in Early Victorian England.* New Brunswick, N.J.: Rutgers University Press, 1979.

Roberts, David. *Victorian Origins of the British Welfare State.* Hamden, Conn.: Archon Books, 1969.

Robson, Ann P. *On Higher than Commercial Grounds: The Factory Controversy, 1830–1853.* New York: Garland, 1985.

Rosen, George. *From Medical Police to Social Medicine: Essays on the History of Health Care.* New York: Science History, 1974.

Rosen, George. *A History of Public Health.* New York: MD Publications, 1958.

Rosen, George. "What Is Social Medicine? A Genetic Analysis of the Concept." *Bulletin of the History of Medicine, 21* (1947): 674–733.

Rosenberg, Charles. "Catechisms of Health: The Body in the Prebellum Classroom." *Bulletin of the History of Medicine, 69* (1995): 175–97.

Rosenberg, Charles. *The Cholera Years: The United States in 1832, 1849, and 1866.* Chicago: University of Chicago Press, 1962.

Rosenberg, Charles. "Introduction: Framing Disease: Illness, Society, and History." *Framing Disease: Studies in Cultural History,* eds. Charles Rosenberg and Janet Golden, xv–xxvi. New Brunswick, N.J.: Rutgers University Press, 1992.

Rosenberg, Charles. "Medical Text and Social Context: Explaining William Buchan's Domestic Medicine." *Bulletin of the History of Medicine,* 57 (1983): 22–42.

Rosner, Lisa. *Medical Education in the Age of Improvement: Edinburgh Students and Apprentices 1760–1825.* Edinburgh: Edinburgh University Press, 1991.

Schwarzkopf, Jutta. *Women in the Chartist Movement.* New York: St. Martin's Press, 1991.

Selleck, R. J. W. *James Kay-Shuttleworth: Journey of an Outsider.* Ilford, Essex: Woburn Press, 1994.

Simey, Margaret. *Charitable Effort in Liverpool in the Nineteenth Century.* Liverpool: Liverpool University Press, 1951.

Smith, Dale. "Afterword: The Study of Continued Fever in Victorian Britain." Budd, William. *On the Causes of Fevers,* ed. Dale Smith, 123–154. Baltimore: Johns Hopkins University Press, 1984.

Smith, Dale. "Introduction: Typhoid Fever Research and the Origin of William Budd's Thackeray Prize Essay." Budd, William. *On the Causes of Fevers,* ed. Dale Smith, 1–39. Baltimore: Johns Hopkins University Press, 1984.

Smith, F. B. *The People's Health, 1830–1910.* New York: Holmes and Maier, 1979.

Smith, F. B. *The Retreat of Tuberculosis 1850–1950.* London: Croom Helm, 1988.

Smith, Frank. *The Life and Work of Sir James Kay-Shuttleworth.* London: John Murray, 1923.

Smith, Kenneth. *The Malthusian Controversy.* London: Routledge and Kegan Paul, 1951.

Spencer, Frederick H. *Municipal Origins: An Account of English Private Bill Legislation Relating to Local Government, 1740–1835; with a Chapter on Private Bill Procedure.* London: Constable and Co., 1911.

Szreter, Simon. "The Importance of Social Intervention in Britain's Mortality Decline, c. 1850–1914: A Reinterpretation of the Role of Public Health." *Social History of Medicine,* 1 (1988): 1–37.

Thompson, E. P. *The Making of the English Working Class.* Harmondsworth, U.K.: Penguin, 1968.

Wallis, Graham. *The Life of Francis Place, 1771–1854,* 4th ed. London: George Allen and Unwin, 1925.

Ward, J. T. *Chartism.* New York: Barnes and Noble, 1973.

Watkin, Dorothy. *The English Revolution in Social Medicine, 1889–1911,* Ph.D. diss., University of London, 1984.

Webb, Sidney and Webb, Beatrice. *English Local Government from the Revolution to the Municipal Corporations Act: The Parish and the County.* London: Longmans, Green, 1906.

Webb, Sidney and Webb, Beatrice. *English Local Government: The Story of the King's Highway.* London: Longmans, 1913.

Webb, Sidney and Webb, Beatrice. *English Local Government from the Revolution to the Municipal Corporations Act: Statutory Authorities for Special Purposes.* London: Longmans, Green, 1922.

Weindling, Paul. "Linking Self Help and Medical Science: The Social History of Occupational Health." *The Social History of Occupational Health,* ed. Paul Weindling, 2–31. London: Croom Helm, 1985.

White, Brenda. "Scottish Doctors and the English Public Health." *The Influence of Scottish Medicine*, ed. Derek Dow, 77–85. Park Ridge, N.J.: Parthenon, 1988.

Wilson, Adrian. "The Politics of Medical Improvement in Early Hanoverian London." *The Medical Enlightenment of the Eighteenth Century*, eds. Andrew Cunningham and Roger French, 4–39. Cambridge: Cambridge University Press, 1990.

Wilson, John F. *Lighting the Town: A Study of Management in the North West Gas Industry, 1805–1880*. London: Chapman, 1991.

Wilson, Leonard. "Fevers and Science in Early Nineteenth Century Medicine." *Journal of the History of Medicine*, *33* (1978): 386–407.

Wohl, Anthony S. *Endangered Lives: Public Health in Victorian Britain*. Cambridge Mass.: Harvard University Press, 1983.

Wohl, Anthony. *The Eternal Slum: Housing and Social Policy in Victorian London*. London: Edward Arnold, 1977.

### PRIMARY SOURCES

Alfred [George Kydd]. *The History of the Factory Movement from the Year 1802, to the Enactment of the Ten Hours' Bill in 1847*, 2 vols. 1857, reprint, New York: Augustus M. Kelley, 1966.

Alison, Somerville Scott. *An Inquiry into the Propagation of Contagious Poisons, by the Atmosphere; as also into the Nature and Effects of Vitiated Air, Its Forms and Sources, and Other Causes of Pestilence; with Directions for Avoiding the Action of Contagion, and Observations on Some Means for Promoting the Public Health*. Edinburgh: Maclachlan, Stewart, 1839.

Alison, W. P. "Further Illustrations of the Practical Operation of the Scotch System of Management of the Poor." *Journal of the Statistical Society of London*, *4* (1841): 288–319.

Alison, W. P. "Illustrations of the Practical Operation of the Scottish System of Management of the Poor." *Journal of the Statistical Society of London*, *3* (1840): 211–57.

Alison, W. P. "Inflammation." *A System of Practical Medicine Comprised in a Series of Original Dissertations*, ed. A. Tweedie, 52–112. *Library of Medicine*, 1. London: J. Whitaker, n.d.

Alison, W. P. "Observations on the Epidemic Fever Now Prevalent among the Lower Orders in Edinburgh." *Edinburgh Medical and Surgical Journal*, *23* (1827): 233–262.

Alison, W. P. "On the Effect of Poverty and Privation on the Public Health." *Transactions, National Association for the Promotion of Social Science*, *1* (1858): 434–443.

Alison, William Pulteney. *Observations on the Management of the Poor in Scotland, and Its Effects on the Health of Great Towns*, 2d ed. Edinburgh: Blackwood, 1840.

Alison, William Pulteney. *Observations on the Epidemic Fever of 1843 in Scotland and Its Connection with the Destitute Condition of the Poor*. Edinburgh: Blackwood, 1844.

Alison, William Pulteney. *Observations on the Famine of 1846–7 in the Highlands of Scotland and in Ireland as Illustrating the Connection of the Principle of Population with the Management of the Poor*. Edinburgh: Blackwood, 1847.

Alison, William Pulteney. *Reply to the Pamphlet Entitled "Proposed Alteration of the Scottish Poor Law Considered and Commented on," by David Monypenny, Esq. of Pitmilly*. Edinburgh: Blackwood, 1840.

Alison, William Pulteney. *Reply to Dr. Chalmers' Objections to an Improvement of the Legal Provision for the Poor in Scotland*. Edinburgh: Blackwood, 1841.

*Answers to Certain Objections Made to Sir Robert Peel's Bill for Ameliorating the Condition of Children Employed in Cotton Factories.* Manchester: R. and W. Dean, 1819.

Anti-Centralization Union. *Public Health Bill; and Nuisances Removal Bill, 1855,* 2d ed. London: Anti-Centralization Union, 1855.

Armstrong, John. *Practical Illustrations of Typhus Fever, of the Common Continued Fever and of Inflammatory Diseases,* 3d ed. London: Baldwin, Craddock, and Joy, 1819.

Arnott, Neil. *On Warming and Ventilating; with Directions for Making and Using the Thermometer-Stove or Self-Regulating Fire.* London: Longman, Orme, Brown, Green, and Longmans, 1838.

Austin, Henry. "On a Few Points in Relation to the Drainage of Towns." *Transactions, National Association for the Promotion of Social Science,* 1 (1857): 422–29.

Ayre, Joseph. *Practical Observations on the Nature and Treatment of Marasmus.* London: Baldwin, Craddock, and Joy, 1818.

Barker, F. and Cheyne, J. *An Account of the Rise, Progress, and Decline of the Fever Lately Epidemical in Ireland,* 2 vols. London: Baldwin, Craddock, and Joy, 1821.

Bateman, Thomas. *Reports on the Diseases of London and the State of the Weather from 1804 to 1816 Including Practical Remarks on the Causes and Treatment of the Former; and Preceded by a Historical View of the State of Health and Disease in the Metropolis in Times Past.* London: Longman, Hurst, 1819.

Bateman, Thomas. *A Succinct Account of the Contagious Fever of This Country Exemplifed in the Epidemic Now Prevailing in London.* London: Longman, Hurst, 1818.

Baxter, G. R. W. *The Book of the Bastilles; or the History of the Working of the New Poor-Law.* London: John Stephens, 1841.

Bentham, Jeremy. "Outline of a Work Entitled Pauper Management Improved." *The Works of Jeremy Bentham Published under the Superintendence of His Executor, John Bowring,* 11 vols., VIII, 363–439. Edinburgh: William Tait, 1843.

Bernard, Thomas. "An Extract from a Further Account of the London Fever Institution." *Report of the Society for Bettering the Condition and Increasing the Comforts of the Poor,* 5 (1808): 138–50.

Bernard, Thomas. "An Extract from a Further Account of the London Fever Institution." *Report of the Society for Bettering the Condition and Increasing the Comforts of the Poor,* 6 (1815): 1–9.

Bernard, Thomas. "Extract from an Account of the Progress of the Dublin House of Recovery." *Report of the Society for Bettering the Condition and Increasing the Comforts of the Poor,* 6 (1815): 147–54.

Blane, Gilbert. *Reflections on the Present Crisis of Publick Affairs, with an Enquiry into the Causes and Remedies of the Existing Clamours, and Alleged Grievances, of the Country, as Connected with Population, Subsistence, Wages of Labourers, Education, etc.* London: Ridgway, 1831.

Blane, Gilbert. *Elements of Medical Logick,* 2d ed. London: Underwood, 1821.

*The Book of Murder! A Vade-Mecum for the Commissioners and Guardians of the New Poor Law throughout Great Britain and Ireland, Being an Exact Reprint of the Infamous Essay on the Possibility of Limiting Populousness, by Marcus, One of the Three. With a Refutation of the Malthusian Doctrine.* London: William Dugdale, 1839.

Boott, Francis. *Memoir of the Life and Medical Opinions of John Armstrong, M.D. to Which Is Added an Inquiry into the Facts Connected with Those Forms of Fever Attributed to Malaria or Marsh Effluvium,* 2 vols. London: Baldwin and Craddock, 1833.

Buchanan, Andrew. "Report of the Diseases Which Prevailed among the Poor of Glasgow, During the Summer of 1830." *Glasgow Medical Journal*, 3 (1830): 435–50.

Budd, William. "On the Causes and Mode of Propagation of the Common Continued Fevers of Great Britain and Ireland." *On the Causes of Fevers*, ed. Dale Smith, 41–122. Baltimore: Johns Hopkins University Press, 1984.

Chadwick, Edwin. *Health of Towns. Report of the Speeches of E. Chadwick, Esq., Dr. Southwood Smith, Richard Taylor, Esq., James Anderton, Esq. and Others . . . to Promote a Subscription in Behalf of the Widow and Children of Dr. J. R. Lynch, Who Died of Fever, Caught in the Course of Exertions to Alleviate the Sufferings of the Poor, and to Promote the Cause of Sanitary Improvement of the Metropolis; with a List of the Names of Those Who Have Already Subscribed.* London: Chapman, Elcoate, 1847.

Chadwick, Edwin. *Report on the Sanitary Condition of the Labouring Population of Great Britain. A Supplementary Report on the Results of a Special Inquiry into the Practice of Interment in Towns.* London: Clowes, 1843.

Chadwick, Edwin. *Report on the Sanitary Condition of the Labouring Population of Great Britain*, ed. M. W. Flinn. Edinburgh: Edinburgh University Press, 1965.

Chadwick, Edwin. *Report to Her Majesty's Principal Secretary of State for the Home Office, on the Sanitary Condition of the Labouring Population of Great Britain.* London: Clowes, 1842.

Chadwick, Edwin. " Subsequent Progress of the Principle of Circulation since 1856." *Circulation or Stagnation, Being a Translation of a Paper by F. O. Ward Read at the Sanitary Congress Held at Brussels in 1856 in the Arterial and Venous System for the Sanitation of Towns, with a Statement of the Progress Made for Its Completion Since Then by Sir Edwin Chadwick, Formerly Chief Executive Officer of the First General Board of Health.* eds. F. O. Ward and Edwin Chadwick, 18–48. London: Cassell, 1889.

Christison, Robert. *Treatise on Poisons in Relation to Medical Jurisprudence, Physiology, and the Practice of Physic*, 1st American ed. from the 4th Edinburgh ed. Philadelphia: Barrington and Haswell, 1845.

Clark, Sir James. *A Treatise on Pulmonary Consumption Comprehending an Inquiry into the Causes, Nature, Prevention and Treatment of Tuberculosis and Scrofulous Diseeases in General.* London: Sherwood, Gilbert and Piper, 1835.

Clutterbuck, Henry. *Observations on the Prevention and Treatment of the Epidemic Fever at Present Prevailing in the Metropolis and Most Parts of the United Kingdom.* London: Longman, Hurst, Rees, Orme, and Brown, 1819.

Collignon, Charles. *Medicina Politica, or Reflections on the Art of Physic as Inseparably Connected with the Prosperity of the State.* London: J. Bentham, 1765.

Copland, James. *A Dictionary of Practical Medicine, Comprising General Pathology*, 3 vols. London: Longman, Brown, 1858.

"Copy of Certificate from Several Physicians of Hospitals and Dispensaries in London, Dated April 9th, 1801, as to the Prevalence of Infectious Fever in the Metropolis." *Report of the Society for Bettering the Condition and Increasing the Comforts of the Poor, 3* (1801): 307–9.

Cowan, Robert. "Vital Statistics of Glasgow, Illustrating the Sanatory Condition of the Population." *Journal of the Statistical Society of London*, 3 (1840): 257–292.

Cullen, William. *First Lines of the Practice of Physic*, 2 vols. Philadelphia: Dobson, 1816.

Davidson, William. "Essay on the Sources and Mode of Propagation of the Continued Fevers of Great Britain and Ireland." *Essays on the Sources and Mode of Action of Fever*, eds. William Davidson and Alfred Hudson. 1–93. Philadelphia: A. Waldie, 1841.

Davis, J. B. *A Popular Manual of the Art of Preserving Health.* London: Whittaker, 1836.

Disraeli, Benjamin. *Sybil, or the Two Nations,* intr. Walter Sichel. London: Oxford University Press, 1926.

Engels, Frederick. *The Condition of the Working Class in England,* trans. and eds. W. D. Henderson and W. H. Chaloner. Oxford: Blackwell, 1971.

*Engineers and Officials: An Historical Sketch of the "Health of Towns Works" (between 1838 and 1856) in London and the Provinces, with Biographical Notes on Lord Palmerston, the Earl of Shaftesbury, Lord Ebrington, Edwin Chadwick, F. O. Ward, John Thwaites.* London: Edward Stanford, 1856.

"Epidemic Fever." *Edinburgh Medical and Surgical Journal,* 14 (1818): 528–549.

Farr, William. "Vital Statistics." *A Statistical Account of the British Empire: Exhibiting Its Extent, Physical Capacities, Population, Industry, and Civil and Religious Institutions,* ed. J. R. McCulloch, 521–90. London: Charles Knight, 1839.

Faust, Bernhard. *The Catechism of Health, trans from the German and Carefully Improved by Dr. Gregory of Edenburg [sic],* 3d American ed. Raleigh: Thomas Henderson, 1812.

Ferriar, John. *Medical Histories and Reflections,* 1st American ed., 4 vols. in 1. Philadelphia: Dobson, 1816.

Fielden, John. *The Curse of the Factory System.* London: A. Cobbett, [1836].

Good, J. M. *A Dissertation on the Diseases of Prisons and Poor-Houses.* London: C. Dilley, 1795.

Good, J. M. *The Study of Medicine,* 2d ed., 5 vols. London: Baldwin, Craddock, and Joy, 1825.

Graham, Robert. *Practical Observations on Continued Fever, Especially That Form at Present Existing as an Epidemic with Some Remarks on the Most Efficient Plans for Its Suppression.* Glasgow: J. Smith and Son, 1818.

Grainger, R. D. *Unhealthiness of Towns: Its Causes and Remedies, Being a Lecture Delivered at the Royal Institution of Liverpool and the Atheneum, Manchester.* London: Charles Knight, 1845.

Green, James. "The Sewerage of Bristol." *Minutes of Proceedings, Institution of Civil Engineers,* 7 (1848): 76–107.

[Greg, R. H.]. *The Factory Question, Considered in Relation to Its Effects on the Health and Morals of Those Employed in Factories.* London: J. Ridgway, 1837.

[Greg, W. R.]. *An Enquiry into the State of the Manufacturing Population and the Causes and Cures of the Evils Therein Existing.* London: J. Ridgway, 1831.

Hale, William. *An Appeal to the Public in Defence of the Spitalfields Act: with Remarks on the Causes Which Have Led to the Miseries and Moral Deterioration of the Poor.* London: Justines, 1822.

Hales, Stephen. *A Treatise on Ventilators.* London: Manby, 1753.

Harrison, John Thornehill. "On the Drainage of the District, South of the Thames." *Minutes of Proceedings, Institution of Civil Engineers,* 13 (1853–54): 64–120.

Hawkins, F. Bisset. *Elements of Medical Statistics.* intr. James H. Cassedy. Canton, Mass.: Science History, 1989.

Haygarth, John. *A Letter to Dr. Percival on the Prevention of Infectious Fevers and an Address to the College of Physicians in Philadelphia on the Prevention of the American Pestilence.* Bath: R. Cruttwell, 1801.

Health of Towns Association. *Abstract of the Proceedings of the Public Meeting Held at Exeter Hall, December 11, 1844.* London: Charles Knight, n.d. [1845].

Health of Towns Association. *Report of the Committee to the Members of the Association on Lord Lincoln's Sewerage, Drainage, etc., of Towns' Bill.* London: Charles Knight, 1846.

Health of Towns Association. *Report of the Sub-Committee on the Answers Returned to Questions Addressed to the Principal Towns of England and Wales, and on the Objections from Corporate Bodies to the Public Health Bill.* London: Clowes, 1848.

Heberden, William. *Observations on the Increase and Decrease of Different Diseases.* London: T. Payne, 1801.

Helps, Arthur. *The Claims of Labour: An Essay on the Duties of Employers to the Employed, the 2nd ed., to Which Is Added, An Essay on the Means of Improving the Health and Increasing the Comfort of the Labouring Classes.* London: Pickering, 1845.

Henry, William. "Report on the State of Our Knowledge of the Laws of Contagion." *4th Report of the British Association for the Advancement of Science* (1834): 67–93.

Holland, G. C. *An Inquiry into the Principles and Practice of Medicine Founded on Original Physiological Observations.* London: Longman, Rees, 1834.

Horner, Miss. "Extract from an Account of a Contagious Fever at Kingston upon Hull." *Report of the Society for Bettering the Condition and Increasing the Comforts of the Poor,* 4 (1805): 96–110.

Howard, Richard Baron. *An Inquiry into the Morbid Effects of Deficiency of Food Chiefly with Reference to Their Occurrence amongst the Destitute Poor.* London: Simpkin, Marshall, and Co., 1839.

Hudson, Alfred. "An Inquiry into the Sources and Mode of Action of the Poison of Fever." *Essays on the Sources and Mode of Action of Fever,* eds. William Davidson and Alfred Hudson. 95–178. Philadelphia: A. Waldie, 1841.

*Information Concerning the State of Children Employed in Cotton Factories Printed for the Use of the Members of Both Houses of Parliament.* Manchester: J. Gleave, 1818.

*An Inquiry into the Principle of the Bill Now Pending in Parliament for Imposing Certain Restrictions on Cotton Factories.* London: Baldwin, Craddock and Joy, 1818.

Jackson, Robert. *A Sketch, (Analytical) of the History and Cure of Contagious Fever.* London: Burgess and Hill, 1819.

Johnson, James. *The Influences of Civic Life, Sedentary Habits, and Intellecutal Refinement, on Human Health and Human Happiness, Including an Estimate of the Balance of Enjoyment and Suffering in the Different Conditions of Society.* London: Underwood, 1818.

*The Justice, Humanity and Policy of Restricting the Hours of Children and Young Persons in the Mills and Factories of the United Kingdom, Illustrated in the Letters, Speeches, etc., of Persons of the Highest Respectability and the Most Correct and Extensive Information, of Various Religious Creeds, and Political Views, and of Various Stations in Life, Many of Them Resident in the Midst of Those Districts, Where the Evils Exist, Which It Is Sought to Mitigate by Mr. Sadler's Ten Hour Bill.* Leeds: R. Inchbold, 1833.

Kay (-Shuttleworth), James Phillips. "Physical Condition of the Poor. I. Diet. Gastralgia and Enteralgia, or Morbid Sensibility of the Stomach and Bowels." *North of England Medical and Surgical Journal,* 1 (1830): 220–30.

Kay (-Shuttleworth), James Phillips. *The Moral and Physical Condition of the Working Classes Employed in the Cotton Manufacture in Manchester,* 2d ed. with a new preface by W. H. Chaloner. London: Frank Cass, 1970.

Knight, Arnold. "On the Grinders' Asthma." *North of England Medical Journal,* 1 (1830): 85–91, 167–79.

Leslie, James. "Observations on the Flow of Water through Pipes, Conduits, and Orifices." *Minutes of Proceedings, Institution of Civil Engineers, 14* (1854–55): 273–317.

Lewis, Gilbert Cornwall. *Letters of the Rt. Hon. Sir George Cornwall Lewis, Bt. to Various Friends,* ed. Gilbert Frankland Lewis. London: Longmans, Green, 1870.

Lovett, William. *Life and Struggles of William Lovett in His Pursuit of Bread, Knowledge, and Freedom with Some Account of the Different Associations He Belonged to and of the Opinions He Entertained,* 2 vols. New York: Knopf, 1920.

MacCormac, Henry. *An Exposition of the Nature, Treatment, and Prevention of Continued Fever.* London: Longman, Rees, Orme, Brown, Green, and Longman, 1835.

Malthus, T. R. *An Essay on the Principle of Population; or A View of Its Past and Present Effects on Human Happiness; with an Inquiry into Our Prospects Respecting the Future Removal or Mitigation of the Evils Which It Occasions. The Version Published in 1803, with the Varioria of 1806 1807, 1817, and 1826,* ed. Patricia James. Cambridge: Cambridge University Press/Royal Economic Society, 1989.

Martineau, Harriet. *How to Observe Morals and Manners,* ed. Michael R. Hill. New Brunswick, N.J.: Transaction, 1989.

Marx, Karl and Engels, Frederich. *Capital: A Critical Analysis of Capitalist Production,* 3 vols., trans. from the 3d German ed. Samuel Moore and Edward Aveling. New York: International Publishing Co., 1939.

Mills, Thomas. *A Comparative View of Fever and Inflammatory Complaints with Essays Illustrative of the Seat, Nature, and Origin of Fever.* Dublin: Cumming and McArthur, 1824.

Moss, William. *A Familiar Medical Survey of Liverpool.* Liverpool: Hodgson, 1784.

Parnell, Sir Henry. *A Treatise on Roads; Wherein the Principles on Which Roads Should Be Made Are Explained and Illustrated by the Plans, Specifications, and Contracts Made Use of by Thomas Telford, Esq. on the Holyhead Road.* London: Longman, Rees, Orme, Brown, Green, and Longman, 1833.

Poor Law Commission. *Official Circulars of Public Documents and Information Directed by the Poor Law Commissioners to Be Printed, Chiefly for the Use of Boards of Guardians and Their Officers,* 10 vols. in 2, 1840–1851. New York: Augustus M. Kelley, 1970.

Rawlinson, Robert. "The Drainage of Towns." *Minutes of Proceedings, Institution of Civil Engineers, 12* (1852–52): 25–109.

Reid, D. B. *Illustrations of the Theory and Practice of Ventilation.* London: Longman, Brown, Green, and Longmans, 1844.

Reid, John. *The Philosophy of Death, or a General Medical and Statistical Treatise on the Nature and Causes of Human Mortality.* London: S. Highly, 1841.

Richardson, B. W. *The Health of Nations: A Review of the Works of Edwin Chadwick, with a Biographical Dissertation,* 2 vols. 1887, reprint, London: Dawson, 1965.

Roberton, John. "An Inquiry Respecting the Period of Puberty in Women." *North of England Medical Journal, 1* (1830): 69–85, 179–91.

Roberton, John. *Observations on the Mortality and Physical Management of Children.* London: Longman, Rees, Orme, Brown, 1827.

Rumsey, Henry. *Essays on State Medicine.* London: Churchill, 1856.

Sincere Friends of Industry, to the Mutual Advantage of Master and Labourer. *Remarks on the Objections Which Have Been Urged against the Principle of Sir Robert Peel's Bill.* 1818.

Slaney, Robert. *An Essay on the Employment of the Poor.* London: Hatchard, 1819.

Slaney, Robert. *An Essay on the Employment of the Poor,* 2d. ed, with additions, with a letter by James Scarlett, M.P. London: Hatchard, 1822.

Slaney, Robert. *Reports of the House of Commons on the Education (1838) and on the Health (1840), of the Poorer Classes in Large Towns: With Some Suggestions for Improvement.* London: Knight, Longman, Hatchard, n.d. [1841].

Smith, Thomas Southwood. *The Common Nature of Epidemics, and Their Relation to Climate and Civilization. Also Remarks on Contagion and Quarantine,* ed. T. Baker. London, Trübner and Co, 1866.

[Smith, Thomas Southwood]. "Contagion and Sanitary Laws." *Westminster Review* (1825): 134–67, 499–530.

Smith, Thomas Southwood. *Illustrations of Divine Government;* 1st American from the last London ed. Boston: B Mussey, 1831.

Smith, Southwood. *Results of Sanitary Improvement Illustrated by the Operation of the Metropolitan Societies for Improving the Dwellings of the Industrious Classes, the Working of the Common Lodging Houses Act, etc.* London: Charles Knight/Cassell, 1854.

Smith, Thomas Southwood. *A Treatise on Fever.* Philadelphia: Carey and Lea, 1830.

Southey, Robert. *Essays, Moral and Political.* 2 vols. London: John Murray, 1832.

[Tait, William]. "Dr Alison, etc. on the Causes of Typhus Fever." *British and Foreign Medical Review, 11,* no. 21 (1841): 1–36.

Taylor, W. Cooke. *Notes of a Tour in the Manufacturing Districts of Lancashire,* 3d ed., ed. W. H. Chaloner, 1842; reprint, New York: Augustus M. Kelley, 1968.

Thackrah, Charles Turner. *The Effects of the Arts, Trades, and Professions and of the Civic States and Habits of Living, on Health and Longevity: With Suggestions for the Removal of Many of the Agents Which Produce Disease, and Shorten the Duration of Life.* London: Longmans, Rees, Orme, Brown, 1832.

Thomas, Robert. *The Modern Practice of Physic, Exhibiting the Characters, Causes, Symptoms, Prognostics, Morbid Appearances, and Improved Method of Treating Diseases of All Climates,* 6th ed. London: Longman, Hurst, Rees, Orme, Brown, 1819.

Ward, F. O. "Circulation or Stagnation." *Circulation or Stagnation, Being a Translation of a Paper by F. O. Ward Read at the Sanitary Congress Held at Brussels in 1856 in the Arterial and Venous System for the Sanitation of Towns, with a Statement of the Progress Made for Its Completion Since Then by Sir Edwin Chadwick, Formerly Chief Executive Officer of the First General Board of Health,* eds. F. O. Ward and Edwin Chadwick. 11–17. London: Cassell, 1889.

Watson, Thomas. *Lectures on the Principles and Practice of Physic,* 4th ed., 2 vols. London: Parker, 1857.

Williams, Alfred. "Description of the Sewerage and Drainage Works of Newport, Monmouthshire." *Minutes of Proceedings, Institution of Civil Engineers,* 22 (1862–63): 273–304.

Williams, Charles. *Principles of Medicine Comprising General Pathology and Therapeutics,* ed. Meredith Clymer. Philadelphia: Lea and Blanchard, 1848.

Wing, Charles. *Evils of the Factory System Demonstrated by Parliamentary Evidence.* London: Saunders and Otley, 1837.

Yelloly, John. *Observations on the Arrangements Connected with the Relief of the Sick Poor; Addressed in a Letter to the Rt. Hon. the Lord John Russell, Secretary of State for the Home Department.* London: Longman, Rees, Orme, Brown, Green, and Longman, 1837.

# INDEX

Aberdeen, 188
Accrington, 285, 290
Ackerknecht, Erwin, 113
Adamson, John, 193, 214
aged persons, 12, 29, 80–81, 91, 171, 193, 207–8
air (*see also* atmospheric constitution; malaria; miasma; ventilation)
  as medium of contagion, 23, 60–61, 65–66, 113–17, 119, 124, 130, 169, 211
  relation to nutrition, 225–29, 297
  as required for health, 48, 59, 131, 143, 162, 180, 206, 210, 253, 296, 299
  vitiated or impure, 26, 40–41, 61–62, 64, 76, 100–2, 115–16, 123–25, 129–30, 141, 148, 161–62, 165, 173, 183, 192, 203, 212, 225–29, 250–51, 295–97
Alfreton, 294, 297
Alison, Archibald, 74
Alison, Somerville Scott, 189, 193, 199, 202, 204, 207–8
Alison, William Pulteney, 74, 112, 132, 250, 338–40
  campaign to reform Scottish poor law, 75–76, 78–80, 132–42
  relations with Chadwick, 82–83, 110, 135–42, 158, 184
  social views, 78–82, 150, 195, 199, 201, 208–9, 212–13, 215, 247
  theory of disease, 71, 82–83, 114, 127–30, 154, 214, 224, 226
Ampthill, 169
Andover, 92, 94, 152
anxiety, as cause of disease, 19, 62, 65, 66, 68, 69, 76, 154, 197, 215
architects, 218, 223, 242
Arnott, Neil, 17, 85, 86, 102, 105, 106, 110, 111, 121, 123, 126, 128, 136, 139, 141, 148,160, 189, 190, 205, 206, 224–27, 326, 327
Ashley, Lord, *see* Shaftesbury
Ashton under Lyne, 104, 223, 231, 237, 261

Association for Obtaining an Official Inquiry into the Poor Laws of Scotland, 79, 135
atmosphere as cause of disease, *see* air
atmospheric constitution as cause of disease, 60–61, 65 113–15, 325
Austin, Henry, 283, 310, 316–17, 319, 325, 327–31
Ayr, 189, 196, 201, 206
Ayre, Joseph, 57

Babbage, Benjamin, 283, 285, 288, 290
back drainage, 316, 331
Baines, Edward, 44
Baird, Charles, 189, 192, 200
Baker, Robert, 169, 189, 199, 203, 207
Baker, William, 162–63, 199
Barnard Castle, 313, 322
Barry, David, 97–99, 101, 102
Bateman, J. F., 307
Bateman, Thomas, 58, 73, 114, 116, 125
Bath, 21, 54, 67, 151, 167, 230, 249
Bazalgette, Joseph, 305, 322, 324, 325, 327, 328, 330, 331
beds, 74, 86, 169, 194, 200, 206
Bell, Charles, 37–39
Bentham, Jeremy, 9, 22, 29–31, 84, 85, 88, 113
Benthamite policies, 3, 29, 87, 88, 110, 160, 164, 170, 179, 246, 264, 266
Bentinck, Lord George, 269
Bernard, Thomas, 69, 125
Bethnal Green, 104–5, 117, 119
Bill, Thomas, 37
Birkenhead, 291
Birmingham, 150, 166, 188, 199, 207, 212, 258–59, 267, 272
Black hole of Calcutta, 64, 115
Blackpool, 282
Blane, Gilbert, 37
Blomfield, Bishop Benjamin, 86, 121
boards of health (*see also* General Board of Health), 149, 182, 230